Optimizing Radiographic Positioning

OPTIMIZING RADIOGRAPHIC POSITIONING

Angeline M. Cullinan, RT(R), FASRT
HENRIETTA, NEW YORK

Illustrations by

Arnold L. Gómez

J. B. Lippincott Company Philadelphia
New York London Hagerstown

To my husband Jack. Without his encouragement, suggestions, support, and generous sharing of his time, I would not have been able to accomplish this book.

Acquisitions Editor: Charles McCormick, Jr.
Developmental Editor: Kimberley Cox
Indexer: Patricia Couser
Production Manager: Janet Greenwood
Production Service: Hockett Editorial Service
Compositor: Graphic Sciences Corporation
Printer/Binder: Arcata Graphics/Halliday

1   3   5   6   4   2

Library of Congress Cataloging-in-Publication Data

Cullinan, Angeline M.
    Optimizing radiographic positioning / Angeline M. Cullinan ;
illustrations by Arnold L. Gómez.
        p.   cm.
    Includes bibliographical references and index.
    ISBN 0-397-51050-0
    1. Radiography, Medical—Positioning.   I. Title.
    [DNLM: 1. Posture.   2. Radiography—methods.   WN 200 C967o]
    RC78.4.C85   1992
    616.07′572—dc20
    DNLM/DLC
    for Library of Congress   91-4892
                                                                            CIP

The authors and publisher have exerted every effort to ensure that drug selection and dosage set forth in this text are in accord with current recommendations and practice at the time of publication. However, in view of ongoing research, changes in government regulations, and the constant flow of information relating to drug therapy and drug reactions, the reader is urged to check the package insert for each drug for any change in indications and dosage and for added warnings and precautions. This is particularly important when the recommended agent is a new or infrequently employed drug.

Preface

This book is not a positioning manual and is not intended to replace a favorite positioning atlas.[1-4] I felt that it would be redundant to rewrite material that is available either in widely accepted radiographic positioning manuals or from life experiences. This endeavor goes beyond "how to" perform a study to explain specific options and to offer suggestions for optimizing radiographic positions. Whenever possible, the similarities rather than the differences between basic projections and modifications have been accentuated. This approach differs from most positioning books, in which in-depth instructions are repeated for each routine or modified projection.

Tables are used to show how many projections vary only by slight angulation in the direction of the central ray and/or the position of the patient or part. This synopsis of basic radiographic positioning concepts and projections should make it easier to recall information when special or seldom-requested projections are needed.

Descriptions of the routine positions and projections intentionally are made as brief as possible in order to keep this book to a manageable size. An effort was made to integrate radiographic positioning with radiographic technique and anatomical and pathological observations.

Preparation for this book required an extensive literature search, which revealed many unique modifications in routine projections. These publications may not be readily accessible to all radiographers, and even a familiar paper may be difficult to locate, particularly if needed in an emergency. A portion of this book thus is devoted to describing these previously published modifications. They are included in sections labeled "Conditions or Diseases Meriting Special Consideration" and "Supplementary Projections." I hope that when you need specific information about a special projection or technical concept, you will turn to this book.

Positioning and technical contributions by radiographers made up a large segment of the early literature. Some of our colleagues are now directing more of their writing efforts toward the newer modalities, such as ultrasound, computed tomography, and magnetic resonance imaging, which have become the primary imaging techniques for selective examinations—for example, the use of ultrasound for the biliary system and fetal measurements. In some hospitals and physicians' offices, however, these modalities may not be available and conventional radiography is needed to make a diagnosis.

Conventional radiography is still widely used for most medical imaging studies. Radiographers often modify routine procedures, but are unaware of the uniqueness of their innovations and so do not publish descriptions of their work. An author of a textbook must rely heavily on contributions from many sources. It is not practical or advisable to expose patients to radiation in order to obtain illustrations for an article or textbook. Images made using radiographic phantoms do not approach the quality of clinical images. If you have a unique modification of a standard projection that you are willing to share, I would appreciate the opportunity to review your work for possible inclusion in a future edition of this book. Original images will be returned to you and credit for your contribution given.

Angeline M. Cullinan

Acknowledgments

My thanks to the many authors and publishers who so generously shared their illustrations and published works with me. Credit for their images will be found in the legends, as well as in the references.

I want Derace Schaffer, MD, Chairman of the Department of Radiology, and Sally Gerling, Chief Librarian of the Stabins Library, both at the Genesee Hospital in Rochester, NY, to know that I appreciate the gracious manner in which they allowed me access to resource and reference material needed for this book. Thanks also to Dawn Beck, Publications Coordinator, Health Science Division, Communications and Public Affairs, Eastman Kodak Company, Rochester, NY for helping me to procure some of the interesting radiographs used in several chapters.

Most of the glossy photographs appearing in this book were the work of Dave Welker and his staff at Campos Photography, Henrietta, NY, and I want to thank them for the time they spent to assure faithful reproduction of the images.

I feel that the illustrator, Arnold L. Gómez of Sizzle ink in Rochester, brought a unique dimension to this textbook with his drawings. Often working with only a technical suggestion or basic anatomical outline, he was able to produce uncomplicated artwork. His careful attention to the anatomical landmarks, positioning angles, and other relationships add greatly to the illustrations.

Many people at the JB Lippincott Company contributed to the coming together and production of this textbook. I would like to say a special "thank you" to Charles McCormick, Medical Editor, for creating a conducive atmosphere in which I was able to give my undivided attention to this endeavor.

Thanks to the radiographers, educators, radiologists, and commercial representatives who motivated me to write this companion book to *Producing Quality Radiographs*. Their kind comments following the publication of that book made it obvious to me that I should address the relationships among radiographic technique, anatomy and pathology, and radiographic positioning, all of which contribute to the optimal radiographic image.

A very special thanks to every radiographer who uses innovative positioning to produce radiographs that influence diagnosis and to every radiologist who encourages this initiative in radiographers.

And most of all, my heartfelt thanks to my husband, Jack Cullinan, for the many hours he spent reading, reviewing, and editing this manuscript and for his work with the illustrator.

Angeline M. Cullinan

Contents

CHAPTER **ONE**

Radiographic Positioning and Technique

Radiographers know that proper positioning cannot compensate for poor radiographic technique. A properly exposed radiograph obtained with poor positioning or a correctly positioned patient examined with an inadequate radiographic technique can influence the diagnosis. Regardless of the source of error, a less than optimal study places the radiologist at a disadvantage, compromising patient care.

Medical imaging does more than simply confirm the presence or absence of disease; it provides information about the range of both normal and disease processes, about the staging of tumors, and about the response of disease to therapy.[5] Even though a radiograph may seem to be acceptable for interpretation, a radiologist may detect a minor anatomical or pathological change and require one or more additional images. A radiologist will often ask for a repeat image because a segment of the radiograph does not provide the information needed for a diagnosis. For example, when looking for a kidney stone on a survey film of the abdomen, a small area of poor screen contact in the region of the kidney might nullify an otherwise acceptable image.

Tube angulation, focal film distance (FFD), grid selection and placement, centering to an au-

tomatic exposure control (AEC) sensor, and other technical considerations influence radiographic positioning. The innovative radiographer must assess all technical options.

IMAGE DIAGNOSIS

Most radiographers work independently, without direct supervision. In a large facility, patient volume and work flow can delay the interpretation of medical images. If patients are to be sent back to their rooms or discharged before the study is interpreted, the radiographer must be able to decide whether the images meet the technical standards of the department.

Some radiographers pride themselves on their ability to make a diagnosis from a radiograph—to determine "what's wrong with the patient." Patients are better served, however, by radiographers who use their skills to determine "what's wrong with the radiograph." Experience and skill entitle the radiographer to a technical opinion—to be able to decide whether an anatomical variant, a pathological influence, or a positioning or technical error exists. A radiographer trying to solve a technical problem needs to take a good technical history, obtaining exact information about these variables. A good techni-

1

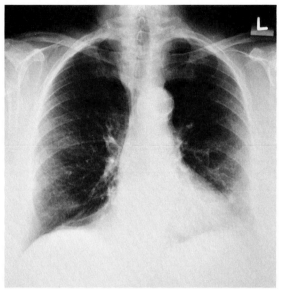

A

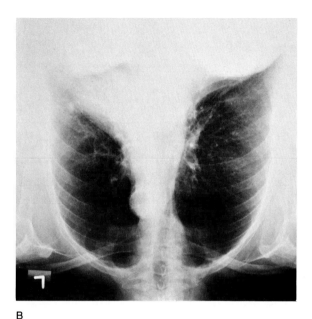

B

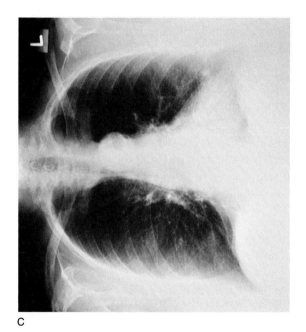

C

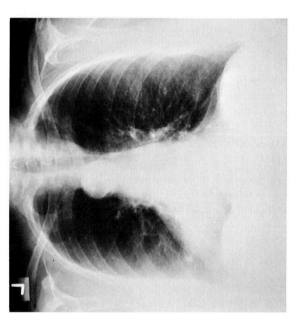

D

FIGURE 1–1 Perception

(A) An x-ray image may be easier to evaluate technically in an unfamiliar presentation, since missing anatomical details are often "filled in" based on previous experiences. A quality assurance check of this image might fail to appreciate the lack of anatomical details in the left lower lung. (B) When the radiograph is positioned upside down, the lack of detail in the left base is apparent when compared with the right base. A cursory viewing with the image

(B) turned upside down, (C) turned sideways, or (D) turned backward and sideways may make it easier to make technical judgments about the radiograph. See Fig 1-2A-D. Since these full-size radiographs are reduced here, this effect may not be fully appreciated. An actual radiograph should be evaluated on a view box to realize how "experience" affects "technical judgment."

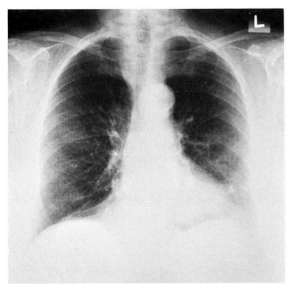

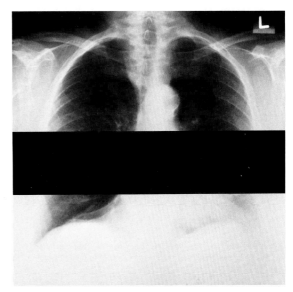

A   B

FIGURE 1–2A,B   Chest Radiograph

A conventional chest radiograph (Fig 1-1) exposed using a high ratio grid and low to moderate kilovoltage. (A) The costophrenic sulci are "seen" only because previous experiences help the viewer to "fill in" the image. (B) When a piece of cardboard is placed on the image to mask anatomical segments, it becomes obvious that a segment of the image (the left costophrenic sulcus) not only is inadequately exposed, but is not diagnostic. When evaluating an image for radiographic technique, inverting the image or masking a portion of it will help to determine whether the radiograph is appropriately exposed.

cal history is as important to an "image diagnosis" as a good clinical history is to a radiological diagnosis. Recording of technical factors helps the radiographer to duplicate an original study and to improve follow-up examinations.

Radiographers should utilize their experience to make a "technical" differential diagnosis. For example, image blur on a radiograph could result from heel effect, poor screen contact, large patient size, or patient motion. An underexposed area on the lateral aspects of an image could be caused by grid cutoff, collimator shutter cutoff, or increased density owing to pathology.

A good radiographer has a knowledge of anatomy and basic pathology. This knowledge, however, can interfere with an image diagnosis. Segmental damage to an image is sometimes not appreciated in an underexposed area of a radiograph. Missing anatomical details are often "filled in" based on previous experiences. Since complex image patterns are difficult to recognize when presented in an unfamiliar orientation, simply placing a radiograph upside down or sideways on a view box disorients the viewer (Fig 1-1).

A piece of cardboard or a film envelope used to mask segments of the image will help to determine whether specific areas are under- or overexposed, show image blur, and so on. Using a cardboard mask, let us look at a routine chest radiograph (Fig 1-2A,B). It becomes obvious that the costophrenic sulci are underexposed; they are almost devoid of radiographic detail. Is this the result of body habitus, inadequate kilovoltage, the use of a higher grid ratio than needed, improper grid focal range, pathology, or some other factor?

In another example, the visualization of bone destruction in the center of a femur could lead to the conclusion that a satisfactory image was made (Fig 1-2C). But when the area of pa-

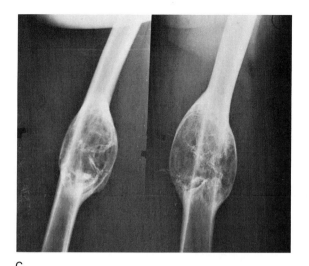

C

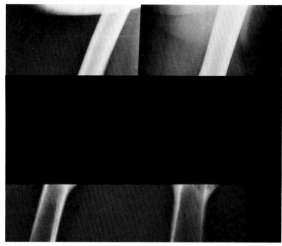

D

FIGURE 1–2C,D Lateral Projection of the Femur

This patient was evaluated for pain in the center of the thigh. Both AP and lateral projections were made. The obvious bone destruction in the center of the femur could lead to the conclusion that a satisfactory image was obtained even though the proximal and distal ends of the femur were not well visualized (C). Using a mask to cover the pathology, note that the proximal portion of the femur is significantly underexposed and the distal portion is overexposed (D). The bone lesion may not be the only concern. Periosteal reaction and/or soft-tissue changes attributable to another disease process might be missed because of an inadequate exposure.

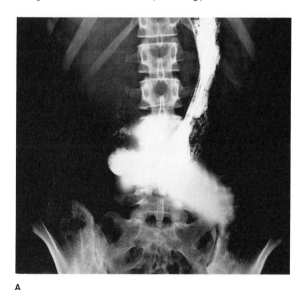

A

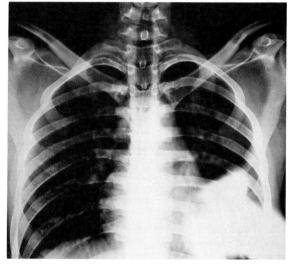

B

FIGURE 1–3 An Unusual Artifact

Supine imaging of a barium-filled stomach resulted in a confusing image. (A) An unsharp "opaque" density masks most of the lower lumbar spine and the left iliac wing. (B) Following the barium study, an AP supine radiograph of the ribs of another patient was made in the same room. The unsharp density also appeared, in the left lower lung field. A metal screw less than 1 in long was found lying on the internal filter of the x-ray tube. In the abdominal film, the slot in the top of the screw and the threads of the screw can be identified. If this type of problem were to occur with mobile equipment, the screw could move around within the housing, producing different configurations and making the artifact harder to isolate. (Courtesy Eastman Kodak Company, Rochester, NY.)

thology is masked, it becomes apparent that the proximal portion of the femur is underexposed and the distal portion overexposed (Fig 1-2D). Demonstration of a fracture or lesion does not absolve the radiographer of the responsibility for imaging the entire segment of the anatomy requested.

Artifacts also represent "image pathology" (Fig 1-3A,B).

TECHNICAL CONSIDERATIONS

This chapter highlights frequently encountered technical difficulties that can affect radiographic positioning. It includes basic information on image blur, filtration, x-ray absorption, screen-film systems, scatter control, and pathology (Fig 1-4). Additional technical considerations are presented in the positioning sections of this book.

Before beginning an x-ray examination, one must recognize the limitations of the patient, of the procedure, and of the equipment. In some departments, the radiographer takes a clinical history before carrying out a study. The selection of technical factors or positioning modifications may be affected by the patient's condition or the type of pathology suspected. A review of a previous study of the patient makes it easier to select a technique. A deformity such as scoliosis or a pathological condition such as bilateral edema of the extremities should be documented for the radiologist. A minor curvature of the spine might

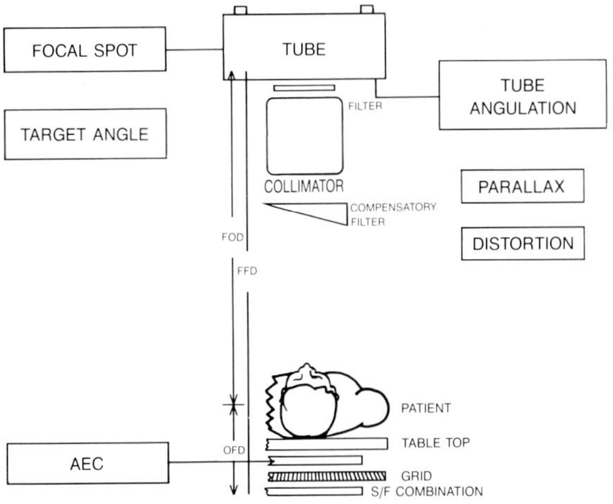

FIGURE 1-4 Diagnostic Imaging Chain

X-ray film records the technical factors and/or the decisions made by the radiographer. While the recording system influences the final image, manipulation of the equipment and selection of technical factors introduce most of the variables that affect the final radiograph. Most modern x-ray tubes using "steep angle" targets (12 degrees or less) have effective focal spot sizes of 0.6 mm (small) and 1 mm or 1.2 mm (large). The use of a steep angle target as opposed to a conventional target (15 to 17 degrees) permits higher instantaneous tube loading while maintaining a smaller effective focal spot. Filtration is added between the tube and collimator. Local, state, and/or federal laws require a specific amount of filtration within the x-ray beam. The mirror in the collimator, used to determine the size of the light/x-ray field, is a part of the filtration system. The combination of inherent and added filtration provides total filtration. When needed, compensatory filtration may be added. In this illustration, a wedge filter is placed at the collimator exit to compensate for the thickness differences of the shoulder. For illustration purposes, the patient is not centered correctly. If the patient were centered properly, this type of compensatory filter would restrict some of the x-ray beam at the lateral aspect of the shoulder, while minimizing undercutting of the image by a primary-beam leak. See Fig 1-11. The x-ray tube may be angled intentionally to distort radiographic anatomy. When the tube is angled more than 25 degrees with a dual emulsion film, image blur increases since the image on the front emulsion of the film is not superimposed exactly on the back emulsion. This may result in an increase in image blur owing to an increased parallax effect.

A 40 in FFD is usually used for table or upright Bucky examinations and a 72 in FFD for chest radiography or that of the lateral cervical spine. The Bucky tray (cassette holder) is a considerable distance (increased OFD) from the tabletop. In this illustration, the screen-film combination is shown at the level of the Bucky tray (6 to 13 cm from the tabletop).

An AEC can be used to control the length of exposure. An entrance type AEC is shown beneath the tabletop, in front of the grid and screen-film combination. Exit type AECs are located behind the cassette. The grid is placed beneath the patient, but above the cassette. Most modern x-ray tables are equipped with a 12:1 ratio grid for use with supine or erect 40-in FFD conventional radiography.

cause a shift in the mediastinal structures. Bilateral edema may indicate a medical condition as opposed to trauma to a single limb.

IMAGE BLUR

Structures or edges of structures are either sharp or not sharp. Some texts describe the poor demonstration of structural borders in an image by the term "unsharpness"; others use the word "blur."[6] Blur and image blur are the terms currently used.

The four basic categories of blur— geometry, the effect of the shape of the structures on absorption—intensifying screen characteristics, and motion—may contribute to loss of detail.

Geometry

Geometric distortion almost always occurs during radiography. The radiographic image is always enlarged when compared with the actual anatomy. Structures further away from the recording medium will appear larger owing to an increased distance between object and film, or object–film distance (OFD) (Fig 1-5). A shortened FFD also increases magnification.

Effect of Object Size, Shape, and Location on Image Blur

The enlargement of an anatomical part or segment of an image may be attributable to the position of the structure within the body, the shape of the structure, or the position or angulation of the x-ray tube. An excellent example of this is the anteroposterior (AP) view of the pelvis. The iliac wings flare outward bilaterally in a curved fashion, magnifying disproportionally. The anterior lateral aspects of the iliac wings enlarge and exhibit significantly more image blur than do the more posterior sacrum and coccyx. See Chapter 4.

Sometimes deliberately distorting a segment of the anatomy is advantageous. For example, the Towne projection elongates the bony vault of

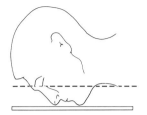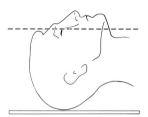

FIGURE 1–5 Geometric Distortion

The positioning of the patient may cause some geometric distortion. Left, With the patient in the conventional Waters position, the lower dotted line represents the level of the orbits, relatively close to the tabletop. Right, With the patient supine, the upper dotted line represents the relationship of the orbits to the tabletop. The PA Waters projection (left) should result in a sharper image of most of the facial structures than the AP Waters projection (right). This illustration does not take into account the increase in the OFD associated with table Bucky imaging. See Fig 1-4.

the skull, projecting the orbits away from the petrous pyramids. See Chapter 5.

The relationship of a body part to its location with regard to the x-ray beam also contributes to image blur. An increased OFD mandates the use of a small focal spot to reduce such blur. For example, some segments of the colon or stomach, particularly in the oblique position, magnify significantly and may be projected away from the receptor.

For a comparison of conventional table Bucky geometry and fluoroscopic spot geometry, see Chapter 6.

Direct Roentgen enlargement techniques benefit from deliberate magnification. Factors contributing to image blur in a magnification study include:

1. An effective focal-spot size larger than 0.3 mm.
2. Focal-spot blooming (an increase in the focal-spot dimension) owing to the use of a high milliampere (mA) setting and/or an extremely low kilovoltage setting.
3. The relationship between the x-ray tube and the detector. For example, if the skull were examined in the AP position using

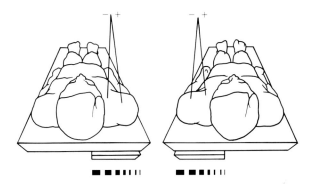

FIGURE 1–6 Effective Focal Spot and Anode-Heel Effect

The anode–cathode relationship affects image blur. The segment of the image produced by the x-ray beam toward the cathode side of the x-ray tube will be less sharp than that toward the anode side. With the x-ray tube positioned transversely (across the table), the lateral aspect of the right shoulder may appear sharper. When the opposite shoulder is examined with the cathode positioned over the lateral aspect of the shoulder, the lateral aspect of the left shoulder may appear less sharp. With reduced field imaging (8 in by 10 in or smaller), this effect might be difficult to see. This variation in sharpness is more apparent in a full field image, particularly when using a steep angle target x-ray tube. In addition to the differences in sharpness caused by the anode–cathode relationship, differences in radiographic density also occur. See Fig 1-8.

an enlargement technique, the orbits might be too close to the tube or too far from the detector, producing noticeable image blur even when using a fractional focal spot (0.3 mm or smaller).

Blur associated with the parallax effect accentuates with tube angle techniques. There is also an increase in image blur toward the cathode side of an x-ray tube as a result of the "heel effect." This change in the effective focal-spot size from the cathode to the anode affects image resolution[7] (Fig 1-6).

Intensifying Screens, X-Ray Film Characteristics, and Blur

Intensifying screen–film combinations contribute to image blur. T-grain, crossover control films produce sharper images at higher speeds than do conventional radiographic films. See "Screen-Film Technology."

Motion

The ability of the patient to cooperate should be determined before starting the examination. Breathing instructions and rehearsal of the procedure help patients understand what is expected. Even with a cooperative patient, the use of restraint and immobilization devices can help to overcome motion, and thus minimize image blur. The time spent on communicating with and immobilizing a patient is usually less than the time that would be required for a repeat examination.

In some radiographic positioning techniques, motion is used intentionally. Breathing sternum and lateral thoracic spine techniques are discussed in Chapter 5.

EFFECT OF ABSORPTION ON RADIOGRAPHIC DENSITY AND CONTRAST

In radiology, the word density has several meanings. Density is sometimes used to describe the light transmission of a translucent film. The radiographer thinks of radiographic density as referring to overall film blackening—the amount of film exposure.

Density also refers to any absorber in the x-ray beam that produces an opacity on a radiograph. The radiologist refers to density on a radiograph as an anatomical or pathological change resulting from the absorption of x-radiation. For example, radiolucent structures such as the lungs absorb very little x-radiation, resulting in increased film blackening, whereas solid mass or fluid within the lung absorbs x-rays, decreasing film blackening in this area. The atomic number and part thickness of a structure determine the degree of x-ray absorption.

The Nomenclature Committee of the Fleischner Society recommends the use of the word opacity in place of density when speaking

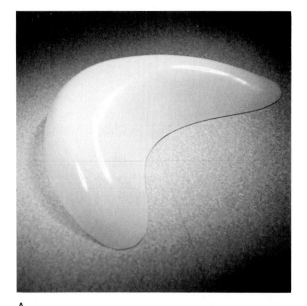

A

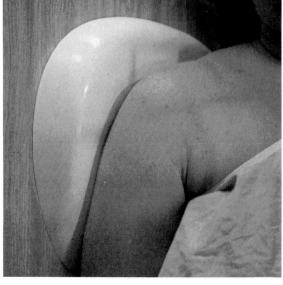

B

FIGURE 1–7   Underpart Filter

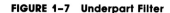

A compensatory filter either can be added to the collimator (see Fig 1-4) or used as an "underpart" filter to avoid a primary beam leak. (A,B) The Boomerang filter will prevent a primary beam leak and undercutting of the soft tissues of the shoulder. Excellent soft-tissue demonstration of areas as anatomically diverse as the face, knee, toes, coccyx, and greater trochanter of the hip are possible with this uniquely configured underpart filter. (C) Note the optimal visualization of calcific densities (tendonitis) in the soft-tissue areas of the shoulder. (Courtesy JA Vezina, Enterprises Octostop Inc, Montreal, Que, Canada.)

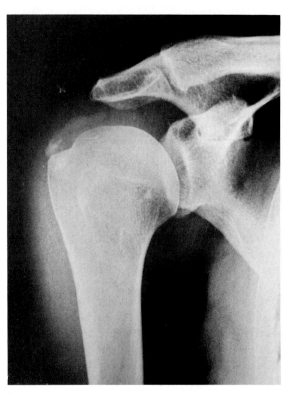

C

of an absorber in the path of the x-ray beam, and the use of the word density only when referring to the light transmission of a radiograph.[8]

Five basic radiographic absorbers—gas, water, fat, minerals (bone), and metal—contribute to density changes in a radiograph. These density differences can be seen in an AP view of the pelvis, which includes gas in the colon, fat stripes adjacent to the hips, soft tissues (water), bones (minerals), and, on occasion, a metallic orthopedic fixation device.

Structures of dissimilar densities in contact with one another are easily imaged, for example, the aerated lungs against the fluid-filled heart.

Structures with similar absorption characteristics are more difficult to image without special technologies or the use of contrast media. In the AP position of the abdomen, the liver, gallbladder, and right kidney are difficult to separate radiographically because of their similar absorption characteristics.

Contrast Media and Absorption

Where significant tissue differentiation does not exist, the introduction of a contrast agent into the body will help delineate anatomical structures. The digestive, biliary, urinary, lymphatic, and vascular systems require contrast media for visualization by x-ray. See Chapter 6.

Kilovoltage and Absorption

The area under study should be sharply outlined and exhibit exposure latitude. For example, in a chest image made with a high kVp/grid technique, the vascular and hilar patterns of the lung should be sharply defined and the ribs "suppressed." A high kVp technique helps one to "see through" the ribs, balancing density differences between mediastinal structures and the aerated lungs. See Chapter 7.

Filtration and Absorption

Low energy x-ray photons have little or no image-making properties, and they increase radiation dosage to the skin. Filters may be used selectively to remove low-energy photons from the x-ray beam, but this may require an increase in x-ray tube loading.

Filters added to the collimator or used at tabletop as "underpart filters" diminish the effect of image undercutting caused by a primary-beam leak[9] (Figs 1-4 and 1-7). An adjustable sliding aluminum filter can help to overcome absorption differences in body parts.[10]

Heel Effect and Absorption and Density

When electrons interact with the target of the x-ray tube, there is a nonuniformity of the intensity of x-ray photons along the long axis of the

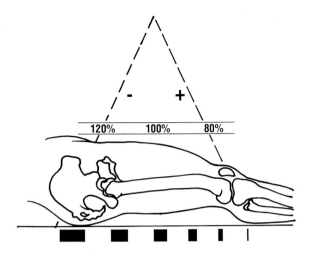

FIGURE 1-8 Anode-Heel Effect and Absorption and Density

When examining a structure of disproportionate thicknesses, for example, from the pelvis to the knee, the positioning of the x-ray tube with the cathode toward the thickest segment and the anode toward the thinnest segment takes advantage of the density differences (anode-heel effect) that occur owing to the line focus principle of the x-ray tube. According to Bushong,[11] these variations in x-ray intensity may be as great as 120% on the cathode side of the x-ray tube and as little as 75% on the anode side. The effect of tube positioning on image sharpness must also be considered. See Fig 1-6.

tube owing to the absorption of x-radiation within the anode.[7,11] With a standard 40 in FFD, there may be variations in x-ray intensity of about 30% measured along the cathode–anode axis of the x-ray tube. The use of a 72 in FFD reduces this variation to approximately 20%.[12]

The forearm, humerus, lower leg, and femur should be positioned to take advantage of the variations in x-ray intensity caused by the anode-heel effect (Fig 1-8).

SCATTER-RADIATION CONTROL

Beam Restriction

Primary and secondary radiation form the x-ray image. A large imaging field (14 in by 17 in) ex-

TABLE 1-1   Effect of Collimation on Exposure Factors

When using conventional techniques with the collimator shutters reduced to a smaller field size (see Fig 1-9), an adjustment in one or more technical factors is required to maintain the original radiographic density. For simplification, only timer adjustments are presented.

Because 50% or more of a full field (238-sq-in) radiograph may be composed of scatter, an adjustment (increase) in technical factors must be made to compensate for the decrease in radiographic density that occurs when tighter collimation is used. If the field size were increased from a tightly collimated field to a full field, a decrease in technical factors would be needed to maintain the original density of the smaller frame.

With an AEC, field size changes are adjusted automatically by an increase or decrease in exposure length. (Courtesy Cullinan AM: *Producing Quality Radiographs.* Philadelphia, JB Lippincott Co, 1987.)

Size	Sq. in.	Field Size	Timer Adjustments, seconds
14 × 17	238	Full	1/10
8 × 10	80	1/3	2/10
4 × 5	20	1/12	3/10

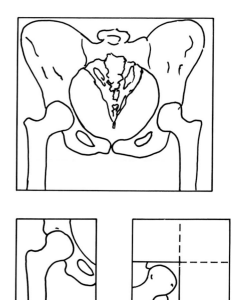

FIGURE 1-9   Field-Size Adjustment

Top, A 14 in by 17 in (238 sq in) radiograph of the pelvis. In a perfectly exposed radiograph with adequate contrast, one half or more of the density may be the result of scatter even when using a high ratio grid. Bottom left, Collimating the x-ray beam to an 8 in by 10 in field for a radiograph of the head and neck of the femur reduces the area to approximately 80 sq in. The exposure must be increased to compensate for the significant change in the primary-to-scatter ratio as field size is reduced. If the beam is further restricted to the head of the femur using one quarter of an 8 in by 10 in film (20 sq in), about 1/12 of the full field pelvis is exposed. Most of the tightly collimated image is produced by primary radiation, thereby requiring an increase in exposure factors. See Table 1-1.

poses a considerable amount of tissue to x-radiation, generating scatter proportionally. Most modern collimators use a positive beam limiting (PBL) system in which the shutters of the collimator automatically adjust to the size of the cassette in use. A change in the FFD also changes the shutter configuration.

Some radiographic views may require tight beam collimation, making it necessary to override the PBL. For example, reducing the field size from 14 in by 17 in to a 6 in by 6 in field exposes less tissue to x-radiation, requiring more primary radiation to produce a satisfactory density. An AEC will extend the exposure length to produce a preselected density[7] (Table 1-1).

With manual techniques, however, significant changes in field size require major technical adjustments—for example, keeping the kilo-voltage constant and adjusting mAs (milliampere seconds), or keeping mAs constant and increasing the kilovoltage (Fig 1-9).

An additional problem arises when the field size is severely restricted to 2 in by 6 in to permit exposure of two or more views of a finger or toe on a single cassette. The shutters in front of the mirror form the light pattern. If a shutter near the x-ray source and within the collimator is out

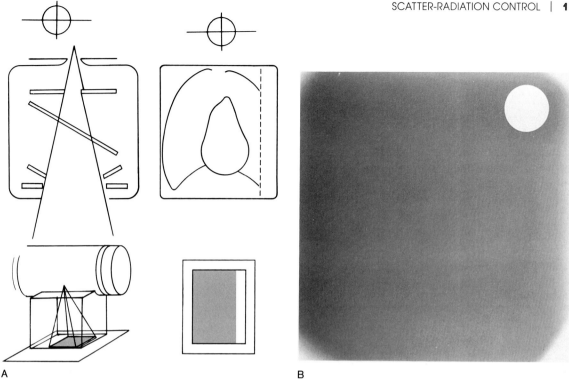

A   B

FIGURE 1–10 Primary Shutter Cutoff

Top left, The internal workings of a collimator, in which an upper shutter is out of alignment A. The x-ray beam is smaller in one dimension than the x-ray shutter light pattern. *Note*: In the collimator, one of the upper shutters has extended into the x-ray beam. The exit shutters form the light-field pattern as well as the x-ray–field pattern. As the light beam exits from the mirror, it forms the light pattern on the patient, theoretically shaping the size of the x-ray field. A chest radiograph made with this shutter defect might have more than a 1 in collimator cutoff on the side of the upper shutter misalignment. Top right, The dotted line represents the segment of the chest not fully exposed owing to the faulty entrance shutter. This line is not sharply imaged on the chest radiograph since

this event occurs almost in contact with the x-ray source. Shutter misalignment should be considered if a radiograph exhibits image blur at its borders.

Scatter and / or extrafocal radiation can "fill in" the image, giving the illusion of proper exposure. Bottom left, To evaluate a collimator for shutter cutoff, set the shutters to the desired field size and tape a sheet of x-ray film in a cardboard or plastic holder to the bottom of the collimator. **Do not use a screen-film combination for this test.** An exposure made at 50 kVp and 20 mAs to 50 mAs (depending on the speed of the film) will produce a black rectangular pattern. Bottom right, If a primary shutter is out of alignment, the shutter will be seen as a less dense area adjacent to the black rectangle. Although this defect is never in sharp focus on a radiograph, it can be seen on the test image since the FFD has been reduced from 40 or 72 in to 12 in or less, as the x-ray film is in contact with the exit segment of the collimator. This image B represents a radiograph made using the test procedure described above. To aid in orientation, a coin was taped to the film holder prior to its placement in position at the bottom of the collimator. Note the sharp outline of the shutters on three sides of the image. The penumbra seen on the fourth side of the image is caused by a primary shutter cutoff. Also note the diagonal cutoff at all four corners owing to the misalignment of a lead iris located external to the top of the collimator to control extrafocal radiation.

of alignment, it may cause the cutoff of a portion of a finger or toe even though the radiographer can see that the light pattern is larger than the size of the part being examined. Unaware of the difference in alignment of the x-ray beam and the light pattern, the radiographer observes only the light pattern on the cassette. A simple test can determine whether a misalignment exists (Fig 1-10A,B).

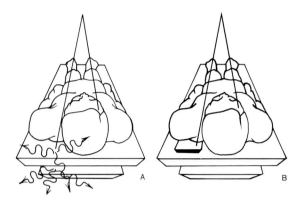

FIGURE 1–11 Primary-Beam Leak

A patient is shown positioned for evaluation of the skull. A primary beam leak is seen on the left side of the skull. Left, The x-ray beam striking the tabletop gives off scatter radiation in all directions. Some of this scatter undercuts the image, masking the soft tissues of the face and scalp. Right, Placing a sheet of lead rubber or a container filled with cornmeal, rice, flour, or water on the tabletop to absorb the unattenuated primary beam will minimize this undercutting effect.

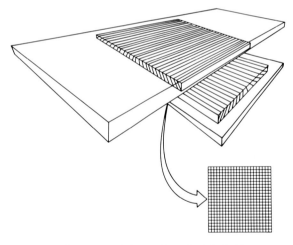

FIGURE 1–12 Improvising a Crosshatch Grid

If a high-ratio grid is needed to examine a large body part, a crosshatch grid can be made by utilizing the existing Bucky grid and a grid cassette with their grid lines positioned at right angles to each other. The grid lines of the Bucky will be blurred by the motion of the grid, but the lines of the grid cassette may be seen on the image. An increase in technical factors is needed to compensate for the increase in ratio of the combined grids. It is better to increase kVp rather than mA or time, within the ratings of the x-ray tube in use, for this change in grid ratio. (Courtesy Eastman Kodak Company, Rochester, NY.)

Primary-Beam Leak

Most segments of the anatomy, at their lateral aspects, do not conform to the shape of a collimated beam. Some of the primary beam may strike the x-ray table or cassette without passing through the patient. This "primary beam leak" (unattenuated x-ray) causes scatter to be emitted in all directions. This scatter undercuts the x-ray image at the peripheral aspects of the part, causing segmental damage to the image. A "tissue equivalent" underpart filter placed in the primary beam not only attenuates unabsorbed primary radiation, but also does not interfere with diagnosis (Fig 1-7). Careful positioning of a sandbag or lead sheet on the x-ray table avoids the masking or obscuring of portions of the anatomy (Fig 1-11).

Segmental scatter can mask the soft tissues (scalp) of the skull, the shoulder, the lateral aspects of the abdomen, the greater trochanter area of the AP hip, the lateral sternum, and the spinous processes of the thoracic, lumbar vertebrae and the sacrum and coccyx in the lateral projection.

Grid Versus Nongrid Technique

A grid or Bucky is recommended when body part measurements exceed 10 cm or when examining dense structures that require high kilovoltage techniques.

Other uses for higher kVp/grid techniques include the imaging of extremities in casts or of body parts with significant variations in thickness, such as the foot in the dorsoplantar position, the AP projection of the ankle, or the AP tangential projection of the calcaneus. See Chapter 4.

Grid Selection

Fiber interspaced grids contain lead lines (metal) bonded to fiber (organic) interspacing materials such as paper, plastic, or cardboard. Temperature changes and absorption of moisture affect organic materials. Aluminum interspaced grids contain metal (lead) bonded to metal (aluminum) and are not affected by environmental changes.

TABLE 1–2 Grid Versus Nongrid Technique Compensation

When a grid technique is substituted for a nongrid technique, some adjustment in kVp and/ or mAs is required. In the early years of radiography, most grids were either 6:1 or 8:1 in ratio. A simple division of the grid ratio by two resulted in the approximate increase in mAs required for the use of a grid over a nongrid exposure. A 6:1 grid required three times the mAs and an 8:1 grid required four times the mAs needed for a nongrid study. With higher-ratio grids, this rule of thumb is not practical. An increase of six or eight times the mAs with a 12:1 or 16:1 grid would significantly increase patient dosage, as well as heat units to the x-ray tube. As grid ratio increases, additional kVp is recommended. Grid focal range is a primary consideration. (Courtesy Cullinan AM: *Producing Quality Radiographs.* Philadelphia, JB Lippincott Co, 1987.)

Type	Ratio	Focal Range (in)	Maximum kVp	+ mAs	+ kVp
Nongrid				1X	
Linear	5:1	28–72	85	2X	+8
Linear	6:1	28–72	85	3X	+8
Linear	8:1	34–44	95	3X–4X	+15
Linear	12:1	36–40	110	5X	+20–+25
Linear	16:1	40	125	6X	+20–+25
Crosshatch	12:1	28–72	110>	5X	+20–+25
Crosshatch	16:1	34–44	125>	6X	+20–+25

Radiographers understand the relationship of grid ratio to the scatter cleanup capability of a grid. However, some misunderstanding may exist regarding the effect on scatter cleanup of the number of lead lines per inch in a grid. Grids with a different number of lines per inch, but all of the same ratio, have similar cleanup capabilities. An 8:1 grid is an 8:1 grid, regardless of the number of lines per inch (60, 80, or 100 lines or more). More lead lines per inch make the lines less visible on the radiograph. Higher ratio grids have severe focus and centering limitations. As grid ratio increases, grid focal range decreases (Table 1-2).

Two linear grids (parallel or focused) superimposed at right angles to each other for maximal scatter cleanup are called crosshatch grids. A high grid ratio effect can be achieved if two low ratio grids are used in a crosshatch configuration. The focal range of this combination is determined by the focal range of the highest-ratio grid. A crosshatch grid can be improvised by using a table Bucky and a grid cassette (Fig 1-12).

Kilovoltage ranges should match the ratio of the grid in use. Higher ratio grids can be used with increased kVp for full-field studies (Table 1-2). Smaller field sizes with lower ratio grids also tolerate higher kilovolt values.

Grid Selection for Pediatric Patients

Pediatric patients vary greatly in size, from neonates to adolescents who are almost adult in size. The same table Bucky grid is often used for patients of all sizes, even though a grid acceptable for an adolescent may exceed the grid ratio needed for an infant. Many departments do not use a grid or Bucky for radiographs of infants.

Grid Artifacts

The movement of a grid in a Potter-Bucky diaphragm blurs grid impurities as well as grid lines. The motion of a grid or Bucky blurs the dense sharp-edged artifacts associated with grid fractures. Unfortunately, these density artifacts within the grid can act as an unwanted "underpart filter" and may mask pathology.

A "striping" artifact occurs when short exposures are used with a conventional speed Bucky and a fiber interspaced grid. Striping of a fiber interspaced grid may mimic a roller mark artifact of an x-ray film processor.

Radiographic evaluation of the grid will demonstrate most grid artifacts.

Grid Centering. Left to right miscentering to a grid results in unilateral grid cutoff. Realignment of the x-ray tube after horizontal beam positioning avoids lateral decentering of the x-ray beam to the grid. An improper FFD can result in a bilateral grid cutoff even when the x-ray tube is properly centered to the grid. See Chapter 7.

> CAUTION: Horizontal beam positioning requires careful alignment of the x-ray beam to the center of the grid. See Chapters 4 through 7.

Placement of Grid for Stereo Radiography. Conventional radiographs are two-dimensional images. However, conventional radiography can be used to produce a three-dimensional effect with two separate exposures and a shifting of the x-ray tube between exposures. The patient must remain in the same position for both exposures. The tube must be moved off center (top to bottom, not side to side) prior to the first exposure. Shifting the tube side to side would result in unilateral grid cutoff of each image (Fig 1-13). After the first exposure, the cassette is changed and another exposure made after the tube has been shifted an equal distance past the center in the opposite direction.

The interpupillary distance, the FFD, and the distance used for stereo viewing all affect the degree of stereo shift. A 40 in FFD needs a tube shift of about 4 in (2 in to either side of center). Chest radiographs made at a 72 in FFD utilize a 6 in shift (3 in off center to the top and 3 in off center to the bottom).

> CAUTION: A problem occurs with beam collimation during a stereo shift. A shutter cutoff can occur at the top of one and at the bottom of the other image. Slight angling of the tube for each exposure rather than opening the collimator to an elongated pattern avoids this problem (Fig 1-13).

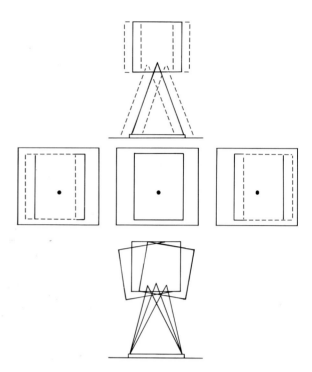

FIGURE 1-13   Tube Alignment for Stereo Radiography

With the patient in the same position for two exposures, a stereo effect can be produced with conventional radiography by shifting the x-ray tube "off center" an equal distance between each exposure. To avoid grid cutoff when using a grid or Bucky, the tube must be moved from top to bottom, never from side to side. Tight beam collimation results in image cutoff in both images unless the shutter pattern is elongated. A slight tube tilt toward center for both exposures is recommended since it will not increase the area of exposure or interfere with the three-dimensional effect.

Grid/high kVp latitude techniques have practically eliminated the need for stereo chest radiography. See Chapter 7.

For many years, stereo radiography of the chest was used to visualize anatomy behind the heart and ribs since the nongrid/lower kVp techniques in use at that time resulted in short scale contrast images—blackened lungs and chalklike osseous structures. Increased scatter generated by the lateral nongrid chest image also resulted in poor-quality lateral images.

See Chapter 5 for special considerations regarding stereo skull radiography.

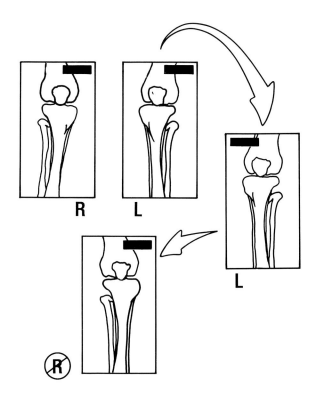

FIGURE 1-14 Use of a Cassette ID Marker to Indicate Patient's Left or Right Side

A lead "R" or "L" is used in radiography to identify the side of the patient being viewed. When, as in an emergency situation, a marker is not available, radiographers know the position of the patient ID blocker in the cassette and can determine whether it is the right or the left side of the patient from this orientation. Unfortunately, the inverting of the cassette changes the location of the patient ID blocker. Since radiographs are transparent, if there is no patient-side indicator, a physician might place the image on the view box as if it were made with the tube side of the cassette up, rather than inverted. Top, Note the position of the ID blocker in the right and left images. If the cassette were to be inverted to image the left leg, the ID blocker would be opposite to its normal position. Bottom, When the inverted cassette image of the left leg is placed on the view box, using the ID blocker as a side indicator, the left leg might be incorrectly identified as the right leg.

Kodak X-Omatic Inverted Cassette as an Improvised Grid. The Kodak X-Omatic cassette contains a thin sheet of lead foil located behind the posterior intensifying screen to absorb backscatter. Sweeney[13] reports that an inverted X-Omatic cassette functions at up to 85 kVp as a 5:1 ratio grid without the focal range restrictions of a grid. With the X-Omatic cassette positioned in a conventional manner (tube side up), the radiographer can see the location of the patient identification (ID) blocker. An inverted cassette changes the location of the patient ID area. The manufacturer did not intend for this cassette to be used in an inverted manner.

CAUTION: This ID marker should never function as a part or side indicator, particularly with the use of an inverted cassette (Fig 1-14).

AUTOMATIC EXPOSURE CONTROL

Most AECs have a density selector that increases or decreases radiographic density by adjusting the exposure length. An adjustment for an underexposed radiograph requires a plus density change; an overexposed radiograph requires a minus density change (Fig 1-15, page 16).

With an AEC, the radiographer usually selects mA, kVp, and focal spot size. A normal AEC setting is generally used to produce a preselected density automatically. The AEC also controls density adjustment caused by changes in field size. Since the phototimer or ionization chamber is a timer, a severe limitation in field size (e.g., from 14 in by 17 in to 6 in by 6 in) automatically increases the exposure length to produce the preselected density. Conversely, converting from a small field to a larger field shortens the exposure owing to the increase in scatter.

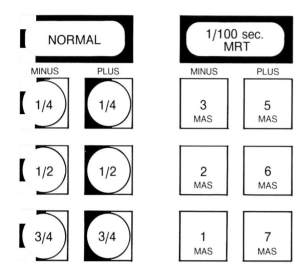

FIGURE 1-15   Adjustment of AEC

The normal AEC density setting is generally predetermined to meet departmental preferences. Occasionally, a radiograph may be lighter or darker than desired and the use of the "minus" or "plus" settings should, in theory, decrease or increase the density. A radiograph repeated using the −1/2 or +1/2 station should produce an image 50% lighter or darker, respectively, than the original image. Many older AEC units have a minimal response time of

1/100 second — the fastest possible exposure that this unit can make. If high kilovoltage (140 kVp), high milliampere (400 mA) chest images are made, with a minimal response time of 1/100 second, every patient will receive an exposure of at least 4 mAs at 140 kVp. Most patients do not require 4 mAs or more at 140 kVp for a PA chest exposure, particularly with a 400 speed screen-film system. If the kVp value were lowered to reduce the density, the AEC would stay on for a longer time. Lowering the kVp would produce a shorter scale of contrast. To overcome the minimal response time, one should lower the mA setting; a small patient might require 50 mA, a medium size patient 100 mA, and so on. It is important that tube rating charts be checked before making changes in the mA setting since the lower mA stations often automatically shift to the small focal spot. For illustration purposes, a density adjustment device is shown (left) with changes in mAs rather than density percentages (right). For this illustration, 400 mA is used at a 1/100 second minimal response time, therefore, the shortest possible exposure would be 4 mAs. On the plus side, the changes result in 5 mAs, 6 mAs, and 7 mAs adjustments. On the minus side, the changes should result in 3 mAs, 2 mAs, and 1 mAs, but this is impossible. Since the unit cannot terminate an exposure faster than 1/100 second, all patients examined using 400 mA would receive a minimum of 4 mAs. If 1 mAs were indicated, the mA setting would have to be lowered to 100 mA or less to give the AEC time to respond beyond its minimal response time.

Exit-type AECs require cassettes containing little or no lead backing. With entrance-type detectors, cassette backing material does not influence AEC factor selection.

AEC and Contrast

A fixed or optimal kVp is generally used with an AEC. The kilovoltage level selected influences the contrast scale in an image.

An increase in kVp automatically lowers mAs to produce a preselected density, resulting in a longer scale of contrast. A decrease in kVp automatically raises the mAs value and produces a shorter scale of contrast.

AEC and Density

An AEC cannot distinguish among primary, scatter, and remnant radiation.

When using manual techniques, miscentering a patient to a cassette has little effect on density. But improper centering of a patient to an AEC sensor often results in an unsatisfactory radiograph. Off-centering may also result in a primary beam leak, with undercutting of the image, and may cause premature termination of an exposure.

Predetermined film blackening will occur even with minimal inspiration when using an AEC for chest radiography. Unfortunately, the elevated diaphragm associated with poor inspiration widens the heart shadow, often making an accurate diagnosis difficult. See Chapter 7.

SINGLE-PHASE OR THREE-PHASE X-RAY EQUIPMENT

Many x-ray departments have single- as well as three-phase equipment. Generator phase (output) has a major effect on technique.

With the exception of angiography and chest radiography, technical-factor recommendations

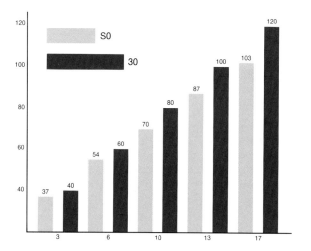

FIGURE 1–16   Single Phase Versus Three Phase

This graph can be used to make technique adjustments from single-phase to three-phase equipment. (Extrapolated from the data of GJ Barrone and ED Trout, reported in *Radiology*, September 1971.)

for specific studies are rarely found in the literature. When kilovoltage is mentioned, almost never is it specified whether it's being generated with single-phase, three-phase, constant-potential, or high-frequency equipment. A significant difference is seen in the radiographic "look" with the same kilovoltage value at single phase, at three phase, and at constant potential, even with a compensatory adjustment in mAs (Fig 1-16). To duplicate the density of a radiograph made in

a single-phase room at 80 kVp would require 70 kVp if a three-phase unit were used at the same mAs value. If the exposure factors were proper for the single-phase equipment and a view were repeated for a positioning change, the use of the same factors in a three-phase room would result in an image overexposed by 10 kVp or more. A true high frequency generator produces up to twice the output of conventional single-phase systems.

Suggestions for optimal kilovoltage values and appropriate ratio grids for specific examinations are discussed in the positioning segments of this book.

SCREEN-FILM TECHNOLOGY

Hundreds of screen-film (single- or double-emulsion) combinations using conventional or rare earth phosphors are available to the radiographer. In the interests of efficiency and economy, some medical imaging departments use only one screen-film combination. While a contrast type of radiographic film is excellent for high contrast images such as bone or radiopaque contrast media studies, the abrupt black and white effect of this film may be less than optimal for chest radiography. Latitude or extended latitude films favor chest imaging, but may not be optimal for visualization of bony trabeculation.

Intensifying screens, when exposed to x-radiation, emit light in the blue, green, and ultravi-

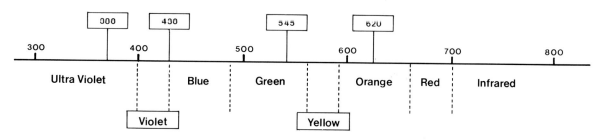

FIGURE 1–17   Electromagnetic Spectrum

A review of the electromagnetic spectrum helps one to appreciate the need for matching specific phosphors to appropriate films. X-ray film responds to specific emissivity ranges of the phosphors used in the intensifying screens. Ultraviolet, blue, and green film-sensitivity ranges must match intensifying-screen light emissions. The electromagnetic spectrum is shown from 300 to 800 nm. (Courtesy Cullinan AM: *Producing Quality Radiographs*. Philadelphia, JB Lippincott Co, 1987.)

olet ranges, with one of these colors being dominant. Therefore, a green-emitting screen emits primarily green light and a blue screen emits primarily blue light.

The color sensitivity of radiographic film should be matched to the type of light emitted by the intensifying screen[7] (Fig 1-17, page 17).

CAUTION: If a blue-sensitive film were used with a primarily green-sensitive screen, the system speed would be reduced to approximately one half. The same result occurs when a green-sensitive film is used with a primarily blue-emitting screen.

The use of more than one film bin in a darkroom to accommodate films of different speeds is an efficient, low-cost option that takes advantage of state-of-the-art screen-film technology.

An automatic cassette loader makes different sizes and types of films easily accessible. The cassette loader minimizes the possibility of accidentally loading a cassette with a film that is not compatible with the screen selected.

Screen and Film Speed and Resolution

Calcium tungstate screens have a linear, nearly flat, response over the range of 50 to 120 kVp. Barium strontium sulfate screens increase in speed from 50 to 80 kVp, and then fall off slightly. Below 65 kVp they can be slower than calcium-tungstate screens.[14] Conventional rare earth intensifying screens (250 speed), when compared with high speed calcium tungstate screens (250 speed), demonstrate a significant increase in sharpness.

A 400 speed rare earth system can have the resolution capability of a high speed calcium tungstate screen (250 speed) owing to improved absorption/conversion phosphor efficiency[7] (Fig 1-18).

Although the term rare earth screen-film combination usually implies an ultrafast screen-film speed, rare earth screen-film technology varies in system speed from 20 to 1,200. Information is available from the manufacturers of screen-film combinations on the speed and image blur characteristics of their products.

In the past, it was generally believed that the diagnostic properties of medical images were synonymous with spatial resolution. The probability of detecting abnormalities depends on both the contrast of the lesion and the complexity of the structures that surround it. Objects of complex shape can be more easily hidden by surrounding structures that possess similar features. Items of very low spatial frequency, such as soft tissue, may be brought into a perceptibly more advantageous frequency range by using a minifying (reducing) lens or by moving further away from the radiographs for viewing.[5] Resolution is influenced by an increased FFD and the selection of a smaller focal spot made possible by the use of high speed intensifying screens.

CAUTION: When comparing screen-resolution limitations, one must be sure that the screens being compared are of the same phosphor type.

Kilovoltage Selection

Some radiographers still appear to be preoccupied with using low kVp to produce short scale contrast—abrupt blacks and whites—a photographic rather than a radiographic look. Rare earth screens are kVp dependent below the 70 kVp range. Some screens function at approximately half speed below the 40 kVp level and may not be appropriate for some examinations.

Some rare earth screens may increase in speed with an increase in kilovoltage from 50 to 120 kVp. Below 60 kVp, they may have no speed advantage over calcium tungstate or barium strontium sulfate. As Logan et al[15] comment, "We were impressed by how little exposure reduction was possible at low kVp using the rare earth screens. The response of screen-film combinations to radiation at different energies is complex and depends on the filtration of the beam, the peak energy of the beam, and the position of the K-absorption edges of the compounds of the screen. Some rare earth intensifying screens when used with low kVp may have little or no advantage over conventional intensifying screens."

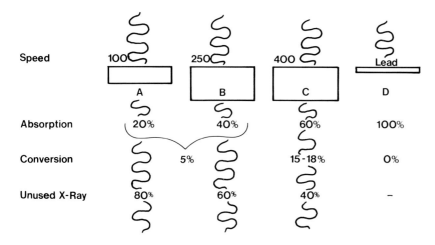

FIGURE 1–18 Intensifying-Screen Absorption / Conversion Ratio

The speed-numbering system associated with screen-film radiography is not related to the International Standards Organization numbering system associated with photography. For many years, all intensifying-screen products were of the same speed. When screen-film combinations were increased in speed in the 1950s, some speed designator had to be provided. Existing systems were labeled speed 100 (A) and the newer system speed, two times faster, labeled 200 speed, etc. Before x-radiation can be converted to light, it must be absorbed by the phosphor in the screen. As the thickness of the phosphor layer of the screen increases, there is increased absorption of x-ray photons (B). Rare earth phosphors (C) absorb more x-rays than conventional calcium tungstate phosphors of equal thickness. However, absorption is not the only characteristic required of an intensifying screen. If this were so, a thin sheet of lead (D), which absorbs 100% of the x-radiation would be efficient for imaging. When x-ray photons are absorbed, they must also be converted into light that can expose radiographic film. Conventional 100 speed (A) and 250 speed (B) calcium tungstate screens absorb approximately 20% and 40% of the x-ray beam, respectively, but convert only 5% of the absorbed photons into useful light. A rare earth screen (gadolinium oxysulfide) that is equal in thickness (C) to the 250 speed calcium tungstate screen (B) will absorb as much as 60% of the primary beam, but will convert 15% to 18% to useful light. Lead (D), which absorbs 100% of the primary beam, converts nothing to light. (Courtesy Cullinan AM: *Producing Quality Radiographs.* Philadelphia, JB Lippincott Co, 1987.)

Quantum Mottle

The effect of quantum mottle on an image and crossover control technology (the reduction of light scatter within the cassette) are two topics that merit comment here. Quantum mottle exists in all screen-film images. It is caused by the variation in optical density resulting from the random distribution of x-ray quanta absorbed by the detector. Visualization of quantum mottle increases with faster screen-film systems of the same phosphor type.

Ordinarily, quantum mottle in a radiograph does not present a problem to the interpreter of the image. It is objectionable, however, in some specific radiographic studies, such as the evaluation of minute osseous structures within the petrous bones, of calculi within the gallbladder, or of the neonatal chest for hyaline membrane disease, known as the respiratory distress syndrome (RDS). Currently, the hearing structures in the petrous areas are usually examined using computed tomography (CT) while ultrasonography is the primary imaging modality for the gallbladder. Fast screen-film combinations, if used for neonatal-chest imaging, may exhibit a high level of quantum mottle and mask an RDS pattern. The neonatal chest is frequently examined using slower systems to overcome timer limitations on bedside units. The shortest possible exposure (1/120th or 1/60th of a second) may result in an overexposed image.

Since many bedside units have a fixed milliampere setting, as well as timer limitations, high speed screen-film systems may force the radiographer to use low kVp values — 50 kVp to 55 kVp.

> C A U T I O N : Most rare earth intensifying screens are kVp dependent and fall off in speeds at the lower levels.

Slow speed, single-emulsion screen-film systems are preferred for extremities: 400 to 600 speed for routine radiography and rare earth 1,200 speed screen-film combinations for follow-up studies of extremities in casts and for scoliotic studies.

Various screen-film combinations should be considered for pediatric radiography because of the wide variations in patient size. A 2 lb neonate compared with a 150 lb adolescent represents a weight ratio of 1 to 75. It is not advisable to use the same screen-film combination for both patients.

Crossover Control

As crossover of light within the cassette produces up to one third of a radiograph's density, control of such crossover greatly reduces image blur (Fig 1-19). The reduction of light within a cassette also permits a radiographer to use a higher kilovoltage than usual for a study. For example, a 10 kVp increase in the 65 to 85 kVp range (at one half the mAs), when employed with a crossover control film at the lower kVp level, exhibits contrast similar to that of a radiograph using conventional high contrast film.

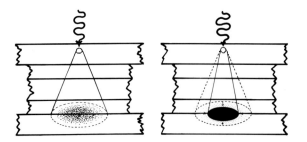

FIGURE 1–19 Crossover of Light

About one third of the density on a radiograph is produced by crossover of light within a cassette. When an x-ray beam strikes an intensifying screen and the absorption/conversion process occurs, light is given off in all directions. In this illustration, a cone of light is shown passing from the screen through the adjacent emulsion and base to the opposing emulsion. Note that the portion of the emulsion of the film exposed adjacent to the screen is larger than the phosphor crystal. Left, A significantly larger portion of the film is exposed on the opposing emulsion. This "blooming" effect adds to image blur. If crossover light control could be added to a screen-film system, the light crossing through to the opposite emulsion could be reduced. Right, Note that, in the illustration representing crossover control, the beam produces a smaller circle of light, resulting in a sharper image. With crossover control, the light that ordinarily would cross through the emulsion is stopped by a dye, usually in the emulsion. The light does not pass easily through the dye and exits forward via the shortest dye path. This cuts the crossover of light approximately in half and reduces image blur as compared with conventional screen-film combinations. Crossover of light can be considered to be "light scatter" that bounces around within the cassette, fogging the image. The reduction of light scatter within the cassette by crossover control has the same effect on the image as does the reduction of x-ray scatter by the use of lower kilovoltage, a grid, or tight beam collimation.

EXAMPLE:

Conventional/high-contrast film

70 kVp at 20 mAs

Crossover control/high contrast film

80 kVp at 10 mAs

Both radiographs will exhibit similar contrast levels. The scatter radiation associated with 80 kVp is present on the crossover controlled radiograph, but light scatter within the cassette is reduced by almost 50%. With crossover control technology, higher kVp can be used to produce a latitude technique.

When examining osteoporitic patients with inherently poor osseous subject contrast, the use of crossover control films results in images with improved radiographic contrast. The lowering of the kilovoltage with a compensatory increase in milliampere seconds can further enhance contrast in osteoporitic structures.

The use of a crossover control system at a higher kVp offers:

1. Improved screen speed response with less chance of a falloff in speed.
2. Greater margin for error (increased technical latitude). If a single type of x-ray film is preferred, a high contrast, crossover control film used with a higher kilovoltage will produce a latitude "look" if needed.
3. Better soft-tissue visualization, with abrupt blacks and whites minimized.
4. Acceptable level of contrast because of the reduced light scatter within the cassette.

DOSAGE REDUCTION

The ALARA (as low as reasonably achievable) concept suggests that there is no threshold dose for radiation injury and that all radiation entails some degree of risk. Furthermore, exposures to radiation produce cumulative effects.

Carbon-fiber materials in tabletops, cassette fronts, grid covers, and grid interspacing materials absorb less radiation than do conventional materials. Carbon-fiber materials can also be used in AEC sensors, image intensifier input phosphor facings, and compression plates for serial film changers.

Dosage can be reduced:

1. Three percent to 15% by changing to a low absorption tabletop.
2. Six percent to 12% by changing to a low absorption cassette front.
3. Twenty percent to 30% by using a grid with carbon-fiber covers and fiber interspacing[16] (Fig 1-20).

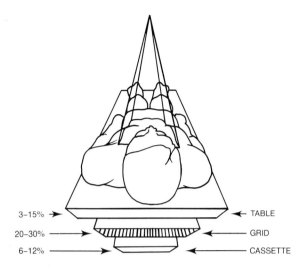

3–15% → TABLE
20–30% → GRID
6–12% → CASSETTE

FIGURE 1–20 Low-Radiation-Absorption Materials

Commercial tabletops and cassette fronts vary in their attenuation characteristics, which is particularly troublesome in the low kVp ranges. When low-absorption products such as carbon-fiber materials are used (at approximately 80 kVp), x-ray dosage reduction can range from 30% to 50%. The low-absorption tabletop, grid, and cassette all absorb significantly less x-radiation than do those made from conventional materials.

> C A U T I O N : Conventional commercial tabletops and cassette fronts vary in their attenuation characteristics owing to the use of different materials and different thicknesses. This attenuation is energy dependent, especially at low kVp values. At approximately 80 kVp with low absorption products, there is an overall reduction in dose in the range of 30% to 50%.

> N O T E : While the interest in low absorption materials is valid, simply converting from a 200 speed to a 400 speed screen-film technology can reduce patient dosage by as much as 100%.

Other Dosage Considerations

The use of a shadow shield for gonadal protection avoids patient embarrassment, and when used in the operating room, helps to avoid contamination of a sterile field.

The posteroanterior (PA) position is sometimes used for skull tomography or a scoliotic evaluation of the vertebral column to reduce radiation to the lens of the eye, thyroid, sternum, and breasts. Equipment calibration also helps to assure image quality and minimizes radiation dosage to the patient and/or radiographer.

QUALITY ASSURANCE

In the practice of radiological technology, one must obtain the greatest amount of useful information possible with the least patient discomfort and radiation risk.

Critically ill patients require highly detailed studies that may contribute more to patient care than some of the newer imaging modalities. The technical expertise of the radiographer affects the management and, in some cases, the survival of the patient.[17] The alertness of the radiographer can make the difference in a diagnostic study and so influence patient care. Understanding the rationale behind a specific examination helps the radiographer to help the interpreter.

Every department should have appropriate testing equipment, as well as personnel who are trained in the performance of tests and the evaluation of the results. Noninvasive testing can be performed by radiographers; complex tests require the services of an x-ray physicist or engineer. Manufacturers of test tools provide instructions for the use of the tools and the evaluation of the test results.

Some basic quality assurance tests to be performed by radiographers are as follows:

1. Tests to assure beam alignment and collimator accuracy.
2. Screen-film–contact testing.
3. Tests of manual timer accuracy.
4. Tests of phototimer reproducibility, so as to include patients of different thicknesses and variations in kilovoltage.
5. Radiography of the grid for defects.
6. Half-value layer test to determine beam filtration.
7. Focal spot size measurements.
8. Measurements of kilovoltage accuracy.
9. Tests of reproducibility of milliampere settings.
10. Processor-control tests.

Carefully maintained records of equipment malfunction make recurrent problems or variations in exposure obvious and help to initiate corrective procedures. Quality assurance goals mandate technically reproducible follow-up studies over an extended period.

As work loads increase, the documentation of technical factors and related information for each study becomes more important. The technical information and the rationale associated with the original technique help the radiographer to make decisions regarding a repeat study.

A clinical history may influence the selection of technical factors since disease or injury affects technique selection. For example, an overexposed chest radiograph might suggest an emphysematous condition, while an underexposed abdomen might indicate the presence of a significant amount of free fluid. If a radiographer has no information about a specific disease process prior to the exposure, an overexposed or underexposed image attributable to pathology is not a technical error.

VIEWING CONDITIONS

Ambient light reflecting off the surface of an image can influence diagnosis and the perception of technical quality. A slightly overexposed radiograph, evaluated on a single, bright view box, may appear greatly overexposed when viewed on a multibank viewing unit in another area. The view boxes at the quality control station or in the processor area or viewing rooms should all have similar light outputs.

PLAIN-FILM RADIOGRAPHY

For most examinations, plain-film radiography is widely available and has many common applications, is characterized by relatively low radiation exposure, and is low in cost.[18]

Any diagnostic examination should yield further information about the patient and thus perhaps alter the treatment of the patient or the outcome of the disease process. A diagnostic examination should have the greatest utility (highest sensitivity and specificity) for a patient while posing as little risk as possible. With these factors being equal, the least costly examination should be chosen.

Cost–benefit considerations will be a major challenge in patient care over the next decade.[18] Cost containment has revitalized an interest in general radiology. When existing equipment can provide similar diagnostic information at a lower cost, the use of an expensive imaging modality must be otherwise justified.

At the University of California, Irvine Medical Center, conventional and new-modality examinations of the chest were evaluated. This study included the likelihood of replacement of conventional screen-film chest x-ray examinations by CT, magnetic resonance imaging (MRI), or digital imaging. According to Eric Milne, MD, of the Irvine Medical Center, CT imaging of the chest has poorer spatial resolution than plain chest radiography, costs approximately ten times more than a PA and lateral chest study, and exposes the patient to up to 200 times more radiation. A CT examination can take four or five times longer than a conventional chest study and perhaps as much as five to ten times longer for its interpretation. Similar drawbacks are seen with MRI, with the exception of the amount of radiation dosage. This procedure requires even more examination time than the CT scan. Five CT scanners dedicated to chest radiography would require eight hour workdays for an entire year to replace 24,000 conventional chest examinations, and ten dedicated MRI units would be needed to replace the conventional chest radiographic examinations.[19]

Cost containment is not a new problem. Complaints are often heard about the number of sheets of x-ray film involved in a study. A lengthy illness or death can be very expensive. A correct diagnosis is always cheapest.[20] This statement, made in 1943, indicates that cost containment has always been a consideration.

Film cost was not the only consideration at that time. Other problems included:

1. Lengthy exposures. Techniques were limited to direct exposure film or 100 speed screen-film systems.
2. Equipment output limitations. An x-ray output of 200 mA was maximal.
3. Large focal spot sizes (2 mm or 4 mm). Slow speed screen-film systems often necessitated the use of a large focal spot.
4. Grid limitations. Low ratio grids (5:1) were needed because of the slow screen-film combinations used at that time.
5. Dosage. The slow speed of the screen-film combination and a lack of national standards for x-ray tube filtration significantly added to patient dosage. Today's high speed screen-film technology, rectangular beam collimation, and high kilovoltage techniques greatly help to reduce radiation dosage.

As a result of these technical limitations, a 100 speed mentality developed—and it is ironic that such a mentality still prevails among some radiographers, physicists, and radiologists who have never used 100 speed screen-film systems or low output, single-phase generators. Today's so-called limited-output mobile units have more film-blackening potential than did the conventional x-ray units of 30 years ago. Increased-speed screen-film combinations (up to 1,200 speed) enhance the film-blackening effect. When comparing a 200 mA, single phase conventional x-ray unit using a 100 speed screen-film combination with a modern 100 mA, three-phase or constant-potential mobile unit using a 1,200 speed screen-film system, a more than sixfold increase in film blackening is possible with a modern mobile unit/high speed screen-film combination.

A 100 speed mentality is acceptable only if one is limited to 100 speed detectors and low-output generators.

CHAPTER TWO

Positioning Concepts

POSITIONING GUIDELINES

Plain-film radiography plays an important part in patient care. In an emergency situation, or in the practice of a primary-care physician, a radiographic examination may be the only diagnostic imaging study available to the critically ill patient. In a large facility, plain radiographs are often a prerequisite to using ultrasonography, CT, or MRI.

Projections or positions traditionally have been named for the person who first described them, the projection of the central ray, or the position of the patient or part. In this book, innovative or unusual positions and projections follow the descriptions outlined by the original authors.

Almost a half century ago, Colson[21] reported in *The X-Ray Technician* (now *Radiologic Technology*) that "cooperation of the technician with his roentgenologist in trying new positions to help establish a diagnosis can give the technician a real feeling of usefulness and justify his profession beyond that of just a 'button pusher'."

An inventive position might be needed to demonstrate a pathological lesion or a fracture not seen on the preliminary study. But before changing a positioning routine, one must thoroughly understand conventional positioning. Deviation from a standardized routine, if needed to accommodate an unusual or difficult situation, should be logical and well thought out. To the innovative, experienced radiographer with a preconceived notion of how the final image will appear, the outcome of the study is predictable.

Basic Guidelines for Optimal Positioning

The following list of positioning concepts documents some of the positioning responsibilities and concerns of radiographers.

- The radiographer must be certain that the patient examined is the one listed on the requisition. A patient will often respond inappropriately to any name.

- It is important that the projection selected suit the patient's condition. Whenever necessary, the patient should be supported with artifact-free pillows, compression bands, or sandbags to limit movement and minimize blur.

- The radiographer must know when to delay or expedite a procedure and how to move an injured patient. The radiographer also must be prepared to step away from the patient if a priority problem develops, such as maintaining an airway. When the radiology department actively participates on the trauma team, time can be saved during the initial examination of severely injured patients. The emergency-room radiographer often has access to a complete clinical history and can ask appropriate questions of the emergency-room physician to help develop innovative positioning techniques. Physical as well as radiographic examinations help to uncover occult injuries.[22]

● All clothing or foreign objects that may absorb x-radiation should be removed, and items such as dentures and jewelry placed in a secure location.

● Before palpating for body landmarks, the radiographer should inform the patient of the objective of and need for the procedure. If the patient is complaining of problems in the area of the left kidney, for example, the patient may not understand the rationale for palpating the symphysis pubis or greater trochanters when the radiographer is positioning the survey film of the abdomen prior to an intravenous urogram.

● Instructions should be clear and concise. Prolonged explanations may confuse the patient. The patient who understands what is expected will be more cooperative, thus making positioning easier. Well-modulated, low-key instructions serve to lessen patient apprehension. A patient with a language barrier may become frightened if spoken to in a loud voice. If the patient has serious concerns about radiation dosage or the results of the study, a supervisor, such as the chief radiographer, a radiation safety officer, or a physician, should be consulted. Patient concerns about radiation dosage merit more than an abrupt explanation.

● The use of the smallest film size possible is not only good economy, but when combined with collimation, also reduces radiation dosage.

● Since a radiograph is a two-dimensional representation of a three-dimensional object, a single projection may not yield adequate diagnostic information. Most positioning routines consist of at least two views, usually at right angles to each other. This requirement is particularly important for localization of foreign bodies or lesions or to demonstrate fracture alignment (Figs 2-1 and 2-2).

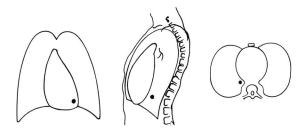

FIGURE 2–1 Foreign-Body Localization

Left, A metallic foreign body represented in this illustration by a small black dot is hidden behind the left border of the heart in the PA projection. Center, In the lateral projection, the foreign body can be seen posterior to the heart in the retrocardiac area. The PA projection demonstrates the foreign body in only one plane. It could be embedded in the skin of the chest or in the front or back of the patient. In the lateral projection, it cannot be determined whether this opaque foreign body is superficial or deep in the chest. If this fragment were more posterior, it could be superimposed over the thoracic vertebrae (behind the heart) and perhaps not be detected. The PA and lateral radiographs localize the foreign body without the use of CT. Right, In a transverse anatomical section such as a CT scan, the foreign body is seen adjacent to the posterior cardiac border.

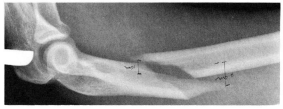

A

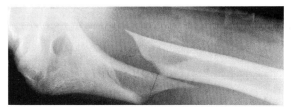

B

FIGURE 2–2 Fracture Alignment

An AP and lateral humerus. (A) Note in the lateral view that the fragments seem to be in good apposition. (B) In the AP view, significant displacement of the fragments is demonstrated. Images made at right angles to each other are essential to determine fracture alignment.

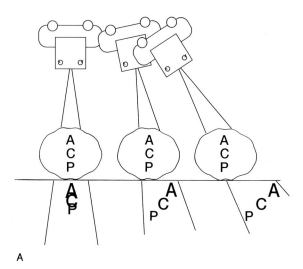

FIGURE 2-3 Effect of Tube Angulation

(A) A schematic representing the body (A, anterior) (C, central), and (P, posterior). Left, A perpendicular beam projection results in superimposition of the A-C-P structures. When the tube is angled across the patient, there is a shifting of the structures, with the anterior segment being displaced more dramatically. Center, The resulting configuration is P-C-A. Right, Increased angulation would result in the same relationship, with the structures more widely separated. (B) Careful attention must be given to tube–cassette–object alignment, particularly at the bedside. The tube and cassette labeled "A" are in proper alignment, with a slight separation of the

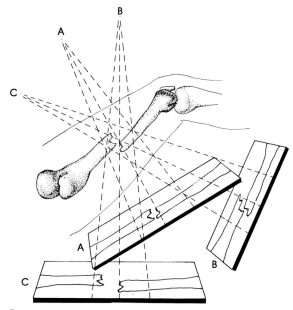

fragments of the femur demonstrated. Tube position "B" in relationship to the cassette gives the illusion of fragment separation. Tube "C" misalignment to cassette "C" gives the illusion of fragment overlapping. Of interest, significant tube angulation requires that the FFD be readjusted to compensate for the increased path of the x-ray beam. The markings on the tube crane do not accurately represent the FFD with tube angled projections. (Courtesy Cullinan AM: *Producing Quality Radiographs.* Philadelphia, JB Lippincott Co, 1987.)

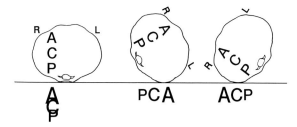

FIGURE 2-4 Effect of Patient Rotation

The schematic representation shown in Fig 2-3 is repeated using AP perpendicular beam projections and various supine positions for three exposures. Left, The A-C-P structures superimpose when a perpendicular beam projection is used without patient rotation. Center, When the patient is rotated to the left, the anterior structures (A) shift to the left and the posterior structures (P) shift to the right. Right, When the patient is rotated to the right, the anterior structures (A) shift to the right and the posterior structures (P) shift to the left.

• Tube angulation and/or patient rotation supplement basic positioning (Figs 2-3 and 2-4). Tube angulation causes a shift in the projection of anatomical structures on the image and can be used to advantage in specific examinations. By using various angles, it is possible to change the projection pattern and to separate superimposed structures in the body. When the tube is angled, the FFD increases. Depending on the degree of tube angulation, this may result in an underexposed radiograph when using manual techniques.

• Sometimes oblique, tangential, or horizontal beam projections are required to make a diagnosis (Fig 2-5). See Chapters 4 through 8.

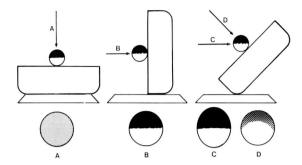

FIGURE 2-5 Horizontal-Beam Imaging for Air — Fluid Levels

A horizontal beam technique (CR parallel to the floor) is required to demonstrate an air–fluid level on a radiograph. (A, top) In this representation of a supine projection, the air in the circular object is represented by the black upper portion of the circle. The white, lower portion represents fluid. (A, bottom) The resultant radiograph would be a diffuse gray object since the air–fluid interface would not be demonstrated in this projection. In the upright position (C, top), the horizontal beam demonstrates the air–fluid interface without distortion (B, bottom). In the semi-erect position (C, D, top), the air–fluid level remains parallel with the floor. If a horizontal beam technique is used (C, top), an air–fluid level is demonstrated with some distortion of the anatomy (C, bottom). If a perpendicular beam technique is used to avoid this distortion (D, top), the air–fluid interface will not be demonstrated (D, bottom). Horizontal beam radiography is used to show free fluid in the chest or sinus cavities or obstruction of the bowels, or in air-contrast barium studies. (Courtesy Cullinan AM: *Producing Quality Radiographs.* Philadelphia, JB Lippincott Co, 1987.)

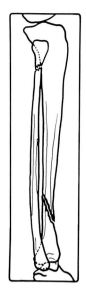

FIGURE 2-6 The Importance of Joint Visualization

It is sometimes difficult to include an entire extremity in a routine examination. In this example, there is a fracture with some displacement of the distal tibia, as well as a fracture of the proximal fibula. If only the ankle were imaged, the fracture of the fibula would not be seen. A similar problem can occur with a displaced fracture of the ramus of the mandible, which is often accompanied by a fracture at the neck of the opposite condyle. See Chapter 5, Fig 5-18.

• Paraprofessionals not familiar with x-ray terminology may request projections not compatible with a departmental routine.

• Although an examination of the extremities should always include the joint nearest to the site of injury, if possible, both the proximal and distal joints should be examined. For example, a displaced fracture of the lower tibia not accompanied by an adjacent fracture of the fibula invariably will demonstrate a fracture somewhere along the fibula, often near its proximal attachment to the tibia (Fig 2-6). Similarly, a displaced fracture of the mandible on one side is often accompanied by a fracture near the neck of the opposing condyle. See Chapter 5, Fig 5-18.

• Radiographs should be evaluated before dismissing the patient to make certain that the images include all related anatomy.

• A laser-positioning device helps to align the patient and cassette with the x-ray beam (Fig 2-7, page 28).

• One corner of a radiograph usually contains an ID area reserved for institution and patient data. The location of the ID marker should not be used to determine which side of the patient is being examined. See Chapter 1, Fig 1-14. Stick-on ID labels, if used, should not cover the area of interest. A routine should be developed for the consistent placement of lead markers to identify positioning indicators.

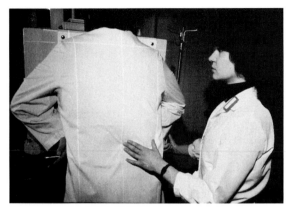

A

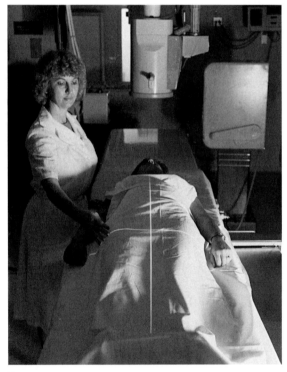

B

FIGURE 2–7   Laser Positioning

The use of a laser-beam system for chest (A), abdominal, or special procedure radiography (B) makes tube–patient–cassette alignment easier, particularly with tube angulation techniques. Exact CR location can be achieved with any x-ray unit when a laser-positioning device is used. (Courtesy Gammex Laser, Milwaukee, Wis.)

Effect of Changes in Position on Technique

The physical appearance of the body gives a general indication of where the internal organs lie within it. With various positions, the anatomy shifts and the location of an organ or foreign body may change. Positioning a metallic marker at the point of entrance of a foreign body can help in its localization.

Changes in the position of the patient affect radiographic technique. In the prone position, the weight of the body flattens the abdominal tissue, necessitating a decrease in exposure factors compared with those used with the supine position. With the decubitus position of the abdomen, tissue thickness increases in its dependent portion. In the erect position, the inferior dependent portion of the abdomen thickens. As the x-ray beam traverses the bodies of patients placed in varying degrees of obliquity, exposure factors require modification (Fig 2-8).

Advantages of the Prone Position in Selective Examinations

Patients with kyphosis may be more comfortable in the prone position. When examining the skull, the prone position reduces primary radiation to the eyes. The use of lead eyeglasses to minimize exposure to the lenses of the eyes during AP intracranial tomography may produce artifacts and a reduction in image quality. When prone, the patient cannot see and, therefore, cannot follow the complex conventional tomographic tube movement (6 seconds' exposure or longer) required, making patient motion less likely to occur.

Scoliotic patients may require long-term follow-up studies, including multiple radiographic examinations. Although one examination may expose the patient to only a small amount of radiation, multiple follow-up studies have a cumulative effect. The PA position for examination of the scoliotic spine reduces radiation to the thyroid, sternum, and breasts.

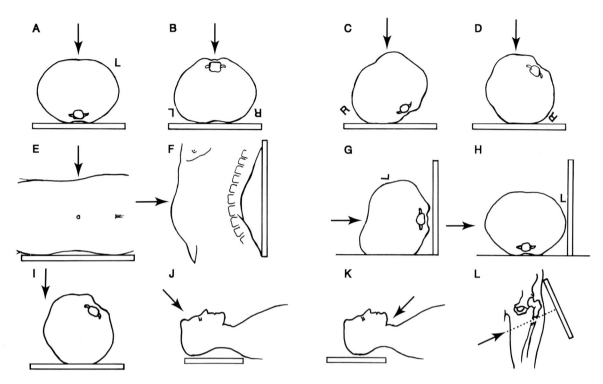

FIGURE 2-8   Effect of Patient or Tube Positioning on Exposure Factors

The configuration of the body may change with changes in the position of the patient. Measurements taken in the supine position (A) for an AP projection or for a dorsal decubitus projection (H) will be greater than those taken in the prone position (B), since in the prone position, there is a flattening of the soft tissues of the abdomen as they spread out bilaterally. In the oblique positions, RPO (C) and RAO (D), changes in configuration may occur as the body is rotated.

If the patient is turned to a lateral decubitus position (G), the dependent portion of the abdomen becomes thicker than the upper segment. The use of a wedge filter, with the thicker portion of the filter positioned to coincide with the upper aspect of the abdomen, may help to overcome absorption differences, particularly with obese patients. When the patient is in the erect position (F), some of the structures in the abdomen may drop, causing a difference in absorption. When the abdomen thickens or flattens, technical factors should be adjusted for conventional imaging. An AEC makes these adjustments automatically.

Projections are sometimes defined by the direction of the CR when it is not perpendicular to the film. Some variations in tube angulation are described. With the patient supine, the CR enters anteriorly and exits posteriorly (A). In the PA position, the x-ray beam enters posteriorly and exits anteriorly (B). A lateral projection is described with reference to the side closest to the x-ray film. This illustration represents the left lateral position, with the x-ray beam entering through the right side of the patient (E). When the patient is in the oblique position and a CR is used for a tangential projection, the image is seen in silhouette and the projection is described as tangential (I). This projection is often used to locate a foreign body in extrinsic tissue or to demonstrate a depressed fracture of the skull. See Chapter 5. The term axial projection is used when the x-ray beam is directed caudad (J) or cephalad (K).

Horizontal beam techniques (F, G, H, L) require that the x-ray tube be horizontal to the floor, regardless of the position of the patient or detector. A horizontal beam projection is often used to radiograph the head of the femur in the axiolateral position (L) or for erect (F) or decubitus (G, H) imaging.

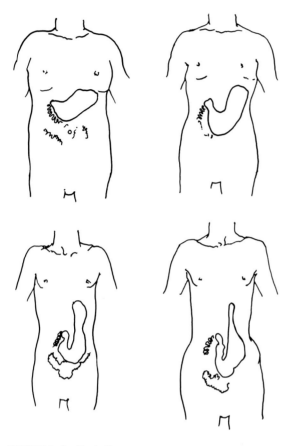

FIGURE 2-9 Body Types

When positioning a patient, body habitus must be considered. Top left, A broad, deep thorax and short, wide lung fields and heart characterize the hypersthenic patient, with the stomach, gallbladder, and transverse colon high in the abdominal cavity. Bottom left, A long, narrow thorax and short abdominal cavity describe the very thin asthenic patient, with a long, narrow heart and lungs and low diaphragm. Sthenic (top right) and hyposthenic (bottom right) body types represent the patients between these two extremes. The position of organs within the body also changes with changes in the position of the patient. The stomach is used in this illustration to remind radiographers of the differences in the locations of organs that may be encountered with different body types.

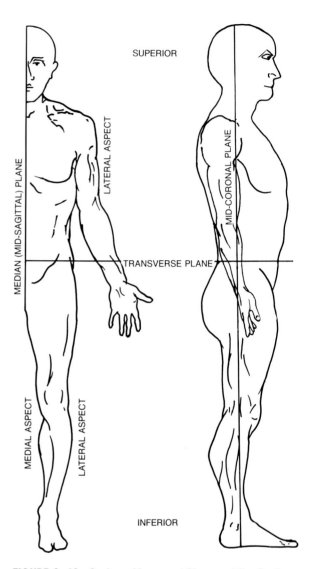

FIGURE 2-10 Surface Lines and Planes of the Body

BODY TYPES

The four major body types—hypersthenic, sthenic, asthenic, and hyposthenic—present wide variations in the location of specific body parts (Fig 2-9). Sthenic and hyposthenic types account for approximately 50% and 35%, respectively, of all individuals.[1] Body habitus, anatomy, the condition of the patient, and the projection of the x-ray beam must be considered when positioning a patient for an examination.

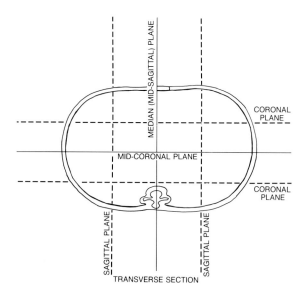

FIGURE 2–11   Transverse Section of the Body

PLANES, LINES, AND SURFACE POINTS

The radiographer needs to know the lines, planes, surface descriptions, and relationships used in radiographic positioning (Figs 2-10 and 2-11).

RELATIONSHIPS OF BODY SEGMENTS TO REFERENCE POINTS

Anterior   The frontal or ventral surface of the body.

Posterior   The back or dorsal surface of the body.

Lateral   The side furthest from the midline of the body.

Medial   The side nearest the midline of the body.

Superior   The portion of the body situated above a reference point.

Inferior   The portion of the body situated below a reference point.

Proximal   The part nearest the center of the body or point of reference.

Distal   The part furthest from the center of the body or point of reference.

Imaginary planes or lines are used as reference points to aid in radiographic positioning (Figs 2-10 through 2-12).

PLANES

Median plane   An imaginary plane that passes in a vertical AP direction, extends through the midline of the trunk, and divides the body into two symmetrical parts. (Often referred to as midsagittal.) There is only one median plane in the body.[23]

Sagittal plane   An imaginary plane or planes parallel to the median plane. A sagittal plane does not have to pass through the sagittal suture any more than a coronal plane has to pass through the coronal suture.[23]

Midcoronal plane   An imaginary plane that passes through the midaxillary area and coronal sutures at right angles to the median plane; it divides the body into anterior (ventral) and posterior (dorsal) segments.

Coronal plane   An imaginary plane or planes parallel to the midcoronal plane.

Transverse (*horizontal*) plane   Imaginary plane or planes that pass in a horizontal direction at right angles to the median and coronal planes. It divides the body into cross sections and superior and inferior segments.

SOME SURFACE POINTS OF THE CHEST AND ABDOMEN (FIG 2-12)

Suprasternal notch   A deep indentation above the superior margin of the sternum.

Midpoint   A point located midway between the suprasternal notch and the symphysis pubis.

Transpyloric line   Imaginary horizontal line halfway between the suprasternal notch and the symphysis pubis, which passes through L-1. When first described, this plane was thought always to pass through the pylorus of the stomach. However, this proved to be not always true since abdominal viscera tend to change shape and position with body habitus, the phase of respiration, and the position of the patient.

Transtubercle line   Imaginary horizontal line across the crests of the ilium at the upper border of L-5.

Anterior superior iliac spines   The uppermost and anterior iliac spines located on the anterior lateral aspects of the ilia.

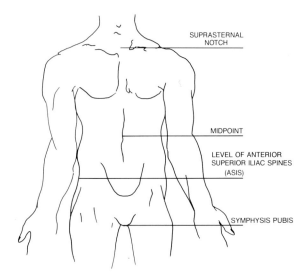

FIGURE 2-12A Surface Points of the Chest and Abdomen

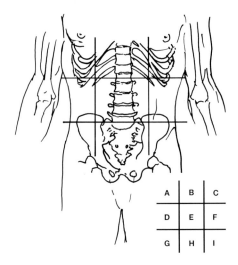

FIGURE 2-12B Regions of the Abdomen

(A) Right hypochondriac
(B) Epigastric
(C) Left hypochondriac
(D) Right lumbar
(E) Umbilical
(F) Left lumbar
(G) Right inguinal
(H) Hypogastric
(I) Left inguinal

Symphysis pubis The anterior junction of the pubic bones, in the midline.

Lateral lines Imaginary lines drawn parallel to the median plane, halfway between the median plane and the anterior superior iliac spines.

SOME LINES, PLANES, AND SURFACE POINTS OF THE SKULL (FIG 2-13)

Supraorbital line (*Supraciliary line*) An imaginary line located above the eyebrows.

Interpupillary line Imaginary line perpendicular to the median plane through the center of the orbits.

Glabellomeatal line Imaginary line that passes through the glabella and auricular points, about 8 degrees above the orbitomeatal line.

Orbitomeatal line Imaginary line lying about 7 degrees above the infraorbitalmeatal line and passing through the orbits and auricular points; referred to as the radiographic base line.

Infraorbitomeatal line Imaginary line that joins the infraorbital point to the external auditory meatus; referred to as the anthropological base line or Reid's base line.

Acanthiomeatal line Imaginary line that passes through the acanthion and external auditory meatus.

Auricular point Center of the external auditory canal.

Glabella A prominence lying between the eyebrows, directly above the bridge of the nose.

Nasion The point at which the nasofrontal suture bisects the median plane and forms a depression at the bridge of the nose.

Acanthion A point at the junction of the upper lip and the tip of the anterior nasal spine.

Gonion The point of angle of the mandible.

Symphysis menti The symphysis of the mandible.

Inion The external occipital protuberance.

LOCALIZATION POINTS

Body habitus affects the position of the stomach, the gallbladder mediastinal structures, the cardiac silhouette, and so on. Other factors include

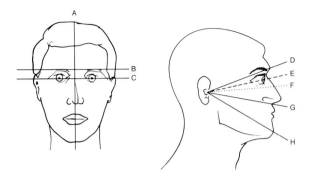

FIGURE 2–13   Lines, Planes, and Surface Points of the Skull

(A) Median plane
(B) Supraorbital (supracilliary) line
(C) Interpupillary line
(D) Glabellomeatal line (solid line)
(E) Orbitomeatal line (dashed line)
(F) Infraorbitomeatal line (dotted line)
(G) Acanthiomeatal line (solid line)
(H) Mentomeatal line (solid line)

posture, position of the patient, degree of respiration, and digestion. Soft-tissue structures, fluid, and foreign bodies may change in location as a result of changes in positioning.

Localization points for a typical adult are listed in Tables 2-1 (below) and 2-2 (page 34).

POSITIONS OF PATIENT OR PART

Radiographic positioning of the patient or body part is described by specific body positions.[24] (See Fig 2-8.)

Recumbent (Basic, Lying Down)

Supine (AP)   Patient is in recumbent position, lying on back (A).
Prone (PA)   Patient is in recumbent position, lying on abdomen (B).
Obliques   Patient is turned diagonally (C, D): right anterior oblique (RAO)*; left anterior oblique (LAO)*; right posterior oblique (RPO)*; left posterior oblique (LPO).*
Laterals   Patient is positioned so that side with area of interest is placed closest to the detector (E).

Recumbent (Modification, Lying Down)

Trendelenburg   Patient's head is lowered; body and legs are elevated on an inclined plane.
Decubitus:
Lateral   Patient is lying on side (G).
Dorsal   Patient is lying on back (H).
Ventral   Patient is lying on abdomen.

TABLE 2–1   Localization Points for Head and Neck

Structures	Localization points
Pharynx and throat cavity	Level of base of skull to C-6
Nasopharynx	Above soft palate
Oropharynx	Between soft palate and C-6
Sella turcica	1 in anterior and 1 in superior to external auditory meatus
Inferior base of the skull; foramen magnum	Mastoid tip; C-1
Hyoid; angle of mandible (with head in neutral position)	C-3
Carotid bifurcation; cartilage of larynx	C-4
Thyroid cartilage	C-5
Pharynx	Base of skull to level of C-6
Esophagus (extends from pharynx to stomach)	C-6 to T-11
Cervical ribs (if present)	C-7

TABLE 2–2   Localization Points for Chest, Abdomen, and Pelvis

Structures	Localization points
	Intercostal spaces
Upper segment of sternum (articulates with clavicle and costal cartilage)	1
Body of manubrium; breast (extends from second to sixth rib and laterally from the sternum to the midaxillary line)	2
Horizontal fissure on right side (seen in PA chest radiograph)	4
Apex of heart (about 5 cm from midline)	5
Spleen (in contact with dome of left hemidiaphragm in left upper quadrant of abdomen; posterior and inferior to stomach)	9
Gallbladder (changes location with posture); upper poles of kidneys (move with respiration; right is about 1 cm lower than left)	11 to L-1 (right side)
Liver (from dome of diaphragm to level of right lower costal margin, varies with position, degree of respiration)	Lower costal margin
Upper margin of scapula	Level of second posterior rib
Lower margin of scapula	Level of seventh posterior rib
Suprasternal notch; upper border of manubrium	T-2, T-3
Sternoclavicular joints	T-3
Sternum	T-3 to T-9
Manubrium	T-4
Bifurcation of trachea; main-stem bronchus (at rest)	T-5
Bifurcation of trachea; main-stem bronchus (at full inspiration)	T-6, T-7
Inferior angle of scapula	T-8
Border of xiphoid process; body of the sternum	T-9
Xiphoid tip; esophageal opening through the diaphragm (lies above and to the left of the aortic opening)	T-10
Cardiac orifice (enters the stomach, 5 cm to left of midline)	T-11
Aortic opening through the diaphragm (lies slightly to the left of the midline)	T-12
Pancreas (from level of L-2 lies obliquely upward to T-12, behind the stomach; head lies within the curve of the duodenum; tail in contact with the spleen)	T-12 to L-2
Kidneys (vary with patient build; right generally 1 cm lower than left)	T-12 to L-3
Stomach (varies in position with body type and posture; fundus lies in close contact with inferior surface of diaphragm)	T-11 to L-2
Transpyloric plane	L-1
Duodenum continuous with jejunum (3 to 4 cm to right of midline); hepatic flexure; transverse colon (runs to left across the abdominal cavity)	L-2
Inferior border of rib cage (lateral aspect formed by tenth rib)	L-3
Iliac crest	L-4, L-5
Transtubercle plane	L-5
Bladder (lies in anterior, inferior portion of pelvic cavity, just above the symphysis pubis; varies with degree of distention; when full, can rise to level of sacroiliac joints); prostate (behind and adjacent to symphysis pubis; surrounds neck of bladder in males)	Symphysis pubis
Hip joint	1.5 in below a point bisecting an imaginary line formed by ASIS and symphysis pubis

Erect (Basic)

Frontal (AP) Patient is facing forward, with dorsal surface closest to detector (F).

Posterior (PA) The ventral surface is closest to the detector.

Obliques Patient is turned diagonally: (RAO) (RPO)*; (LPO) (LAO).*

---

*N O T E : Anatomy seen in RAO view is similar to that of LPO; anatomy seen in LAO view is similar to that of RPO.

N O T E : In the supine or prone oblique position, anterior or posterior structures shift medially or laterally. Midline structures move very little (Fig 2-4).

Laterals Patient is positioned so that the side with the area of interest is placed closest to the detector.

Lordotic (AP) The patient is tilted backward so that the apices of the lungs are projected free of the clavicles.

PROJECTION OF CENTRAL RAY

It is always correct to describe a projection by the direction of the central ray (CR) and the placement of the patient in relationship to the detector. For example, with the patient in the AP position, for a study of the abdomen, the x-ray beam enters the abdomen anteriorly (A), exiting posteriorly (P), thus, it is an AP projection. With the patient in the RPO position, the x-ray beam enters the body anteriorly and exits posteriorly; thus, it is an AP (oblique) projection. (See Fig 2-8.)

Anteroposterior (AP) X-ray beam enters anteriorly and exits posteriorly (A, C, F).

Posteroanterior (PA) X-ray beam enters posteriorly and exits anteriorly (B, D).

Lateral X-ray beam enters laterally, right or left, and exits at the opposite side (E).

Horizontal-beam technique The CR is horizontal to the floor regardless of the position of the patient or film (F, G, H).

N O T E : Projections are sometimes defined by the angle made by the CR when it is not perpendicular to the film; for example, cephalad, caudad, tangential.

Tangential X-ray beam enters an obliquely positioned part to produce a silhouette (profile) of a surface (I).

Axials (AP) (PA) X-ray beam is directed to intersect the long axis of the body.

Caudad X-ray beam is projected toward the feet (J).

Cephalad X-ray beam is projected toward the head (K).

Axioloateral X-ray tube is adjusted to direct the CR at a right angle to the body part (L).

The effect of tube or cassette angulation on image blur must be considered. The use of a perpendicular beam technique, whenever possible,

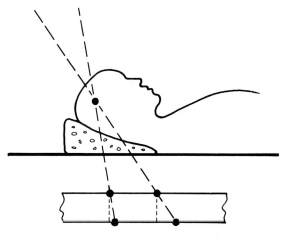

FIGURE 2-14 Parallax

Image blur increases when an x-ray tube is angled while using dual emulsion x-ray film. A small black dot represents the area of interest in this illustration. With a shallow tube angle (10 degrees), the dot is projected onto the dual emulsion film with a slight separation of the image on the anterior and posterior emulsions. When the tube angle is increased to 25 degrees or more, a greater separation of the image is seen. If the patient's head were elevated on a 15 degree sponge and a tube angle of 10 degrees maintained, the parallax effect could be minimized. A small focal spot (0.6 mm or smaller) can help to reduce image blur.

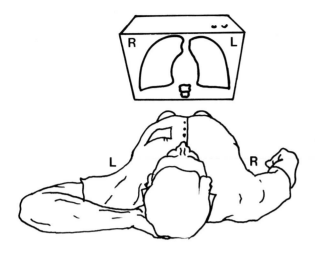

FIGURE 2-15 View of an Image

A radiograph is placed on a view box as if the patient were facing the viewer in the anatomical position. Therefore, the right side of the patient would be on the left side of the viewer. In a textbook, side indications may be confusing. When you look at this radiographic image, the right side of the chest is on the left side of the illustration.

minimizes the parallax effect associated with dual emulsion imaging. Rotation of the patient, rather than tube angulation, to separate superimposed body structures also helps to minimize the parallax effect (Fig 2-14).

In certain types of radiography, such as of the sternum, tube or patient angulation is necessary to separate one structure from another. By using different angles, the projection pattern changes, helping to visualize superimposed structures. See Chapters 4 through 8.

VIEWING OF THE IMAGE

For technical evaluation or interpretation, a radiographic image is presented as the patient would appear if facing the viewer (Fig 2-15).

CHAPTER THREE

Skeletal Radiography

The appendicular and axial portions of the skeleton form the bony framework of the body[25] (Fig 3-1). This structure functions to support and protect certain vital organs, and, by interacting with muscles, it allows movement. This chapter will address anatomical/pathological observations, positioning concepts, and technical considerations related to skeletal radiography.

The technical literature documents many variations in skeletal radiographic routines, with some reports suggesting only minor degrees of change in patient obliquity and/or tube angulation. Since it was not practical to include all of these variations, the modifications that appeared to be most useful are described here.

ANATOMICAL / PATHOLOGICAL OBSERVATIONS

Osteology is the study of the bones of the skeletal system and related cartilaginous and membranous structures. Joints, classified according to their structure and function, are formed when two or more bones of the skeleton come together (Table 3-1). In joints with little or no movement, the bones are held together by fibrous tissue. Joints that have more movement (synovial joints) are united by a fluid-filled fibrous capsule. Cartilage covers the ends and facets of the bones and their articulating surfaces.

Bone tissue is either compact (dense) or cancellous (spongy). The periosteum, a thin vascular membrane of fibrous tissue, covers the portions of bone not enveloped by articular cartilage.

Skeletal motion is described according to the direction of motion of the extremity or joint involved in the motion. For example:

Flexion The act or condition of bending two jointed parts, thereby reducing the angle between the parts.

Extension The stretching out or straightening of two jointed parts, thereby increasing the angle between the parts.

Abduction Lateral movement of a limb away from the body or median plane of the body; movement of digits away from the axial line of the limb; lateral bending of the head or trunk.

Adduction Movement of a limb toward the median plane; movement of digits toward the axial line of the limb.

Eversion Stress lateral deviation of the foot and ankle, hand and wrist.

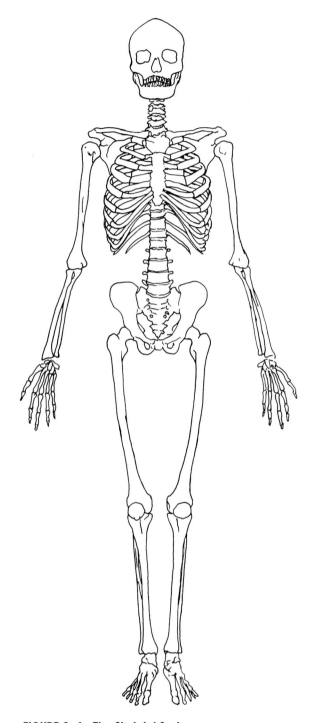

FIGURE 3-1 The Skeletal System

The skeleton is composed of axial and appendicular segments. It is shown intact in this illustration. Appendicular and axial segments are discussed in Chapters 4 and 5.

Inversion Stress medial deviation of the foot and ankle, hand and wrist.

Supination In the hand and wrist, the motion of the arm that places the hand with palm upward; the position of the hand with the thumb away from the middle of the body.

Pronation In the hand and wrist, the motion of the arm that places the palm of the hand downward; the position of the hand with the thumb toward the body midline.

Rotation Movement about a central or long axis.

Circumduction Combination of extension, flexion, abduction, and adduction in a movement that produces a circular motion; occurs in bones composed of a head and articular surfaces.

BONE MARKINGS OR FEATURES

A review of the markings and features of bones includes:

Antrum A nearly closed cavity in bone.

Condyle A rounded knucklelike process forming an articulation at the end of a bone.

Crest A narrow ridge or elongated prominence on a bone.

Fossa A shallow depression in or on a bone.

Head The proximal end of a bone supported on a constricted part or neck.

Process A bony prominence; an outgrowth of bone.

Sinus A cavity within a bone.

Spine A sharp, slender process of bone.

Tubercle A small, rounded process on a bone.

Tuberosity A large elevated process of bone.

POSITIONING CONCEPTS

Musculoskeletal trauma makes up a growing percentage of the work load in most radiology departments.[26] Most skeletal examinations start with routine radiography. Computed tomography, MRI, arthrography, and discography are also used to evaluate the musculoskeletal system.

At least two views are required for skeletal radiography. Whenever possible, the projections should be at right angles to each other. The CR

TABLE 3-1 Types of Joints

Classification	Range	Characteristic	Examples
Fibrous			
Synarthrosis	Immovable	Separated by membrane	Cranial sutures, epiphyseal articulations
Cartilaginous			
Amphiarthrosis	Slightly movable	Fibrocartilaginous disk between bony surfaces of a joint with a ligament uniting the two bones	Symphisis pubis, vertebral articulations, tibiofibular articulation
Synovial (most common)			
Diarthrosis	Freely movable	Adjacent bone ends covered with cartilage, enclosed in a fibrous capsule; joined by ligaments; lined by lubricant-secreting synovial membrane	
	Hinge	Movement occurs on one plane only	Elbow joint, ankle, tibia/fibula articulation
	Condylar	Has two articular surfaces with long axis in line; movement restricted mostly to one plane, with slight movement possible in the second plane	Knee, femoral-tibular articulation
	Ellipsoid	One surface oval, the second surface concave	Radiocarpal articulation
	Saddle	Articular surface saddle shaped; movement occurs in two planes; some rotation possible	Carpometacarpal joint of thumb
	Pivot	Only rotation can occur	Radioulnar joint
	Ball and socket	Hemispherical end of one bone articulates with cup-shaped depression in other bone	Hip, shoulder
	Plane	Flat articular surfaces; only gliding movement possible	Articular processes of vertebrae

should be directed through the center of interest and aligned with the center of the cassette, or, if multiple images are to be recorded on a single film, aligned with the center of an unshielded segment of a lead-divided cassette.

A minor change in the projection of the x-ray beam or position of the patient may alter the perception of the degree of deformity or displacement of a fracture. See Chapter 2, Figs 2-3 and 2-4.

When joints are being evaluated, the CR should be directed through the joint space to minimize distortion of the space by the divergent x-ray beam.

C A U T I O N : Tube angulations and FFD should be standardized so that duplication on repeat examinations is possible. If technical adjustments must be made, they should be documented.

A small lead marker, a lead arrow, or a metallic pointer set on the tabletop pointing to the site of the injury provides the radiologist with a focus for localization and helps in the detection of subtle fractures. If a cast on a lower extremity makes it difficult to localize the center of interest, placing the opposite leg adjacent to the limb in a cast and marking the cast at the joint can help to locate anatomical landmarks. This may be helpful if a repeat radiograph is needed or if a change in centering is indicated.

Because of such factors as injury, discomfort, or the patient's condition, it is not always possible to place the part under study in intimate contact with the screen-film detector. There may be serious injuries above or below the point of obvious trauma. With severe trauma, the lower ribs, lumbar vertebrae, and pelvis should be evaluated for fracture. For example, since the pelvis is a ring, it is commonly broken in two or more places. Dislocations at one of the sacroiliac joints or the symphysis pubis may also occur. Approximately 20% of patients with pelvic arch fractures have ureteral or bladder injuries.[27]

In the presence of bone deformity, joint instability, crepitation, or tenderness, the radiographer must often consider supplementary or in-

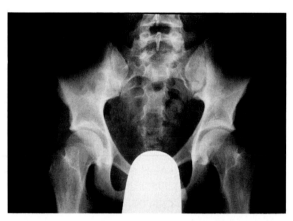

A

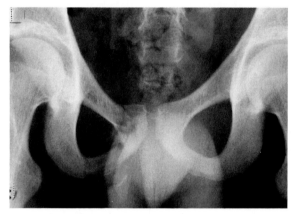

B

FIGURE 3-2 Gonadal Shielding

A radiograph of the pelvis was made of an 18-year-old male. (A) A fracture of the pubic area was not initially suspected and a gonadal shield was used. (B) A repeat examination of the pubic bones demonstrated a fracture. (Courtesy Cullinan AM: *Producing Quality Radiographs.* Philadelphia JB Lippincott Co, 1987.)

novative positions. An obvious fracture does not absolve the radiographer of the responsibility for demonstrating the entire segment of the anatomy requested.

Although swelling is often associated with trauma, it also can be related to a systemic disease. A check of the opposite extremity might show an equal amount of swelling. This finding of bilateral edema should be shared with the radiologist. Collimation should always be restricted to the area of interest.

The use of a male gonadal shield should not interfere with the imaging of the osseous structures of the pelvis (Fig 3-2). However, female gonadal shielding may mask significant pelvic anatomy. If a gonadal shield cannot be applied, high speed screen-film technology and a high kVp/reduced mAs technique help to lower radiation dosage to the patient.

C A U T I O N : Patients of reproductive age, when seated at the end or side of an x-ray table for upper-extremity radiography, must have their gonads shielded from x-radiation.

Comparison Studies

Pain or soft-tissue swelling associated with trauma in a child usually requires radiography of the injured extremity. There is some disagreement as to whether routine comparison views of the uninjured side are needed. Increased radiation dosage and additional costs must be considered. With rapid access x-ray film processing, a comparison image can be made quickly if a fracture is suspected.[27] Within seven to ten days, changes that take place in the bone as a result of interruption of the arterial blood supply make the fracture line more obvious.[28]

DISEASES OR CONDITIONS MERITING SPECIAL CONSIDERATION

Osseous structures are examined for congenital abnormalities, fractures, subluxations, dislocations, and soft-tissue abnormalities. Benign or malignant tumors, as well as bone changes caused by infections, can be evaluated with skeletal radiography. Osseous changes such as seen with arthritis may cause an alteration in bony alignment, articular contours, and joint spaces. Stress radiographs may be used to evaluate joint relationships.[29]

Trauma

Traumatic injuries continue to increase as a result of injuries suffered while riding in automobiles or other vehicles, in urban violence, and during amateur sports activities.[30] Before radiography is performed, the trauma patient should be assessed as to airway and circulatory status and for injury to the thorax or central nervous system. While the presence of an injury can often be ascertained by a physical examination, it is sometimes difficult to determine whether an artery has been damaged. Gunshot or blunt trauma injuries are always suspect for arterial damage.[31] Fracture fragments can damage adjacent blood vessels, perforate a viscus, and cause soft-tissue infection and/or significant blood loss. A common life-threatening condition is a thromboembolism, which can occur in patients with fractures of the pelvis and lower extremities, especially the hip and femur. A fracture through the mastoid air cells, the frontal sinuses, or the cribriform plate of the ethmoids may allow air to enter the subarachnoid space or the ventricular system. There is particular concern if an injury takes place at or near the vertebral column.

Fractures

Four major alterations may occur in the position of the distal fracture fragments in relationship to the proximal fracture fragments: length, angulation, displacement, and rotation.[32]

The parallel bones in the forearm and lower leg are rigid and are secured to each other by ligaments or other structures. A shortening or dislocation of one of these bones will often fracture or dislocate the other bone. The entire forearm and lower leg should be examined in both AP and lateral projections. See Chapter 2, Fig 2-6. A similar problem occurs with the mandible. See Chapter 5, Fig 5-18.

Severe injuries may indicate more than one fracture. With severe trauma, the lower ribs, lumbar vertebrae, and pelvis should be evaluated for fracture. If a patient is brought into a trauma area in the PA position, some creative imaging may be necessary before subjecting the patient to routine positioning.

Even with high quality radiographs and a clinically suspected fracture, it is sometimes difficult to detect a fracture in such bones as the carpal scaphoid, the clavicle, the ribs, the metatarsal bones, or the shaft of the tibia. See Chapter 4. While multiple projections can help to locate a fracture, sometimes a compromise must be reached in the interest of patient comfort, economy, and radiation dosage.

A repeat examination is often ordered ten days to two weeks after the initial radiographic study. Even if little or no new bone has been formed, the fracture line may be easier to see with delayed imaging.

Some of the more common types of fractures are described as follows:

1. An avulsion fracture represents the tearing of a piece of bone by a forceful pull of a muscle, tendon, or ligament.
2. An incomplete fracture travels partway through a bone.
3. A complete fracture extends from one cortex to the other, with neither fragment connected to the other.
4. A comminuted fracture has more than two fragments and is usually splintered into pieces.
5. An open fracture (compound) is associated with an open wound at the fracture site.
6. A greenstick fracture, seen in children, causes a buckling, bending, or partial fracture of a bone.
7. An epiphysial fracture—a separation of the epiphysis from the bone—occurs only in children.
8. An impacted fracture images as an area of increased density rather than as a radiolucent fracture line since the impacted fragments are wedged into one another.
9. A stress fracture (often called a military or march fracture), which is a fine hairline fracture without soft-tissue injury, occurs when a bone is subjected to increased stress, such as in jogging. The original study may appear negative; however, within a few weeks, the healing process produces changes in bone density.
10. A pathological fracture is a fracture through a diseased bone caused by a

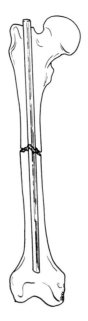

FIGURE 3–3   Intermedullary Nail

An intermedullary nail can be used for fractures of the femoral shaft, tibia, humerus, and so on. Whenever possible, both joints and the entire metallic device should be visualized. This illustration demonstrates an intramedullary nail in the medullary cavity of the femur, used to align a fracture of the central femur A. (Courtesy Kilcoyne RF: *Handbook of Orthopaedic Radiologic Terminology.* Chicago, Year Book Medical Publishers, 1988.)

force that healthy bone should tolerate.
11. A depressed fracture is found when a fragment of the skull is driven inward. Special tangential imaging is sometimes needed to demonstrate this fracture. See Chapter 5.

Ongoing monitoring of fractures as they heal includes follow-up radiographic studies. After treatment of a fracture that may involve reduction, a metallic pin or screw or a cast may be used to stabilize the injured area until healing has taken place. A variety of fixation devices are available to the orthopedic surgeon to treat fractures of the femoral shaft, hand, and so on (Figs 3-3 and 3-4). See Chapter 4, Fig 4-51.

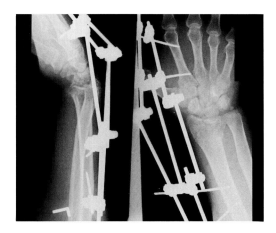

FIGURE 3–4   External Fixation of a Fracture

External fixation devices can be used so that alignment of the fracture can be adjusted following surgery. Shown is an external wrist fixation device used with an unstable fracture of the distal radius. (Courtesy Richardson ML, Kilcoyne RF, Mayo KA, et al: Radiographic evaluation of modern orthopedic fixation devices. *RadioGraphics* 1987;7:685-701.)

C A U T I O N :   Every effort should be made to visualize both joints and as much of the long bones as possible.[33] Both ends of a fixation device should be visualized on the radiograph.

Fat-Pad Signs

Most joints within the body lie in direct continuity with small collections of fat. When these fat pads are obliterated or displaced from their normal positions, joint effusion must be considered. Fractures through a joint surface (intra-articular fractures) sometimes are detected by the presence of fat within the joint[34] (Fig 3-5, pages 44–45).

The presence of a fat-pad sign without an obvious fracture is an important diagnostic indicator. Localized soft-tissue swelling and changes in the normal fat lines may be the only signs of subtle fracture.

In most normal radiographs of the wrist, a radiolucent fat line, seen as increased radiographic density, can be identified along the pronator quadratus muscle, paralleling the radius. The scaphoid fat pad or stripe is seen as a collec-

tion of fat paralleling the scaphoid on normal AP radiographs in over 90% of adults (Fig 3-5). This stripe is not reliably seen in children under the age of 12.[35]

In the elbow, the joint capsule has anterior and posterior layers of fat between its synovial and fibrous layers. On a properly positioned and exposed lateral radiograph of the elbow, the anterior fat pad can be seen hugging the anterior aspect of the humerus. The posterior fat pad normally is not seen on the lateral image. Joint effusion causes the posterior fat pad to be seen on the lateral view and the anterior fat pad is elevated. If there is distortion of the elbow joint capsule by hemorrhage or effusion, the fat pads are forced upward and outward[27] (Fig 3-5).

In children, almost all elbows that have been subjected to trauma and show a positive posterior fat-pad sign will have a fracture. In adults, fat pads of the elbow are not as easily displaced.[35]

Effusion

Intra-articular injuries, including ligament strains, rupture, cartilage tears, and fractures, can be diagnosed by a post-traumatic effusion of the knee, best demonstrated on the lateral radiograph with the joint in less than 15 degree flexion. Increased flexion may obliterate an effusion.[3] Elastic support bands or tightly rolled-up pants legs can have a similar obliteration effect.

C A U T I O N :   In the presence of a recent or suspected fracture of the patella, the knee should not be flexed.

The lateral view should be obtained with an overhead tube instead of by a cross-table lateral study so that fluid will not gravitate over the femur, masking the effusion.

A horizontal beam image may be required to demonstrate a fat–fluid level in a suprapatella bursa. This indicates a fracture that has permitted fat from the marrow to enter the joint[27,30] (Fig 3-6, page 46).

Similar changes in the fat densities of the ankle and heel pad occur with trauma.

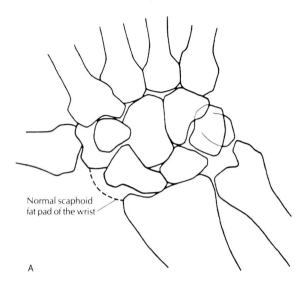

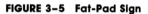

Normal scaphoid
fat pad of the wrist

A

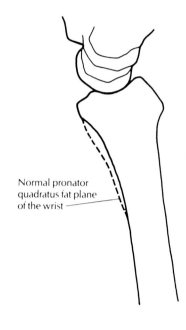

Normal pronator
quadratus fat plane
of the wrist

FIGURE 3–5 Fat-Pad Sign

Fracture through a joint can sometimes be detected
by the presence of fat within the joint. Most joints are
accompanied by small collections of fat, which, when
obliterated or displaced from their normal position,
suggest joint effusion. To demonstrate changes in the
position of fat pads, soft tissues of the extremities and
pelvis must not be overexposed. Low kVp/high mAs
techniques blacken the soft-tissue structures, making
fat-pad evaluation difficult.

Fat-pad locations for the wrist (A, B), elbow (C),
hip (D), knee (E), and ankle (F) are shown. The normal
anterior fat pad in the elbow hugs the anterior aspect
of the humerus. The posterior fat pad is seen only
when fluid is present. The abnormal anterior fat pad
(known as a "sail sign") takes a more perpendicular
position in relation to the humerus. An abnormal
posterior fat pad is shown with fluid pushing the joint
capsule posteriorly (C). (Courtesy Alexander JE,
Holder JC: Fat pad signs in the diagnosis of subtle
fractures. *Am Fam Physician* 1988;37:92-102.)

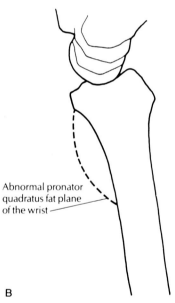

Abnormal pronator
quadratus fat plane
of the wrist

B

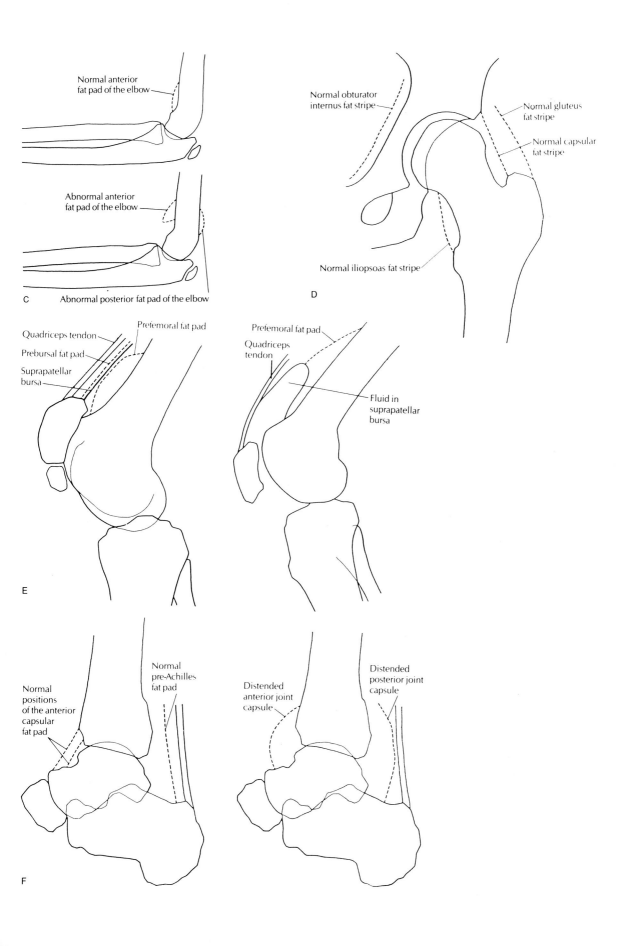

Normal anterior
fat pad of the elbow

Abnormal anterior
fat pad of the elbow

C

Abnormal posterior fat pad of the elbow

Normal obturator
internus fat stripe

Normal gluteus
fat stripe

Normal capsular
fat stripe

Normal iliopsoas fat stripe

D

Quadriceps tendon

Prefemoral fat pad

Prebursal fat pad

Suprapatellar
bursa

E

Prefemoral fat pad

Quadriceps
tendon

Fluid in
suprapatellar
bursa

Normal
positions
of the anterior
capsular
fat pad

Normal
pre-Achilles
fat pad

Distended
anterior joint
capsule

Distended
posterior joint
capsule

F

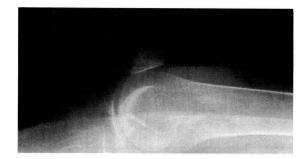

FIGURE 3–6   Horizontal-Beam Imaging for Knee Effusion

A fat–fluid level that indicates the presence of an intra-articular fracture can be demonstrated with a horizontal beam radiograph. (Courtesy M Mitchell, MD, Dalhousie University, Halifax, Nova Scotia.)

Subluxations and Dislocations

Subluxation, a partial or incomplete dislocation of a joint, can result when a normal joint relationship is slightly exceeded. Dislocation is a displacement of a bone from its normal position in a joint (Fig 3-7). Careful attention to positioning is important since minute shifts in the relationship of the bones to each other may be the only sign of subluxation or a dislocation.

Mechanical stress helps to determine whether there is a looseness in a joint and aids in the evaluation of joint relationships and the degree of instability in a joint caused by ligament or muscle injuries. Examples include inversion and eversion stress applied to the ankle, a weight-bearing view of the acromioclavicular joint, and standing or weight-bearing views of the knees and feet.[36]

A weight-bearing study must be truly weight bearing. Patients should not shift their weight during the study. Disruption of the ligaments can be demonstrated with a stress view of the knee; however, the injured structure or an existing condition may be aggravated by stress maneuvers.

Stress procedures are almost always carried out in the presence of a physician, with the exception of weight-bearing upright imaging of the shoulder for acromioclavicular joint separation. Stress AP views of the acromioclavicular joint to determine the degree of acromioclavicular separation require that 10 lb weights hang independently from each wrist, which must be comfortable for the patient.[28] In some cases, the department or physician may prefer weights of up to 20 lb.[3]

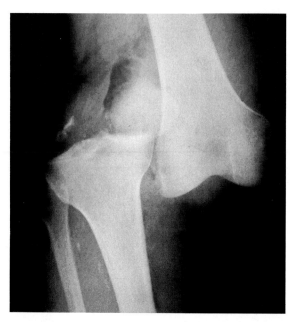

FIGURE 3–7   Lateral Dislocation of the Knee

This injury was the result of a motor vehicle accident. The osseous fragments of the lateral aspect of the leg above the tibial plateau arose from the lateral femoral condyle. Note the air in the soft tissue, denoting an open wound. (Courtesy Mitchell M: Diagnostic imaging of lower extremity trauma. *Radiol Clin North Am* 1989;25:909-928.)

> CAUTION: Often patients will splint their arms during a procedure to relieve discomfort, thus negating the weight-bearing effect.

Bone Disease

In this book, only osseous changes that have an influence on radiographic contrast and density are discussed.

Bone lesions can be categorized into two groups: osteolytic and osteoblastic. Bone tumors, inflammatory processes, degenerative changes, and/or disuse may reduce the amount

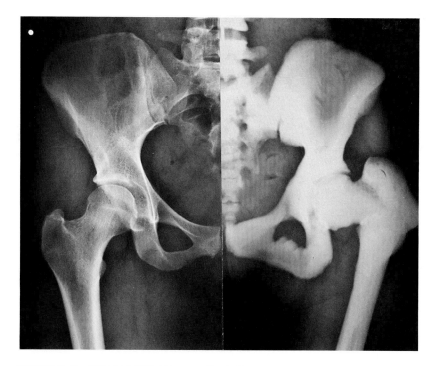

FIGURE 3-8   Effect of Pathology on Technique

Normal pelvic bony anatomy is seen (left) compared with a pelvis with osteopetrosis (right). An increase in bony density requires an increase in x-ray exposure. Conversely, an osteoporitic condition would require a decrease in the exposure needed for normal bone.

of calcium within a bone, resulting in an osteolytic condition. An overall decrease in bone density (demineralization) is often seen in bone that has been immobilized in a cast or in braces.

Osteoblastic conditions result in the formation of additional bone (Fig 3-8). Metabolic changes may also cause new bone formation. Healing fractures first decalcify at the fracture site, and then begin to form new bone.

Paget's disease, a bone disease common in the skull, spine, and long bones of the elderly, can occur in two stages—early, or osteolytic; and late, or osteoblastic.

A clinical history or a review of a previous radiograph helps to determine the need for a change in exposure factors.

Periosteal new bone may be found in association with abnormalities, such as infection or tumor. Periosteal changes are not ordinarily seen on a radiograph unless an underlying pathologi-

cal change has occurred. A periosteal reaction may be the result of subperiosteal extensions of blood, pus, or tumor. Periosteal new-bone formation includes solid, laminated, or spiculated patterns and is difficult to demonstrate radiographically. The term "onion-skin peeling," used to describe the laminated elevation of the periosteum from the cortex, serves to describe minute changes in this important diagnostic sign.[29]

TECHNICAL CONSIDERATIONS

Image Sharpness

If possible, the part under study should be placed against the detector. Injury, discomfort, or the condition of the patient may require a change in the positioning routine. For example, in the presence of trauma, the clavicles and pelvis are difficult to image in the PA position.

A small focal spot (0.6 mm or smaller) helps to minimize image blur caused by an increased OFD. See Chapter 1.

The heel effect should be considered in the positioning of a long bone since both density and image blur may be influenced by the anode–cathode relationship. See Chapter 1, Figs 1-6 and 1-8.

Effect of Pathology on Technical-Factor Selection

Technical factors have to be adjusted when imaging significant bony changes. For example, osteolytic lesions require a low kVp technique, whereas osteoblastic lesions may require a large increase in kVp and the use of a higher ratio grid (Fig 3-8). Osteoporosis may require an increase in mAs with a reduction in kVp to produce adequate radiographic contrast.

Kilovoltage Selection

Lower kilovoltage values (55 kVp or less), if used with most rare earth screen-film combinations, may cause a falloff of system speed. See Chapter 1.

Scatter Control

Tight beam collimation restricts the primary ray, which minimizes interaction with tissue and results in less radiation to the patient. Most distal extremities are examined using nongrid techniques. Nongrid cassettes can be divided into segments by lead-rubber sheeting or tight beam collimation for multiple views.

> C A U T I O N : Subdivision of a grid cassette by lead dividers for multiple exposures on a film may result in grid cutoff (Fig 3-9). Larger body parts, such as the hip or shoulder, require a grid or Bucky to clean up scatter. See Chapter 1.

Screen-Film Versus Nonscreen Techniques

There are a number of references in the literature to the use of screen film or nonscreen film in cardboard or plastic holders for extremity radio-

graphy—a direct exposure technique. More silver (a thicker emulsion) is used in nonscreen film. Nonscreen direct exposure film is difficult to use with automatic roller-film processors and predetermined cycle times. The length of the automatic processing cycle must be increased in order to process most nonscreen films properly. Direct exposure technology is rarely used in modern radiography. High detail rare earth screen-film combinations minimize image blur and permit the use of small or fractional focal spots for studies of the extremities, as well as of larger body parts.

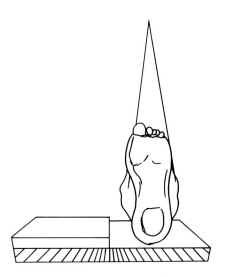

FIGURE 3–9   Grid Placement for Radiography of an Extremity in a Cast

Most distal-extremity studies utilize nongrid techniques. In the AP projection, the ankle mortise is difficult to penetrate because of the thickness of the ankle joint in its relationship to the foot. If a grid technique is used, the patient should be centered either to a table Bucky or to a grid cassette for an individual exposure. In this illustration, it can be seen that dividing a cassette into segments would result in the x-ray beam's striking an out-of-focus grid. An extremity that is in a cast can benefit from a moderate to high kVp grid technique.

Single emulsion film/single screen rare earth systems use one tenth or less the radiation needed for direct exposure studies. Occasionally, a foreign body might require a direct exposure image to verify or rule out the presence of a small dust artifact on a screen-film study.

> C A U T I O N : A screen type film used in a direct exposure technique requires three to four times more x-radiation than does a nonscreen film.

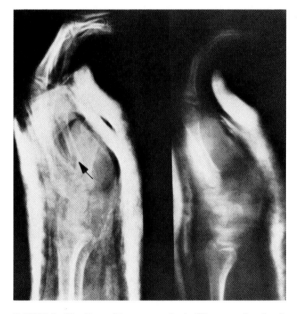

FIGURE 3–10   Use of Tomography to "Remove" a Cast

Cast material may mask small anatomical details in a radiograph. The use of a tomographic unit to blur out or "remove" the cast is recommended. Note the poor visualization of the fracture (arrow) in the conventional cast study. With employing a linear tomographic study a 20 degree exposure angle, the fracture alignment is more easily visualized. Since the cast did not have to be removed physically, healing and alignment of the fracture were not jeopardized. If linear tomography is used to evaluate long bones, the part must be positioned tangential to the x-ray tube/cassette path to minimize parasitic artifacts—linear striations that might interfere with interpretation. (Courtesy Cullinan JE, Cullinan AM: *Illustrated Guide to X-Ray Technics.* Philadelphia, JB Lippincott Co, 1980.)

The use of slow speed, high detail single screen/single emulsion film combinations (speed 20 to speed 40) is suggested to demonstrate periosteal new bone, calcifications, minor degenerative changes, or densities within joint spaces.

High speed screen-film combinations (600, 800, 1,200 speed) should be considered when examining extremities in casts, particularly when a considerable amount of cast material has been used or Bucky images are required. Some structural details can be obscured by cast material, suggesting that the use of a slow speed system is of no advantage and results in increased patient exposure. In a casted body part that is less than 2 cm thick, such as a finger or thumb, a slower speed screen-film combination may be helpful.[37]

With conventional screen-film technology, approximately one third of the density of a radiograph is the result of the crossover of light within the cassette. See Chapter 1, Fig 1-19. The use of crossover control imaging technology reduces the crossover of light (light scatter) within the cassette by approximately one half. Most crossover control images made using contrast film exhibit short scale contrast. Higher kilovoltage values with reduced mAs factors can be used with crossover control, high contrast technology to increase technical latitude. See Chapter 1.

Tomography

The use of conventional tomography to "remove" a cast radiographically is an innovative application of an established technology (Fig 3-10). If linear tomography is used, the extremity should be positioned so that the long bones are not parallel to the linear movement of the tomographic unit. The cast material, separated from the osseous structures, will blur out easily. Narrow angle (up to 10 degrees) tomography (zonography) is acceptable for this procedure.[7] Improper placement of the part in the x-ray tube path can result in less than optimal images. Parasitic artifacts, known as linear striations, may interfere with interpretation. High speed screen-film receptors are recommended for use with tomography of structures in casts.

Soft-Tissue Demonstration

Demonstration of bony details at the expense of the soft tissues of the skeleton may require viewing under bright light for soft-tissue evaluation. A proper technique has been achieved when soft-tissue and bony structures are both visible. Soft-tissue structures are easy to overexpose owing to either the thinness of the part or the shape of the x-ray field.

An overexposed radiograph can fail to demonstrate a soft-tissue lesion. There is a one-to-four difference in thickness from the tip of the fingers to the wrist and an even greater difference in thickness from the toes to the tarsal area of the foot. See Chapter 4. It is also difficult to balance density from one end of the humerus to the other, since the shoulder is usually examined using a Bucky technique and the elbow with a nongrid technique. A significant difference in thickness in the femur and in the lower leg presents similar exposure problems. See Chapter 4. The lateral aspect of the shoulder, because of its thinness, is easily overexposed. This makes it difficult to visualize calcified tendonitis, bursitis, the acromioclavicular joints, or the distal end of the clavicles. A primary beam leak may undercut an image, masking soft-tissue detail. See Chapter 1, Fig 1-11. If possible, the humerus should be kept away from the body so that the soft tissues of the chest will not superimpose on the soft tissues of the upper arm.

Despite these differences in densities, all soft-tissue structures should be seen. An underpart filter can be positioned beneath the shoulder, even for upright radiographs. See Chapter 1, Fig 1-7.

If subcutaneous fat or fat between muscle planes is infiltrated by edema (water density), the fat will not contrast sharply with adjacent structures that have the density of water.

Soft-tissue structures are also evaluated for swelling, gas in tissue planes (Fig 3-11), calcifications, or opaque foreign bodies. Wood, glass, and metal are foreign bodies commonly associated with soft-tissue injuries[39] (Figs 3-12 and 3-13). Ultrasound is useful in detecting nonopaque foreign bodies such as wood, which is visible radiographically only 15% of the time.[28]

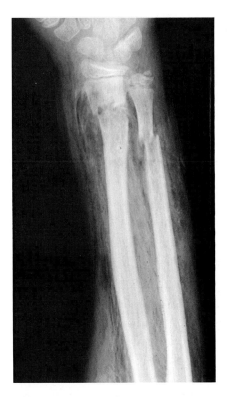

FIGURE 3-11 Gas Gangrene

Radiolucent linear streaks are seen, representing gas shadows in the soft tissues of the forearm.

There is considerable discussion in the literature as to whether glass fragments embedded in a patient's hand or foot can be demonstrated on screen-film radiographs. All commonly available glass should be easily seen on standard radiographs of the hand or foot. An elaborate experiment, using 66 varieties of glass embedded in the leg muscles of a chicken cadaver, was performed by Tandberg, who found that overlying bone can mask small (0.5 to 1.0 mm) or thin glass fragments. Larger fragments (2 mm or greater) can be seen even if overlying bone.[40]

The resolution capability of a screen-film system determines whether an opaque foreign body can be detected. Single screen/single emulsion systems used for mammography are an ideal choice to demonstrate foreign bodies. Xeroradiography, suggested as the method of

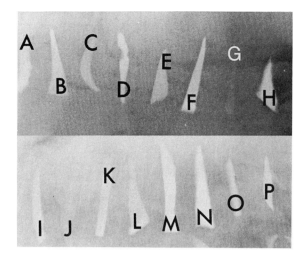

FIGURE 3–12   Imaging of Glass and Plastic Fragments

Thin glass slivers (not greater than 3.5 cm in thickness) placed at a depth of 2 cm in a 5 cm piece of pork: (A) beer glass; (B) beer bottle; (C) wine glass; (D) wine bottle; (E) milk bottle; (F) laminated windscreen; (G) light bulb (60 W); (H) nonlaminated windscreen; (I) head lamp cover (glass); (J) rear-light housing (plastic); (K) window (standard); (L) window (bullion); (M) window (frosted); (N) window (Elizabethan); (O) window (greenhouse); (P) optical glass. (Courtesy de Lacey G, Evans R, Sandin B: Penetrating injuries: How easy is it to see glass (and plastic) on radiographs? *Br J Radial* 1985;58:27-30.)

choice in detecting foreign bodies of low radiopacity, is not readily available in many institutions. While wood splinters are slightly radiolucent, they become equivalent to tissue density as they absorb body fluids.[41]

The use of a rare earth screen film combination with a dedicated mammographic unit for radiography of the hand is an accepted technique. For many years, prepackaged direct exposure industrial film was used for this purpose. With single screen/single emulsion rare earth screen-film imaging, the entrance dose is reduced from 1.20 R to 0.15 R. Excellent rendition of bone detail, soft-tissue detail, and, in particular, calcification in soft tissue is possible.[42]

> CAUTION: When multiple images are made on one cassette to save time and film costs, soft-tissue structures should not be sacrificed.

While CT can demonstrate soft-tissue masses, soft-tissue contrast is more clearly defined with MRI.[38]

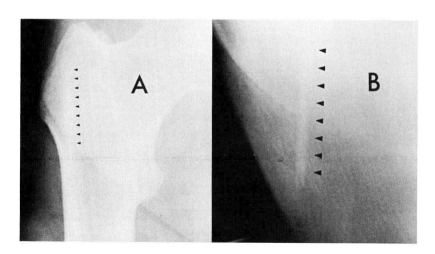

FIGURE 3–13   Clinical Example of a Glass Foreign Body

(A) A puncture wound 6 cm inferior and lateral to the greater trochanter. The silver (4 cm long) was not detected. Five weeks later, an oblique projection was made with the buttocks projected off of the bone. (B) This view clearly demonstrates the dense sliver of glass. (Courtesy de Lacey G, Evans R, Sandin B: Penetrating injuries: How easy is it to see glass (and plastic) on radiographs? *Br J Radiol* 1985;58:27-30.)

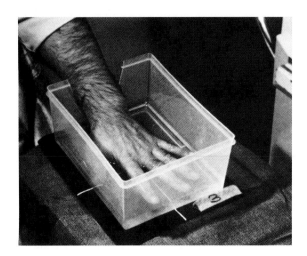

FIGURE 3–14   Immersion Imaging of the Hand

Immersion hand radiography can be performed to outline the skin, the subcutaneous fat layers, and the fat layers between muscle planes. With the film holder placed beneath the liquid-filled tray, the hand is shown immersed in the liquid. (Courtesy Ngo C, Yaghmai I: The value of immersion hand radiography in soft tissue changes in musculoskeletal disorders. *Skeletal radiol* 1988; 17: 259-263.)

Immersion Imaging of the Hand

Immersion radiographs help to outline the skin in order to visualize subcutaneous fat layers and the fat layers between muscle planes. The tendons and soft-tissue components of the joint can also be seen with this technique. Inner and outer margins of the skin are sharply outlined, with the subcutaneous fat layer clearly differentiated from the adjacent skin and soft tissues.

Periarticular soft tissue can be seen through the periarticular fat layers in greater detail than seen on conventional studies. The patient's hand must be immersed in a solution of 50% alcohol and 50% water in a plastic tray on the top of a cassette. A mammographic x-ray unit with a molybdenum target (0.3 mm) focal spot is a prerequisite for this technique. A low kilovoltage range (approximately 32 kVp) is suggested[43] (Fig 3-14).

CHAPTER FOUR

The Appendicular Skeleton: Upper and Lower Extremities, Shoulder, and Pelvic Girdles

The appendicular skeleton consists of the upper and lower extremities and the shoulder and pelvic girdles (Fig 4-1).

ANATOMICAL / PATHOLOGICAL OBSERVATIONS

Anatomical/pathological observations related to the extremities can be found in Chapter 3.

POSITIONING CONCEPTS

Positioning concepts related to skeletal radiography are also presented in Chapter 3.

Basic positioning routines for the extremities may vary with departmental preferences. Tables 4-1 through 4-19 (pages 56-63) are summaries of routine projections and are presented to show that often only slight modifications are required to obtain similar views of adjacent areas.

THE UPPER EXTREMITIES AND SHOULDER GIRDLE

Projections suggested for routine radiography of the upper extremities and shoulder girdle include:

1. AP, oblique and lateral thumb (Tables 4-1 through 4-3).
2. PA, oblique and lateral fingers (Tables 4-1 through 4-3).
3. PA and oblique hand (Tables 4-1 and 4-3).
4. PA, lateral and both obliques of the wrist (Tables 4-1 through 4-3).
5. AP and lateral forearm (Tables 4-4 and 4-5).
6. AP and lateral elbow (Tables 4-4 and 4-5).
7. Axial elbow (Table 4-6).
8. AP and lateral humerus (Tables 4-4, 4-5, 4-7, and 4-8).
9. AP shoulder, internal and external rotation (Table 4-7).
10. AP/PA axial shoulder (Table 4-9).
11. AP and lateral scapula (Tables 4-7 and 4-8).
12. AP/PA and axial clavicle (Table 4-9).

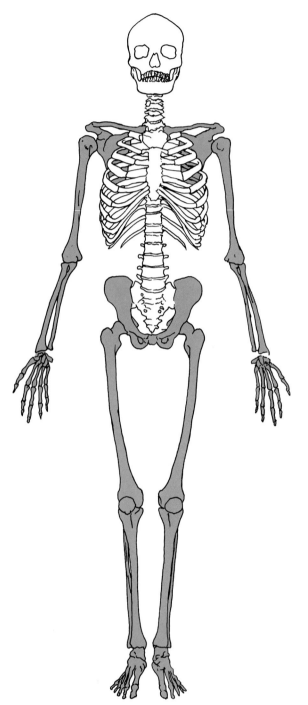

FIGURE 4–1   Appendicular Skeleton, Shown in Relationship to the Full Skeleton

SUPPLEMENTARY IMAGING OF THE UPPER EXTREMITIES AND SHOULDER GIRDLE

Modified AP Projections of the Thumb

The base of the first metacarpal and carpometacarpal joint should be demonstrated when examining the thumb in the AP position. While the AP view demonstrates the distal structures, it is often inadequate for visualization of the base of the thumb, even if the patient retracts the extended fingers with the opposite hand.

A modified projection of the x-ray beam directs the CR 15 degrees toward the palm of the hand (along the long axis of the thumb) centered to the base of the first metacarpal. This technique avoids underexposure resulting from the increased tissue thickness in the area, as well as the superimposition of the fifth metacarpal bone[44] (Figs 4-2, and 4-3).

C A U T I O N :   Care must be taken not to rotate the thumb from the AP position when the fingers are retracted.

Another modification of the standard AP position of the hand, with the dorsum of the thumb against the cassette, requires that the x-ray beam be directed at a 10 to 15 degree angle (along the long axis of the thumb) toward the wrist, centered to the first metacarpophalangeal joint. An increased rotation of the hand (dorsum toward the tabletop) minimizes muscular overshadowing[45] (Figs 4-4 and 4-5).

Imaging of the First Carpometacarpal Joint

For a clear projection of the first carpometacarpal joint, the patient's hand and wrist are hyperextended, similar to the position used for the carpal-tunnel projection of the wrist. (See

(Text continues on page 63)

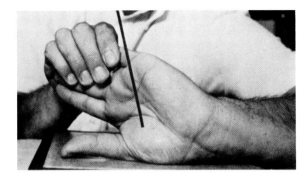

FIGURE 4-2   Modified AP Projection of the Thumb

(Courtesy Gratale P, Turner GW, Burns C: A modified AP projection of the thumb. *Radiol Technol* 1985; 56:320-321.)

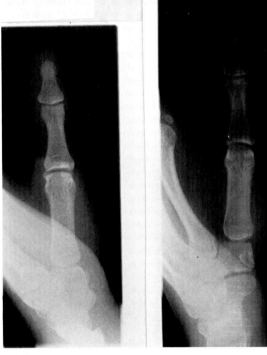

FIGURE 4-4   Modified Position of Hand and Thumb, to Provide a Clearer Visualization of a Greater Length of the Thumb

(Courtesy Lewis S: New angles on the radiographic examination of the hand II. *Radiography Today* 1988;54:29.)

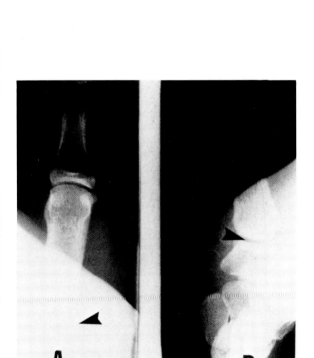

FIGURE 4-3   Comparison Radiographs

(A) Standard AP view and (B) modified AP view of the thumb. The proximal end of the carpometacarpal joint and the trapezium are better demonstrated with the modified projection. (Courtesy Gratale P, Turner GW, Burns C: A modified AP projection of the thumb. *Radiol Technol* 1985;56:320-321.)

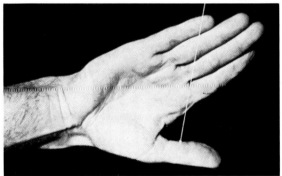

FIGURE 4-5   Modified AP Projection of the Thumb with Increased Rotation of the Hand

(A) Standard technique compared with (B) modified technique, with increased rotation of the hand (dorsum turned more toward the tabletop). (Courtesy Lewis S: New angles on the radiographic examination of the hand II. *Radiography Today* 1988;54:29.)

TABLE 4–1 PA / AP Thumb, Fingers, Hand, and Wrist

Area	Position of Part	Projection of Central Ray	Demonstrates (View)
Thumb (AP)	Posterior surface of thumb adjacent to film plane, hand in extreme internal rotation	CR directed perpendicular to film plane to enter at first metacarpophalangeal joint	Thumb from distal tip to trapezium (greater multangular)
Thumb (PA)	Hand lateral, thumb abducted, dorsal surface parallel with film plane; thumb and wrist elevated and supported	See Thumb, AP projection	See Thumb, AP view
Fingers	Hand in PA position	CR directed perpendicular to film plane to enter at proximal interphalangeal joint	Phalanges; interphalangeal joint
Hand	PA, fingers slightly separated	CR directed perpendicular to film plane to enter at third metacarpophalangeal joint	Carpals; metacarpals; phalanges of digits 2 to 5; oblique view of thumb; wrist joint and distal radius and ulna
Wrist (PA)	Wrist PA	CR directed perpendicular to film plane to enter at midcarpals	Carpals; distal ends radius and ulna (the ulna being slightly oblique); upper ends of metacarpals
Wrist (AP)	Wrist AP	See Wrist, PA projection	Carpal interspaces better seen; distal end of radius; distal end of ulna without rotation

TABLE 4-2 Lateral Thumb, Fingers, Hand, and Wrist

Area	Position of Part	Projection of Central Ray	Demonstrates (View)
Thumb	True lateral	CR directed perpendicular to film plane to enter at first metacarpophalangeal joint	Thumb from distal tip to trapezium (greater multangular)
Finger	True lateral (fingers 2, 3 radial side down; fingers 4, 5 ulna side down)	CR directed perpendicular to film plane to enter at proximal interphalangeal joint	Phalanges; interphalangeal joint
Hand	True lateral (fingers completely extended, thumb slightly abducted and parallel to film plane, ulnar or radial side adjacent to film holder)	CR directed perpendicular to film plane to enter at metacarpophalangeal joint	Foreign body
Hand	True lateral (fingers flexed to maintain natural arch; thumb parallel to film plane)	See Hand (above)	Anterior or posterior displacement of metacarpals
Wrist	True lateral (rest arm and forearm on table; flex elbow 90 degrees	CR directed perpendicular to film plane to enter through wrist joint	Carpals, upper ends of metacarpals, lower ends of radius and ulna

TABLE 4-3 Oblique Thumb, Fingers, Hand, and Wrist

Area	Position of Part	Projection of Central Ray	Demonstrates (View)
Thumb	Palmar surface of hand adjacent to film holder	CR directed perpendicular to film plane to enter at first metacarpophalangeal joint	Distal tip of thumb to trapezium (greater multangular); phalanges and metacarpal will appear rotated
Finger	45 degree oblique	CR directed perpendicular to film plane to enter at proximal interphalangeal joint	Oblique projection of finger
Hand	Rotate the hand medially from the lateral position, ulna side adjacent to film holder; flex fingers slightly, tips touching the cassette; foam-sponge supports used to support fingers when joint spaces are to be imaged	CR directed perpendicular to enter at third metacarpophalangeal joint	Oblique projection of bones and soft tissue
Wrist	PA oblique; rotated 45 degrees from prone; ulnar surface adjacent to the film holder	CR directed perpendicular to film plane, to enter distal to the radius at the scaphoid	Carpals on lateral side of wrist; scaphoid; distal radius and ulna; proximal half of metacarpals
	AP oblique; rotated 45 degrees from supine	CR directed perpendicular to film plane, to enter at midcarpal area	Carpals on medial side; pisiform; proximal half of metacarpals

TABLE 4–4 AP Forearm, Elbow, and Distal Humerus

Area	Position of Part	Projection of Central Ray	Demonstrates (View)
Forearm	Elbow fully extended, hand supinated; body turned laterally to place anterior surface of elbow and humeral epicondyles parallel to the film plane	CR directed perpendicular to film plane, to enter at midpoint or forearm	Radius, ulna; proximal carpal bones; elbow joint
Elbow	See AP forearm	CR directed perpendicular to film plane, to enter at midpoint of elbow joint	Elbow joint; distal humerus; proximal forearm
Elbow (internal rotation)	See AP elbow; hand pronated; adjust extremity to place anterior surface of elbow 40 to 45 degrees to plane of film (medial oblique position)	See AP elbow projection	Coronoid process; elbow joint
Elbow (external rotation)	See AP elbow; hand supinated; adjust extremity to place posterior surface of elbow 40 to 45 degrees to plane of film (lateral oblique position)	See AP elbow projection	Radial head and neck; elbow joint
AP elbow	Elbow extended; see AP forearm position	If patient cannot rotate arm medially or laterally, CR is directed 45 degrees medially for first exposure and 45 degrees laterally for second exposure	Radial head, separated from olecronon process
Distal humerus	Forearm partially flexed (degree of flexion depends on patient's condition); hand supinated as far as possible without patient discomfort; support elevated hand and forearm; humeral epicondyles parallel to film plane	CR directed perpendicular to film plane, to enter at humeral epicondyles	Distal humerus; elbow joint (closed)

TABLE 4-5 Lateral Forearm, Elbow, and Distal Humerus

Area	Position of Part	Projection of Central Ray	Demonstrates (View)
Forearm	Elbow flexed 90 degrees; long axis of forearm aligned to long axis of film; hand lateral, thumb side up; adjust shoulder to allow humerus to rest on tabletop; humeral epicondyles super-imposed, perpen-dicular to film plane	CR directed perpendicular to film plane, to enter at midforearm	Proximal row of carpal bones to distal end of humerus
Elbow, Distal Humerus	See Forearm	CR directed perpendicular to film plane, to enter at midelbow joint	Elbow joint; proximal forearm; distal humerus
Elbow	See Forearm Four positions: 1. Hand supinated, externally rotated 2. Rotate hand to lateral position (thumb up) 3. Rotate hand to pronation (palm down) 4. Rotate hand to extreme internal rotation (resting on thumb surface)	See Lateral elbow projection	See Lateral elbow, view; radial head
Elbow	Elbow flexed 90 degrees, hand pronated	CR directed 45 degrees toward shoulder, to enter at radial head	Radial head, capitellum; see Lateral elbow
Elbow	Elbow flexed 80 degrees, hand pronated	CR directed 45 degrees toward brachial crease (away from the shoulder)	Coronoid process, trochlea; see Lateral elbow view

TABLE 4-6 Elbow — Axial Projection

Area	Position of Part	Projection of Central Ray	Demonstrates (View)
Elbow	Acute flexion; lateral aspect of humerus parallel to film plane	CR directed perpendicular to film plane; to enter slightly above humeral condyles	Olecranon process; distal humerus; radius and ulna superimposed over humerus
Elbow	Acute flexion; posterior surface of forearm parallel to film plane	CR directed perpendicular to film plane; to enter at a point just medial to olecranon process	Epicondyles; trochlea; ulnar sulcus; olecranon fossa

TABLE 4-7 AP Humerus, Shoulder, and Scapula

Area	Position of Part	Projection of Central Ray	Demonstrates (View)
Humerus	Patient AP (erect or recumbent); imaginary line passing through medial and lateral epicondyles parallel to film plane; hand supinated (if possible)	CR directed perpendicular to film plane, to enter at midpoint of humerus	Entire humerus
Shoulder (neutral position)	Patient AP (erect or recumbent); shoulder in contact with tabletop; imaginary line connecting medial and lateral epicondyles at 45 degrees to film plane; hand at side	CR directed perpendicular to film plane, to enter at coracoid process	Proximal humerus; glenoid fossa of scapula: humeral head slightly superimposed on glenoid fossa; greater tuberosity superimposed on humeral head (except for lateral border)
Shoulder (internal rotation)	See Neutral position; imaginary line connecting medial and lateral epicondyles, perpendicular to film plane; rotate palm of hand medially (thumb side down)	See Neutral projection	See Neutral view; humeral head superimposed on about one half of glenoid fossa; greater tuberosity overlies head of humerus; profile of lesser tuberosity overlies glenoid fossa
Shoulder (external rotation)	See Neutral position; imaginary line connecting medial and lateral epicondyles parallel to film plane (rotate palm of hand laterally; extreme supination)	See Neutral projection	See Neutral view; humeral head nearly in profile; greater tuberosity seen in profile on lateral border of humerus, lesser tuberosity overlies humerus
AP Shoulder (oblique)	Patient supine or erect; body rotated 45 degrees toward affected side; arm abducted (slight internal rotation)	CR directed perpendicular to film plane, to enter at a point 2 in medial and 2 in distal to the upper outer border of the shoulder	Joint space between humeral head and glenoid fossa; glenoid fossa in profile
Scapula	Patient erect or supine; arm abducted 90 degrees; hand supinated	CR directed perpendicular to film plane, to enter at midscapula (2 in below coracoid process)	Scapula; lateral border free of rib superimposition

TABLE 4–8 Lateral Humerus and Scapula

Area	Position of Part	Projection of Central Ray	Demonstrates (View)
Humerus	Patient erect (PA or AP); arm flexed; hand on abdomen; imaginary line connecting medial and lateral epicondyles perpendicular to film plane	CR directed perpendicular to film plane, to enter slightly above midpoint of humerus	Humerus; shoulder joint; elbow joint greater tuberosity superimposed on humeral head; lesser tuberosity seen in profile; lateral and medial epicondyles superimposed
Humerus	Patient supine; elbow flexed; forearm rotated medially to place the imaginary line connecting the medial and lateral epicondyles perpendicular to film plane; posterior surface of hand resting against patient's side	See Erect humerus position	Humerus
Humerus (transthoracic)	Patient erect; lateral surface of affected extremity adjacent to film holder; rotate body, placing humeral head between sternum and vertebral column; imaginary line connecting medial and lateral epicondyles perpendicular to film plane, if possible; opposite arm raised, elbow flexed and forearm resting on top of head	CR directed perpendicular to midportion of film plane, to enter through the chest and exit at the affected extremity	Proximal humerus and shoulder joint without superimposition of opposite shoulder, vertebrae or sternum
Scapula	Patient erect in anterior oblique position (rotated 30 degrees from lateral); scapula in true lateral position; arm on side of interest crossed over chest of patient; hand resting on opposite shoulder	CR directed perpendicular to film plane, to enter at midvertebral border	Lateral scapula projected away from rib cage
Scapula	Patient recumbent; posterior oblique position (rotated 60 degrees from lateral); for position of arm and hand, see erect scapula position	See erect scapula projection	See erect scapula view

TABLE 4-9 AP Shoulder, PA Axial Shoulder and Axial Clavice

Area	Position of Part	Projection of Central Ray	Demonstrates (View)
AP Shoulder (Axial)	Patient supine, arms at sides of body; arm abducted slightly, hand supinated	CR directed 15 degrees to 30 degrees cephalad (the degree of angle depends on patient habitus) to enter at the coracoid process	Coracoid (free of self-superimposition); scapular notch
PA shoulder (Clavicle)	Patient prone or erect; arms at sides, head turned away from affected side	CR directed perpendicular, to enter midway between the median plane of the body and the lateral edge of the shoulder at the level of the coracoid process	Clavicle; acromioclavicular joint; sternoclavicular joint
PA Shoulder (clavicle axial)	See above	CR directed 25 to 30 degrees caudal, to enter midway between the median plane of the body and the outer border of the shoulder at the level of the coracoid process.	See PA shoulder view

"Wrist, Carpal-Tunnel Imaging.") The hand is then rotated to place the thumb in the horizontal position. The CR, directed 45 degrees toward the elbow, enters a point about 1 in distal to the first carpometacarpal joint.[1] With the hand placed in the dorsipalmar position, with the thumb rotated slightly toward the palmar aspect, the second to fifth digits and their metacarpals are not parallel with the film surface. The resulting radiograph shows different degrees of obliquity of the joints of the phalanges and metacarpals[46] (Fig 4-6).

Modified Position for the PA Hand

A modified position, with the forearm rotated at the elbow to raise the ulnar border of the hand off the cassette, brings the plane of the dorsum of the hand parallel to the image detector. The thumb is then in the lateral position and the planes of the second to fifth digits, including

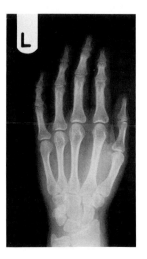

FIGURE 4-6 Dorsipalmar Radiograph of the Hand, Using Standard Positioning Technique

(Courtesy Lewis S: New angles on the radiographic examination of the hand I. *Radiography Today* 1988;54:44-45.)

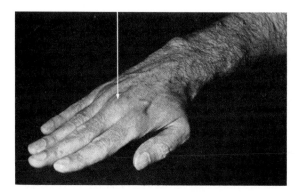

FIGURE 4-7 Modified Dorsipalmar Position of the Hand

(Courtesy Lewis S: New angles on the radiographic examination of the hand I. *Radiography Today* 1988;54:44-45.)

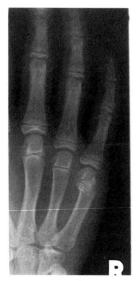
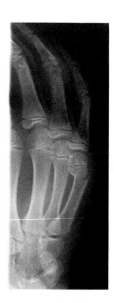

FIGURE 4-9 Radiographs of the Fifth Metacarpal

(A) Dorsipalmar and (B) dorsipalmar oblique. (Courtesy Lewis S: New angles on radiographic examination of the hand III. *Radiography Today* 1988;54:47-48.)

their metacarpals and the carpus, are parallel to the cassette. The CR is directed to the head of the third metacarpal.

Several advantages result with this modification. The thumb is turned to the true lateral position, the phalanges and metacarpals of the second to fifth digits are in the true dorsipalmar position, and the scaphoid (navicular) is separated from adjacent carpal bones[46] (Figs 4-7 and 4-8).

> NOTE: The joint between the proximal second and third metacarpals, however, is not as clearly seen in the modified projection.[46]

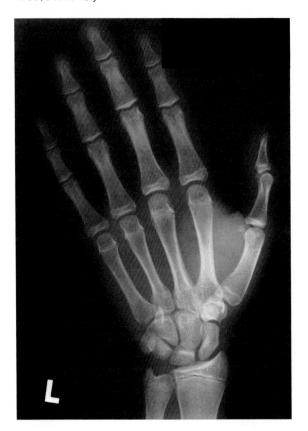

FIGURE 4-8 Dorsipalmar Radiograph, Modified Technique

(Courtesy Lewis S: New angles on the radiographic examination of the hand I. *Radiography Today* 1988;54:44-45.)

Modified Oblique Position for the Fifth Metacarpal

The routine dorsipalmar oblique position of the hand does not offer a deep oblique or lateral view of the fifth metacarpal area (Fig 4-9).

A modified position, with the hand externally rotated to 5 degrees backward beyond the lateral position, avoids superimposing the second to fourth metacarpals on the fifth. The thumb is extended fully, with the hand relaxed (slightly cupped) to remove the unwanted metacarpals. The CR is directed to the center of the fifth metacarpal. A slight angulation of the x-ray tube (parallel to the extended thumb) is required for the CR to pass parallel to the extended thumb[47] (Figs 4-10 and 4-11).

Magnified Oblique Imaging of the Wrist

A unique four-oblique-projection study with 1.4× magnification can be used to supplement standard radiographs of the wrist. With the forearm resting on the table, a foam wedge is placed beneath the hand so that the wrist is in 10 degrees of extension with no radioulnar deviation. The CR is directed to the scaphoid and four exposures are made, with the following variations in the direction of the ray: 25 degree ulnar (U-25), 20 degree radial (R-20), 10 degree distal (D-10), and 10 degree proximal (P-10) (Figs 4-12 through 4-14). These unusual beam angulations project all parts of the scaphoid (navicular) free of the other carpal bones.[48]

A fractional focal spot (0.3 mm or smaller) helps to reduce image blur with direct enlargement techniques.

Flexion Studies of the Wrist

The ulnar flexion position is used to demonstrate the scaphoid (navicular) without distortion. The adjacent carpal interspaces should be open. After the hand and wrist have been positioned for a conventional PA projection of the wrist, the hand is turned outward. The CR directed perpendicular to the film plane enters the midcarpal area.[1,3]

NOTE: An angle of from 10 to 15 degrees (proximal or distal) may be required to demonstrate some fractures.[1,3]

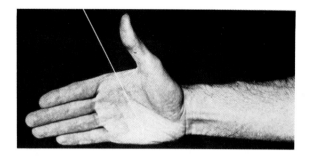

FIGURE 4-10 Position of Hand for Modified Technique to Demonstrate Fifth Metacarpal

(Courtesy Lewis S: New angles on the radiographic examination of the hand III. *Radiography Today* 1988;54:47-48.)

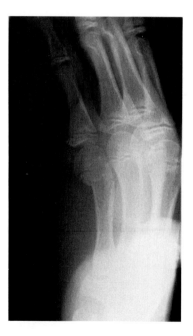

FIGURE 4-11 A Steep Oblique Radiograph (Near Lateral) of the Fifth Metacarpal

(Courtesy Lewis S: New angles on the radiographic examination of the hand III. *Radiography Today* 1988;54:47-48.)

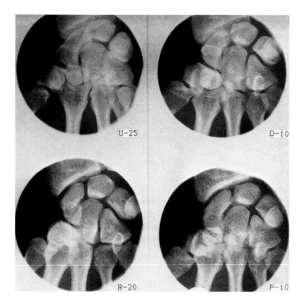

FIGURE 4-12 Oblique Projections of the Carpal Scaphoid

Four normal oblique scaphoid radiographs using unique x-ray tube angulations. Upper left, U-25. Upper right, D-10. Lower left, R-20. Lower right, P-10. (Courtesy Just SL, Sloth C, Amundsen P-O; Diagnosis of fracture of the carpal scaphoid with 4 oblique projections. *Eur J Radiol* 1989;9:152-154.)

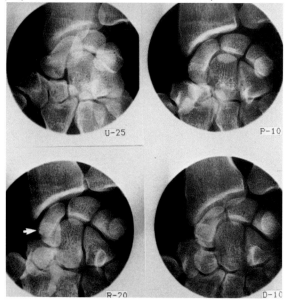

FIGURE 4-13 Fracture of the Carpal Scaphoid

Fracture through the scaphoid waist laterally, visible in the R-20 view (lower left, arrow). (Courtesy Just SL, Sloth C, Amundsen P-O: Diagnosis of fracture of the carpal scaphoid with 4 oblique projections. *Eur J Radiol* 1989;9:152-154.)

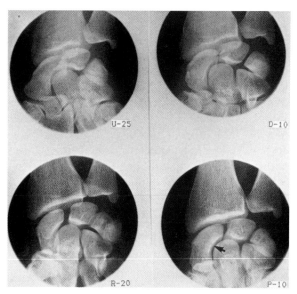

FIGURE 4-14 Oblique Projection of the Carpal Scaphoid

Fracture (incomplete) of the ulnar margin of the scaphoid waist. This fracture is visible only in the P-10 view (lower right, arrow). (Courtesy Just SL, Sloth C, Amundsen P-O: Diagnosis of fracture of the carpal scaphoid with 4 oblique projections. *Eur J Radiol* 1989;9:152-154.)

The positioning for radial flexion studies requires that the hand be turned inward. Radial flexion studies open the interspaces between the carpals on the medial side of the wrist and demonstrate the distal radius and ulna, carpals, and proximal metacarpals.[1,3]

Scaphoid (Navicular) Imaging

Demonstration of the scaphoid in the PA position can be obtained by (1) elevating one end of the cassette on a 20 degree support inclined toward the elbow (thereby achieving angulation of the part) and directing the CR perpendicular to the tabletop, (2) keeping the wrist and film plane horizontal and directing the CR 20 degrees toward the elbow, or (3) elevating the distal end of the scaphoid to lie parallel to the film plane by having the patient make a fist and directing the CR perpendicular to the film plane.[1]

Modified Angled Projections of the Scaphoid (Navicular). Posteroanterior, lateral, and oblique positions are usually used to demonstrate the carpo-scaphoid area.

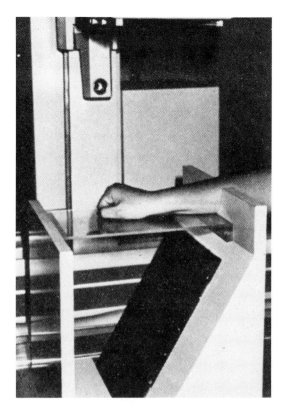

FIGURE 4–15 Device Used to Hold Cassette at an Angle of 60 Degrees to Long Axis of Forearm for Angled Projection of the Wrist

(Courtesy Proubasta I, Lluch A, Celaya F, et al: Angled radiographic view of the wrist for diagnosis of fractures of the carpal scaphoid. *AJR* 1989; 153: 196.)

A modified angled projection is often helpful in visualizing a fracture of the scaphoid. An elaborate process was used to evaluate the angulation between the longitudinal axis of the scaphoid and the horizontal plane (S-H angle). A series of images were made on three human cadaver specimens in the PA position with central-beam angulation adjusted from +60 degrees proximally to −60 degrees distally. It was determined that the projections in the proximal directions were of no value and that the PA position with the CR directed about 40 degrees distally should always be included as part of a scaphoid study.[49]

In a clinical study of the wrist in moderate extension, and ulnar deviation, the cassette was placed on the volar side of the wrist at an angle of 60 degrees to the forearm, thus putting the scaphoid in better alignment with the long axis of the forearm, perpendicular to the x-ray beam. An elongated magnified image of the scaphoid resulted owing to the oblique position of the cassette in relationship to the scaphoid[50] (Figs 4-15 and 4-16).

The use of a fractional focal spot (0.3 mm or smaller) helps to minimize image blur.

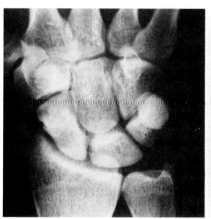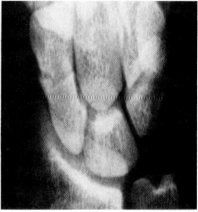

FIGURE 4–16 Conventional Versus Angled Radiograph of the Wrist for Diagnosis of Fracture of the Carpal Scaphoid

Left, In the standard AP view of the wrist, no fracture is seen. Right, On the radiograph of the same patient made with a cassette at a 60 degree angle, the fracture is clearly demonstrated. (Courtesy Proubasta I, Lluch A, Celaya F, et al: Angled radiographic view of the wrist for diagnosis of fracture of the carpal scaphoid. *AJR* 1989; 153: 196.)

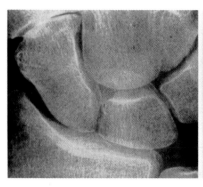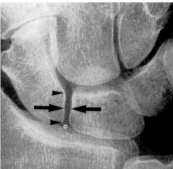

FIGURE 4–17 Demonstration of the Scapholunate Space

Left, Conventional PA view with partial overlapping between the scaphoid and lunate. Right, The PA view with 10 degree angulation toward the radius demonstrates the scapolunate space. (Courtesy Kindynis P, Resnick D, Kang HS, et al: Demonstration of the scapholunate space with radiography. *Radiology* 1990; 175: 278-280.)

Imaging of the Scapholunate Space. In the routine PA radiograph, the scaphoid (navicular) and lunate bones often overlap, making it difficult to demonstrate the scapholunate space. To do so, the hand is placed in the PA position, with the x-ray tube angled 10 degrees from the ulna toward the radius[51] (Fig 4-17).

Carpal-Tunnel Imaging

Tangential Projection (Inferosuperior). To demonstrate the carpal canal, hamular process (hook of the hamate), scaphoid tuberosity, and palmar aspect of the carpal bones, the wrist is hyperextended and traction used to hold the hand as nearly perpendicular to the film plane as is tolerable while rotating the hand slightly toward the radial side. The CR, directed 25 to 30 degrees toward the long axis of the hand (the palmar surface), enters 1 in distal to the base of the fourth metacarpal. This angle may have to be increased if the patient cannot hyperextend the wrist adequately.[1,3]

Alternative Method (Superoinferior). If the patient cannot assume the position required for the inferosuperior projection of the carpal canal, the superoinferior projection is recommended as an alternative method. With the patient standing beside the table and leaning forward with the wrist in extreme dorsiflexion, the palmar surface of the hand is placed on the film holder. The CR, directed perpendicular to the film holder, enters through the carpal bones.[1,3] The patient may be required to lean forward to raise the hand off the film in order to align the carpal tunnel perpendicular to the film plane.[52]

A modification of the superoinferior projection requires that the patient's palm be in contact with the cassette and the forearm adjusted perpendicular to the film. The CR, directed at a 45 degree angle toward the fingers, enters though the carpal tunnel[52] (Figs 4-18 and 4-19).

Tangential Imaging of the Carpal Bridge

A tangential view of the carpus is sometimes needed to demonstrate a fracture of the scaphoid, chip fractures of the dorsal aspect of the carpal bones, lunate dislocations, or foreign bodies or calcifications in the dorsum of the wrist. The dorsal surface of the hand, forming a right angle with the forearm, is placed against the cassette. The CR, directed at a superoinferior angle of 45 degrees, enters at a point about 1.5 in proximal to the wrist joint.[1]

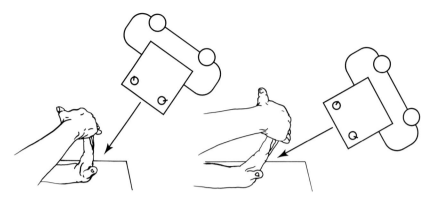

FIGURE 4–18 Carpal-Tunnel Evaluation

Left, Routine projection for the inferosuperior projection of the carpal tunnel. Right, A modification of this projection for use if patients are unable to extend their wrists adequately. (Redrawn from Fodor J III, Malott JC, Merhar GL: Carpal tunnel syndrome: The role of radiography. *Radiol Technol* 1987;58:497-502.)

Imaging of the Distal Ulna

An extended pronated view of the wrist is useful when evaluating the distal ulna. The forearm is placed flat on the cassette and the hand is pronated until the thumbnail bed is flat on the cassette. The patient's shoulder is brought well forward, with the wrist dorsiflexed as far as possible. The CR is directed perpendicular to the cassette and enters at the wrist joint (the distal ulnar area) to demonstrate the distal ulna head and styloid.[53]

Modified Lateral View of the Radial Head

A conventional lateral view of the elbow demonstrates the anterior fat pad. The posterior fat pad of the elbow is not usually seen on a negative study. If there are changes in the elbow joint, the normal shape and position of the fat pad or pads will be altered.[34] See Chapter 3, Fig 3-5.

The radial head–capitellum view is a modified lateral view of the elbow joint with the CR directed 45 degrees toward the radial head. This projection differs from the conventional lateral in that it eliminates the overlap of bones at the humeroradial and humeroulnar articulations, separating the cornoid process and radial head,

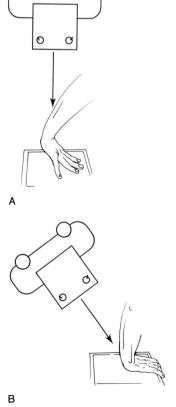

A

B

FIGURE 4–19 Carpal-Tunnel Evaluation

(A) Superoinferior projection of the carpal tunnel. (B) Variation in position for superoinferior projection of the carpal tunnel. (Redrawn from Fodor J III, Malott JC, Merhar GL: Carpal tunnel syndrome: The role of radiography. *Radiol Technol* 1987;58:497-502.)

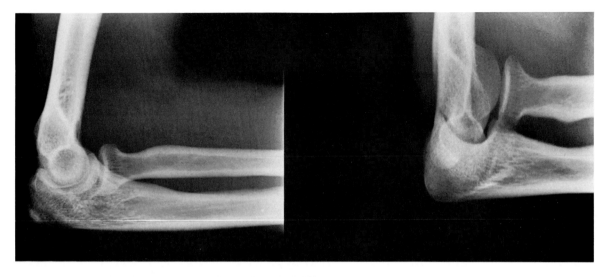

FIGURE 4-20 Modified Lateral Projection of the Radial Head

Left, Conventional lateral of the elbow. Modified lateral of the radial head (capitellum view) projects the radial head ventrad, eliminating bony overlap. Right, With this projection, the articular surface of the capitellum is slightly elongated.

and projecting the radial head ventrad. Demonstration of the coronoid process is important since a fracture in this area can put the elbow at risk for recurrent dislocation[54] (Fig 4-20).

Tangential Projection of the Elbow

When examining an injured elbow in complete flexion, a lateral and tangential projection, with the patient positioned with the elbow in full flexion and the humerus parallel to the cassette, should be attempted. The tangential projection may also be made with the forearm parallel to the film, if this is more comfortable for the patient.

Modifications of the tangential projection, in which two separate exposures are employed and the entire arm (humerus parallel to the film plane) is rotated from the shoulder 45 degrees internally and 45 degrees externally, may provide additional information before attempts are made to extend the arm for conventional views.[55]

Imaging of the Humerus

As with all body parts, one must attempt to get two opposing right angle views, and not just settle for internal and external rotations of the humerus. Any rotation of the hand rotates the humerus in its joint. While internal and external rotations of the humerus provide right angle views of the humerus, they do not furnish additional views of adjacent structures.[27]

A fracture or dislocation of the shoulder (humerus) is a surgical emergency. Pain may make routine positions difficult to accomplish.

Imaging of Intermedullary Pins

An intermedullary pin is sometimes needed to stabilize a fracture of a long bone. See Chapter 3. A radiograph with an intermedullary pin adjacent to the uninjured arm or leg may be made to show the orthopedist the relationship of the pin to the length of the injured long bone. With the cassette placed diagonal to the uninjured extremity to include both joints, a tightly collimated image of the proximal end of the uninjured long bone is made. The x-ray tube is then centered over the distal end of the long bone and a second exposure made. (See "Lower Extremities: Preoperative Bone Measurement.")

CAUTION: The patient must not move between exposures.

Transthoracic Lateral View of the Humerus

With the patient standing or sitting, the injured arm is positioned against the upright Bucky. The opposite arm is raised and the forearm placed on the head, depressing the opposite shoulder and thus minimizing superimposition. If possible, the humeral epicondyles should be perpendicular to the film plane. The CR is directed perpendicular to the film plane and enters the chest at the level of the surgical neck of the humerus being examined. A 10 degree or greater cephalad tube tilt may be used to project the uninjured shoulder superiorly.

Lung markings may be blurred out by using a low mA long exposure time (5 seconds or more) technique. A patient with a dislocation or fracture may find it difficult to cooperate in this technique. A high kVp (100 kVp or greater)/grid chest technique with full inspiration is suggested[55] (Fig 4-21).

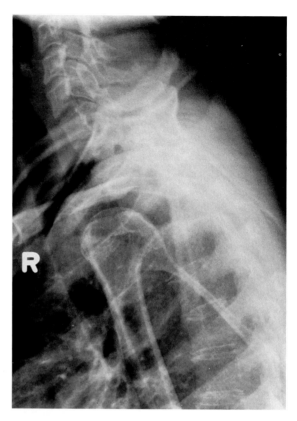

FIGURE 4-21 Transthoracic Lateral View of the Humerus

An image was obtained with the patient in the erect position using a high kVp technique (125 kVp) and deep inspiration. This projection also can be used to demonstrate cervicodorsal alignment. (Courtesy Eastman Kodak Company, Rochester, NY.)

Axillary View of the Shoulder

A 30 degree or greater abduction of the arm at the glenohumeral junction is required for the axillary position. The x-ray beam is directed cephalad through the axilla.[56]

Modified Transaxillary Projection of the Shoulder. In the presence of an injured shoulder, the axillary view can be accomplished with minimal abduction.

A modification of the transaxial projection requires that the patient lie on the unaffected side with the arm of the affected shoulder in 90 degree abduction. The palm of the hand faces the x-ray tube. The cassette can be positioned against the patient's neck and held in place by the other hand. If the patient has difficulty abducting the arm, a moderate degree of abduction, with the arm supported by a foam sponge, can result in a satisfactory transaxial projection[57] (Fig 4-22).

CAUTION: If a grid cassette is used for this procedure, the lead lines should be positioned perpendicular, not parallel, to the tabletop.

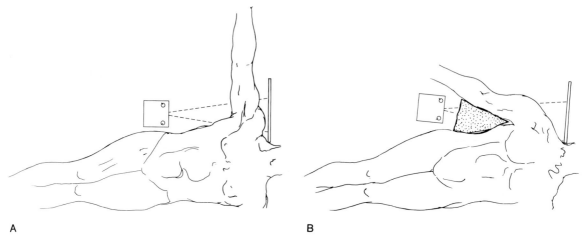

A   B

FIGURE 4-22   Modified Transaxial Projection

(A) A conventional transaxial projection is shown with the patient's arm abducted at a right angle to the body, with the palm of the hand facing the x-ray tube. This position demonstrates the lesser tuberosity in profile. If the patient were unable to abduct the arm to the full 90 degrees, a moderate degree of abduction would be acceptable. (B) With the arm abducted to the degree tolerable to the patient, a foam-rubber sponge can be used to maintain the position. The arm may be flexed at the elbow if necessary. (Drawn from Clements RW: Adaption of the technique for radiography of the glenohumeral joint in the lateral position. *Radiol Technol* 1979;51:305-312.)

Bicipital-Groove Imaging

The bicipital groove is examined to demonstrate calcific deposits within the muscle sheath projected within the groove. Bony spurs, bridges, or irregular erosions of the groove attributable to degenerative changes can also be seen.[58]

Most reports describe the patient in the erect position, with the x-ray tube inverted. The cassette is placed above the patient's shoulder and the CR is directed (inferosuperior) perpendicular to the film plane.

A modified projection requires that the patient be seated at the table with the elbow flexed at 90 degrees and the hand supine. The patient is asked to move slightly forward (approximately 10 to 15 degrees from the upright position). The radiographer, using one hand to palpate the shoulder, can identify the bicipital groove by moving the patient's forearm back and forth, causing the humerus to rotate internally and externally. The CR is directed (superoinferiorly) perpendicular to the cassette positioned on the tabletop (Fig 4-23). An alteration of the patient's position (less forward angulation of the trunk)

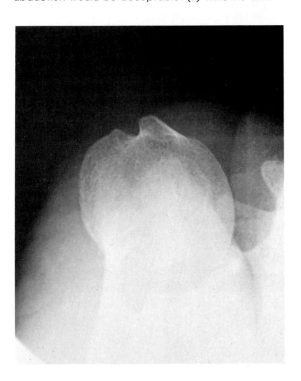

FIGURE 4-23   Radiograph of the Bicipital Groove

(Courtesy Eastman Kodak Company, Rochester, NY.)

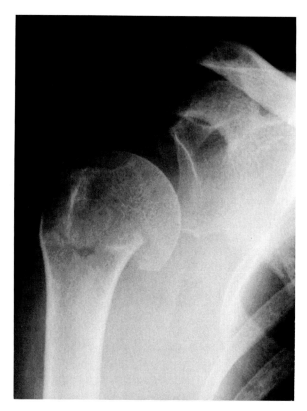

FIGURE 4–24 Transverse Fracture of the Surgical Neck of the Humerus with an Inferior Subluxation of the Humeral Head

(Courtesy Bangert BA, Pathria MN, Resnick D: Advanced imaging of the shoulder. *Surg Rounds Orthopaed* June 1989, pp 48-57.)

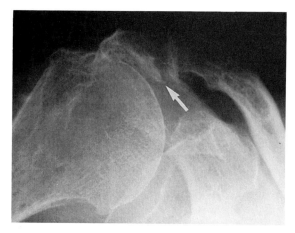

A

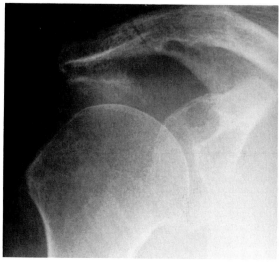

B

FIGURE 4–25 Comparison Radiographs to Demonstrate a Subacromial Spur

(A) A frontal radiograph demonstrating narrowing of the humeral acromial distance and a subacromial spur (arrow). (B) A radiograph obtained with a caudad angled projection more accurately reflects the size of the spur. (Courtesy Bangert BA, Pathria MN, Resnick D: Advanced imaging of the shoulder. *Surg Rounds Orthopaed* June 1989, pp 48-57.)

may be required if the acromion process is superimposed on the bicipital groove, which occurs in approximately 10% of the patients examined.[58]

Modified AP Projections of the Shoulder

The shoulder impingement syndrome results from entrapment of the periarticular soft tissues between the humeral head inferiorly, the acromion superiorly, and the fibrous coracoacromial arch anteriorly. The conventional AP radiograph of the shoulder underestimates the size of subacromial spurs, which are best seen on an erect AP image with a 30 degree caudad tube tilt[56,59] (Figs 4-24 through 4-28).

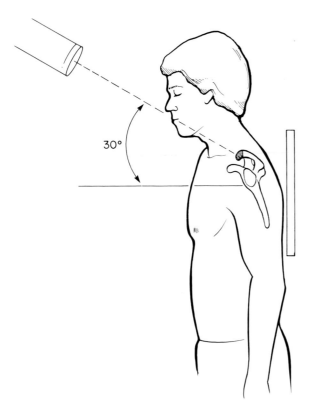

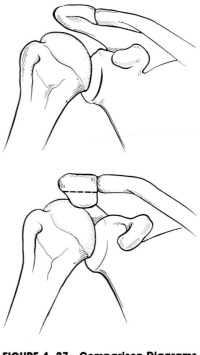

FIGURE 4–26 Position of Patient for AP Projection with 30 Degree Caudad Angle to Demonstrate the Anterior Part of the Acromium

(Courtesy Kilcoyne RF, Reddy PK, Lyons F, et al: Optimal plain film imaging of the shoulder impingement syndrome. *AJR* 1989; 153: 795-797.)

FIGURE 4–27 Comparison Diagrams of Conventional AP Projection and Superspinatus Outlet View

Top, No abnormality is seen. Bottom, An abnormally long acromial spur is seen in the 30 degree caudad projection. The dotted line represents the abnormality. (Courtesy Kilcoyne RF, Reddy PK, Lyons F, et al: Optimal plain film imaging of the shoulder impingement syndrome. *AJR* 1989; 153: 795-797.)

Modified Transscapular Lateral Shoulder

A modified transscapular lateral projection utilizing a 5 to 10 degree caudal angle, known as the supraspinatus outlet view, will also demonstrate the extent of the anterior projection of the acromium[59] (Fig 4-29).

Another modification, the "zero" projection, is used to demonstrate recurrent, transient subluxation of the shoulder. A posteroinferior subluxation of the shoulder joint can be seen on an AP radiograph made following active elevation of the shoulder ("zero" position) (Figs 4-30 through 4-32, page 76). The patient, rotated to the affected side, stands with the back against the erect Bucky. The blade of the affected scapula is parallel to the film plane (30 to 45 degrees). The affected arm is raised and the palm of the hand is placed on the occiput. The axis of the humerus is adjusted parallel to the film plane. The hand is then moved down toward the nape of the neck as far as the patient is able to tolerate. This should demonstrate any abnormal movement of the humeral head attributable to the defect in the musculature. A horizontal beam is used, centered over the coracoid process.[60]

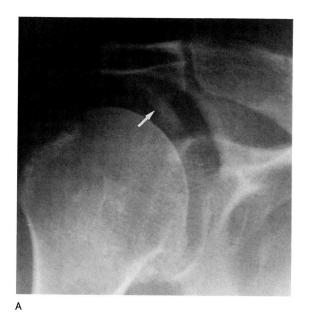

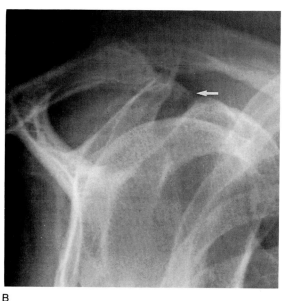

A   B

FIGURE 4–28   Radiographic Demonstration of Subacromial Spur

(A) A subacromial spur (arrows) can be seen on the 30 degree caudad angled AP view. (B) Subacromial spur is also seen on the supraspinatus outlet view. See Fig 4-29 for positioning information. (Courtesy Kilcoyne RF, Reddy PK, Lyons F, et al: Optimal plain film imaging of the shoulder impingement syndrome. *AJR* 1989; 153: 795-797.)

> C A U T I O N :   The patient must not rotate the head and neck. This would produce a tilt toward the affected shoulder.

Comparison images in the "zero" position may help to demonstrate a subtle subluxation.[60]

Apical Oblique Projection of the Glenohumeral Joint

For a true AP projection of the glenohumeral joint, a posterior oblique view must be taken with the extremity rotated 40 degrees posteriorly. The apical oblique projection of the shoulder can be used as a supplemental projection to the AP and transthoracic projections to demonstrate glenohumeral instability.

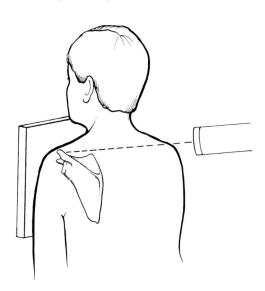

FIGURE 4–29   Supraspinatus Outlet View to Show Anterior Part of Acromium in a Lateral View

Patient is placed in the transcapular lateral position with tube angled 5 degrees caudad. (Courtesy Kilcoyne RF, Reddy PK, Lyons F, et al: Optimal plain film imaging of the shoulder impingement syndrome. *AJR* 1989; 153: 795-797.)

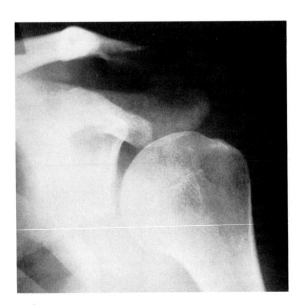

FIGURE 4-30   AP Shoulder: The Zero Projection

Inferior subluxation of the humeral head. (Courtesy Horsfield D, Phillips RR: The zero projection. *Radiography Today* 1990;56:14-16.)

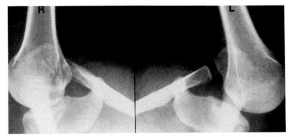

FIGURE 4-32   Zero Projection of the Shoulder

Excessive movement of the humerus of the left shoulder as the result of a muscular defect. (Courtesy Horsfield D, Phillips RR: The zero projection. *Radiography Today* 1990;56:14-16.)

An optional method uses the apical oblique position, in which the patient is rotated 45 degrees posteriorly and the beam is directed 45 degrees caudad. With the patient seated erect in the posterior oblique position, the CR is directed 45 degrees caudad and enters on or just medial to the glenohumeral joint. The patient must flex and rotate his or her neck contralaterally. Glenoid and coracoid fractures, posterior glenohumeral dislocations, acromioclavicular separations, and soft-tissue calcifications are demonstrated with this projection[61] (Figs 4-33 through 4-37).

A retrospective analysis of more than 500 patients using the apical oblique view of the shoulder demonstrated that this projection, combined with the AP view, should be used to detect acute shoulder injuries.[62]

Clavicle Imaging

An AP view with a 15 degree cephalic angulation will demonstrate the middle and lateral portions of the clavicle free of the ribs and scapula. Enhanced visualization of the medial aspect of the clavicle requires a 40 degree cephalad tube angulation.[28]

Frontal radiographs of a fractured clavicle can be misleading. Fragments can be displaced anteriorly, with opposing fragments displaced posteriorly, giving the illusion of reasonable frac-

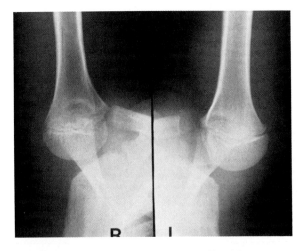

FIGURE 4-31   Zero Projection of the Shoulder

Posteroinferior subluxation of the left shoulder. (Courtesy Horsfield D, Phillips RR: The zero projection. *Radiography Today* 1990;56:14-16.)

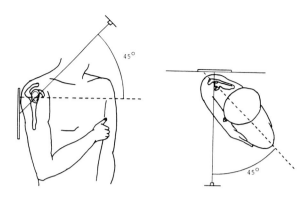

FIGURE 4–33   Apical Oblique Projection of the Glenohumeral Joint

The injured side is rotated 45 degrees posteriorly with the CR directed 45 degrees caudad and centered on the glenohumeral joint. (Courtesy Sloth C, Just SL: The apical oblique radiograph in examination of acute shoulder trauma. *Eur J Radiol* 1989;9:147-151.)

ture apposition. With the patient supine, the x-ray tube can be angled 45 degrees cephalad. A dislocation of a joint anteriorly or an anterior fracture segment will be projected higher than the uninjured clavicle. If the injured clavicle or portion of the clavicle is projected lower than the uninjured clavicle, then a posterior dislocation has occurred.

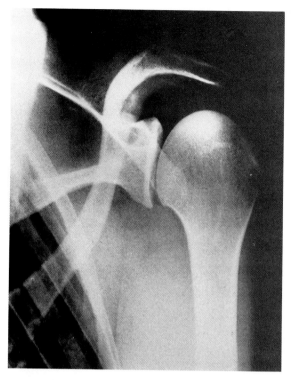

FIGURE 4–34   Normal Apical Oblique Radiograph

The humeral head, glenoid fossa, and scapular neck are free of other structures. The coracoid process is projected from the glenoid rim with the acromioclavicular joint projected cephalad. (Courtesy Sloth C, Just SL: The apical oblique radiograph in examination of acute shoulder trauma. *Eur J Radiol* 1989;9:147-151.)

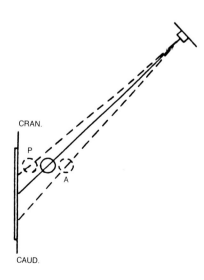

FIGURE 4–35   Schematic Representation of an AP Dislocation

On the apical oblique radiograph, structures dislocated posteriorly (P) project cephalad while structures dislocated anteriorly (A) project caudad. A conventional AP radiograph would not necessarily show a dislocation. (Courtesy Sloth C, Just SL: The apical oblique radiograph in examination of acute shoulder trauma. *Eur J Radiol* 1989;9:147-151.)

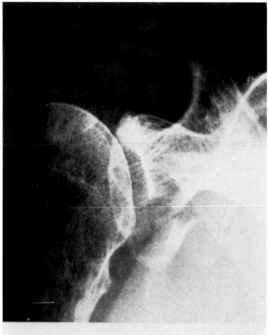

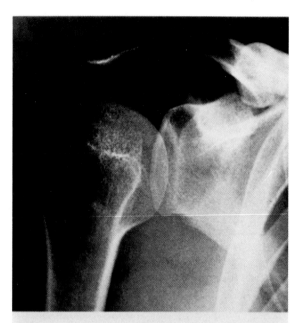

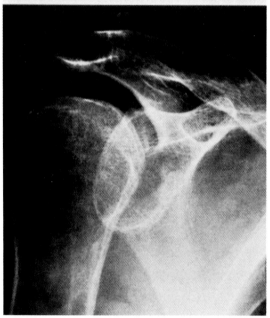

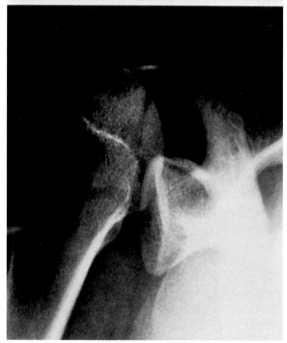

FIGURE 4-36 Fracture of the Glenoid Fossa

Top, A conventional radiograph does not demonstrate a fracture through the glenoid fossa. Bottom, The fracture is seen only in the apical oblique projection. (Courtesy Sloth C, Just SL: The apical oblique radiograph in examination of acute shoulder trauma. *Eur J Radiol* 1989;9:147-151.)

FIGURE 4-37 Posterior Glenohumeral Dislocation

Top, This dislocation is not seen on the AP projection. Bottom, On the apical oblique study, the humeral head is clearly displaced and projected cephalad. (Courtesy Sloth S, Just SL: The apical oblique radiograph in examination of acute shoulder trauma. *Eur J Radiol* 1989;9:147-151.)

Acromioclavicular Joint Imaging

The acromioclavicular joints are easily overexposed owing to the thinness of the anatomical part and the potential for image undercutting by a primary beam leak. See Chapter 1.

Simultaneous Exposure of the Acromioclavicular Joints. Stress radiographs may be needed because some acromioclavicular separations may appear normal on nonstress images. Sandbags or other weights used with studies of these joints must be able to be held comfortably since patients will often splint their arms during a procedure, negating the effect of the weights. The recommended weight for stress imaging is approximately 15 lb per extremity and may vary from 10 to 20 lb, depending on departmental routine.[3]

Because of the divergent effect of the x-ray beam, the lateral aspects of the shoulders may be projected off of a 7 in by 17 in cassette. A pair of 8 in by 10 in cassettes, positioned transversely in a Bucky tray, may provide the additional film coverage needed to overcome this divergent effect.[1-3]

Modified Acromioclavicular Joint Imaging. Since the acromiohumeral window is slightly caudal in the AP view, the x-ray beam should be directed 10 to 20 degrees toward the feet with the patient supine and slightly less with the patient erect. An underpart filter will help to minimize soft-tissue burnout.[9] See Chapter 1, Fig 1-7.

An alternative technique places the patient in the upright position, with the arms relaxed at the sides. The posterior aspect of the shoulder is in contact with the cassette. The CR is directed 25 degrees cephalad and 10 degrees laterally toward the lateral end of the clavicle at the acromioclavicular joint. Both sides are examined for comparison, but a weight-bearing view is not considered necessary since any malalignment of the joint is usually demonstrated by this projection.[63]

> CAUTION: Because of the dual tube angle, this technique should be employed without a grid, using tight beam collimation.

Imaging of Sternoclavicular Dislocations

A clavicle fracture or dislocation may occur in either end of the clavicle as the result of direct trauma. A posterior dislocation of the sternoclavicular joint may pose an emergency since injury to the trachea, esophagus, and major blood vessels is possible.[64]

Sternoclavicular dislocation can be evaluated with an AP view of the chest using a 40 degree cephalad tilt with the CR directed to the manubrium. An anterior dislocated clavicle will be displaced superior to the normal clavicle. With a posterior dislocation, an inferior displacement occurs.

Scapular Imaging

Most scapular fractures result from serious trauma and can be accompanied by rib or clavicle fractures, pulmonary contusion, subcutaneous emphysema, or pneumothoax.

Tangential View of the Scapular Spine. If the spine of the scapula must be visualized because of trauma or disease, the patient is placed in the supine position with the unaffected shoulder elevated on a sandbag and the tube tilted caudad 40 to 45 degrees. The CR enters tangentially through the posterosuperior portion of the scapula.

In the reverse position, with the patient prone, the CR is directed through the scapular spine at an angle of 45 degrees cephalad.[65]

Modified Lateral Projections of the Scapula. A view of the lateral scapula may be obtained with the patient supine and the unaffected arm flexed at the elbow, raised upward, and abducted so that the arm covers the eyes.

If the arm on the affected side cannot be raised, it should be brought forward across the chest so that the scapula is perpendicular to the tabletop. Palpation of the scapula is suggested to determine the degree of rotation.

If the arm cannot be positioned across the chest, it should be abducted until the elbow is located over the anterior surface of the upper abdomen. The patient is then rotated until the scapula is perpendicular to the tabletop. For both projections, the CR is directed perpendicular to the film plane, entering at a point below the head of the humerus.[66]

THE LOWER EXTREMITIES AND PELVIC GIRDLE

Projections suggested for basic radiography of the lower extremities and pelvis include:

1. AP (dorsoplantar) oblique and lateral toes (Tables 4-10 through 4-12).
2. AP (dorsoplantar) oblique and lateral foot (Tables 4-10 through 4-12).
3. Axial (plantodorsal) and lateral calcaneus (Tables 4-11 and 4-19).
4. AP and lateral ankle (Tables 4-11 and 4-13).
5. AP and lateral lower leg (Tables 4-13 and 4-14).
6. AP and lateral knee (Tables 4-13 and 4-14).
7. AP oblique knee and ankle (Table 4-15).
8. PA axial knee (Table 4-16).
9. PA. lateral and tangential patella (Tables 4-14, 4-16, and 4-17).
10. AP and lateral femur (Tables 4-13 and 4-14).
11. AP and lateral hip (Tables 4-13 and 4-14).
12. AP pelvis.

SUPPLEMENTARY IMAGING OF THE LOWER EXTREMITIES AND PELVIS

In the dorsoplantar position, there is approximately a one-to-five difference in the thickness of the foot from the toes to the tarsal area. Despite this difference in density, all soft tissues, as well as osseous structures, must be imaged. A compensatory filter can help to balance radiographic density from the toes to the tarsal area (Fig 4-38).

Tangential Projection of the Toes

A tangential projection is used to free the sesamoids of superimposition by the head (distal end) of the first metatarsal. The distal ends of all five metatarsals should be seen. With the patient in the prone position and the leg extended, the foot rests on the dorsiflexed great toe. The ball of the foot should be perpendicular to the film plane. The CR is directed to the distal end of the second metatarsal.[3]

A modification of this examination is performed with the patient in the supine position. A long strip of gauze placed around the toes is used by the patient to retract the toes to the dorsiflexed position. With the ball of the foot perpendicular to the film plane, the CR is directed to the distal end of the second metatarsal.[3]

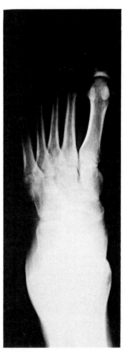 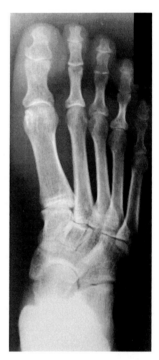

A   B

FIGURE 4–38
Dorsoplantar View of the Foot

Conventional radiograph of the foot. Adequate exposure of the tarsal area results in a "burnout" of the toe anatomy (A). A CLEAR-Pb Filter (compensatory) was used with radiograph B. Image density is similar from the toes to the tarsal area. Excellent soft-tissue detail is also maintained. (Courtesy Nuclear Associates, Carle Place, NY.)

TABLE 4-10   AP (Dorsoplantar) Toes and Foot

Area	Position of Part	Projection of Central Ray	Demonstrates (View)
Toes (AP [DP])	Patient seated on table with knee flexed, foot resting on cassette with no elevation of cassette	CR directed perpendicular to film plane, enters at third metatarsophalangeal joint	Phalanges; of digits; distal metatarsals
	Optional: toes elevated 15 degrees, on foam sponge	See AP projection	See AP view
	Optional: toes resting on cassette, no elevation of cassette	CR directed 15 degrees cephalad	See AP view
Foot	See Toes AP position	CR directed perpendicular to base of third metatarsal (may require angulation of from 5 to 15 degrees cephalad)	Entire foot from distal phalanges to tarsals

TABLE 4-11   Lateral Toes, Foot, Calcaneus, and Ankle

Area	Position of Part	Projection of Central Ray	Demonstrates (View)
Toes	Patient recumbent lateral; toe in question closest to film; traction on toes above and below the toe in question may be required to avoid superimposition	CR directed perpendicular to interphalangeal joint	Lateral phalanges; the toenail should be seen in profile
Foot	Patient recumbent, lateral; foot neutral	CR directed perpendicular to bases of metatarsals	Distal tibia and fibula; tarsals; metatarsals; phalanges
Calcaneus	Patient recumbent lateral; foot dorsiflexed, sole of foot parallel to bottom of cassette and perpendicular to film plane	CR directed perpendicular to film plane, to enter at midcalcaneus	Calcaneus, adjacent tarsals, talus, subtalar joint, ankle joint
Ankle	See Calcaneus position	CR directed perpendicular to film plane, to enter at ankle joint	Distal ends of tibia and fibula; ankle joint; talus; calcaneus

TABLE 4-12 Oblique Toes and Foot

Area	Position of Part	Projection of Central Ray	Demonstrates (View)
Toes (medial oblique)	Patient supine with knee flexed, foot rotated 30 to 45 degrees medially	CR directed perpendicular to film plane, to enter at metatarsophalangeal joints	Phalanges and distal metatarsal bones; interphalangeal joints, metatarsophalangeal joints
Toes (lateral oblique)	See Medial oblique position; foot rotated 30 degrees laterally	See Medial oblique projection	See Medial view
Foot (medial oblique)	See Toes position; foot rotated 30 degrees medially	CR directed perpendicular to film plane, to enter midline of foot at base of third metatarsal	Intertarsal joints, tarsals, metatarsals, tarsometotarsal joints; phalanges; sinus tarsi
Foot (lateral oblique)	See Toes, medial oblique position; foot rotated 30 degrees laterally	See Foot, medial oblique projection	See Foot, medial oblique view

Dorsal Oblique Projection of Tarsals

A dorsal oblique projection of the tarsals provides an excellent demonstration of the articulations between most of the tarsal bones. With the patient prone and the leg extended, the sole of the foot forms an angle of about 45 degrees with the film plane. The CR is directed perpendicular to the film plane to enter the center of the foot.[1]

Weight-Bearing Studies of the Foot

In most patients, there is a different alignment of the bones of the feet in weight-bearing as compared with non–weight-bearing positions. Weight bearing puts the skeleton in contact with the ground, using a natural structural relationship as the body weight passes through the foot. To complete the weight-bearing function, the feet must be placed in the base and angle of gait.

The base is defined as the distance between the feet as a patient walks and the angle of gait as the angle of one foot relative to the other.[67]

Each foot must be centered and imaged separately. A tube tilt of 15 degrees toward the patient is recommended for the dorsoplantar image, with the CR entering the foot between the third cuneiform and the navicular on the dorsal surface of the foot.

If weight-bearing images of the foot cannot be made, non–weight-bearing projections should be taken with the patient sitting and the lower leg positioned at a right angle to the foot. This reproduces the weight-bearing position. The CR is directed parallel to the long axis of the foot. A 15 degree tube tilt toward the patient helps to duplicate weight-bearing alignment.[67]

(Text continues on page 86)

TABLE 4-13 AP Ankle, Lower Leg, Knee, Femur, and Hip

Area	Position of Part	Projection of Central Ray	Demonstrates (View)
Ankle	Patient supine; leg extended, foot slightly inverted (do not rotate leg)	CR directed perpendicular to film plane, to enter midpoint of ankle joint	Distal tibia and fibula; talus; ankle joint
Leg (tibia and fibula)	Patient supine; leg extended, foot slightly inverted (do not rotate leg or pelvis)	CR directed perpendicular to film plane, to enter midpoint of lower leg	Tibia; fibula; ankle joint; knee joint (if both joints cannot be included on the survey film, a second radiograph should be made)
Knee	Patient supine; leg extended and rotated 5 degrees medially (do not rotate pelvis)	CR directed perpendicular to film plane, to enter about 1 cm below apex of patella	Distal end of femur; proximal ends of tibia and fibula
Knee (joint space)	See Knee position	CR directed 5 to 7 degrees cephalad	Knee joint; see knee view
Femur	Patient supine; leg extended and rotated 15 degrees medially with toes inverted (do not rotate pelvis)	CR directed perpendicular to film plane, to enter at midpoint of film	Femur to include hip and/or knee joint
Hip	Patient supine; leg extended and rotated 15 degrees medially with toes inverted (do not rotate pelvis)	CR directed perpendicular to film plane, to enter at superior margin of greater trochanter	Hip joint; proximal femur
Pelvis	See Hip	CR directed perpendicular to film plane, to enter midway between symphysis pubis and iliac crests	Hip joints; sacrum; coccyx; femoral heads and necks; greater trochanters

TABLE 4–14 Lateral Lower Leg, Knee, Patella, Femur, and Hip

Area	Position of Patient	Projection of Central Ray	Demonstrates (View)
Leg (tibia and fibula)	Patient recumbent; leg lateral, foot dorsiflexed, patella perpendicular to film plane	CR directed perpendicular to film plane, to enter at midpoint of lower leg	Tibia and fibula; ankle joint; knee joint
Knee	Patient recumbent; leg lateral, knee flexed 45 degrees	CR directed 5 degrees cephalad, to enter 1 cm below apex of patella, perpendicular to the joint space	Distal femur; proximal tibia and fibula
Patella	See Knee; knee flexed 5 to 10 degrees, patella perpendicular to film plane	CR directed perpendicular to film plane, to enter midportion of patella	Patella; knee joint; distal femur proximal tibia and fibula
Femur (upper portion)	Patient recumbent; affected leg rotated to lateral aspect	CR directed perpendicular to film plane, to enter above midthigh	Proximal femur; hip joint
Femur (lower portion)	See Femur	CR directed perpendicular to film plane, to enter below midthigh	Distal femur; knee joint

TABLE 4–15 Oblique Ankle, Knee, and Patella

Part	Position of Patient	Projection of Central Ray	Demonstrates (View)
Ankle (medial oblique)	Patient supine; leg rotated, intermalleolar line at 45 degree angle with film plane; foot dorsiflexed to place ankle at nearly right-angle flexion	CR directed perpendicular to film plane, to enter at midankle joint	Distal tibia and fibula; lateral malleolus; distal tibiofibular joint; ankle joint
Knee (anterolateral)	Patient supine; elevate hip of affected side to rotate extremity 45 degrees laterally	CR directed perpendicular to film plane, to enter at knee joint	Femoral condyles; patella; tibial condyles; head of fibula
Knee (anteromedial)	See Knee position; rotate extremity 45 degrees medially	See Knee projection	See Knee view; proximal tibiofibular articulation
Patella	See Knee position	See Knee projection	See Knee view

TABLE 4–16 PA Patella

Area	Position of Part	Projection of Central Ray	Demonstrates (View)
Patella	Patient prone; plane surface of patella parallel to film plane	CR directed perpendicular to film plane, to enter posterior surface of knee, exits at midportion of patella	Patella; distal femur; proximal tibia and fibula; knee joint

TABLE 4–17 Tangential Patella

Area	Position of Part	Projection of Central Ray	Demonstrates (View)
Patella	Patient prone; knee flexed; patellar surface is perpendicular to film plane, if tolerable (no rotation of leg)	CR directed perpendicular to film plane, to enter through patellofemoral space	Patella, femoropatellar space

TABLE 4–18 Intercondylar Fossa (Axial)

Area	Position of Part	Projection of Central Ray	Demonstrates (View)
Knee	Patient prone; knee flexed; lower leg forms an angle of 40 degrees with film plane	CR directed 40 degrees caudad, to enter posterior surface of knee, 1 cm below apex of patella	Intercondylar fossa; tibial eminences; knee joint

TABLE 4–19 Axial Calcaneus

Area	Position of Part	Projection of Central Ray	Demonstrates (View)
Calcaneus (Plantodorsal PA)	Patient seated or supine on table; leg extended, ankle flexed until plantar surface of foot is perpendicular to film plane	CR directed 40 degrees cephalad, to enter plantar surface at base of third metatarsal	Calcaneus
Calcaneus (Dorsoplantar AP)	Patient prone; plantar surface of foot in contact with cassette (supported perpendicular to tabletop)	CR directed 40 degrees caudad, to enter above heel; exits at base of fifth metatarsal in midline of plantar surface of foot	Calcaneus

The lateral weight-bearing projection is made with the medial portion of the foot positioned against the detector. This differs from the routine recumbent lateral position in which the lateral portion of the foot is placed against the cassette. If lateral non–weight-bearing images must be made, the patient should be placed in a sitting position with the foot at an angle of 90 degrees to the leg, using a mediolateral position.[67]

Imaging of Stress Fractures of the Sesamoids of the Great Toe

Foot and ankle injuries, including stress fractures of the sesamoids of the great toe, are common in both competitive and recreational athletes. Repetitive forces (cumulative microtrauma), which by themselves will not cause a fracture, may ultimately lead to bone failure. Unfortunately, 5% to 30% of normal asymptomatic individuals have bipartite great-toe sesamoids. Obvious injuries can be diagnosed and treated promptly, but some subtle injuries may be difficult to detect.

Radiographs of the opposing foot are of little value since 75% of the population with bipartite sesamoids have unilateral involvement. A radionuclide bone scan will confirm the diagnosis of a stress fracture of the sesamoids of the great toe.[68]

Stress-Fracture Imaging of the Tarsal Navicular

If patient history and a clinical examination of a fracture of the tarsal navicular are not supported by conventional AP, lateral, and oblique radiographs, a tomogram in the AP position may be helpful. A radionuclide scan of both feet may also demonstrate increased activity in the tarsal navicular area.[68]

Imaging of the Transchondral Talar Dome

Conventional AP projections of the ankle are used to demonstrate transchondral talar-dome fractures, usually caused by inversion and eversion injuries to the ankle. If initial radiographs do not demonstrate a fracture, delayed images (six weeks or longer) after the initial injury may demonstrate a fracture of the talar dome.[68]

Imaging of the Os Trigonum

Conventional AP, lateral, and mortise views of the ankle are used to demonstrate the os trigonum, which is located posterior to the posterior tubercle of the talus. This structure, one of the 21 accessory bones of the body present in 5% to 20% of the population, is unilateral in two thirds of these patients. Because of this frequency of unilateral findings, comparison views of the other ankle are not helpful.[68]

Subtalar Joint Imaging

Excellent demonstration of the talocalcaneal joint, including the sinus tarsi and lateral malleolus, is obtained with the patient lying on the affected side in the lateral position with the knee of the opposite leg flexed and the leg under study extended. The leg is then rolled slightly forward from the lateral position to raise the heel 1.5 in from the true lateral position. The CR is directed 5 degrees anteriorly (toward the toes) and 23 degrees distally to enter at the ankle joint.[1]

In a modified true lateral position, the CR is directed 25 degrees anteriorly (toward the toes) with a simultaneous 25 degree tube angle distally (toward the talocalcaneal joint)[69] (Fig 4-39).

Oblique Projection of the Calcaneus

With a conventional plantodorsal axial view of the calcaneus, the CR is directed 45 degrees cephalad through the calcaneus. In the axial projection, the heel varies greatly in thickness, making it difficult to expose the entire structure equally.

Images taken with 45 degree internal and external rotations, in addition to the axial projection, show the relationship of the calcaneus to the subtalar joint. The obliquity of the foot evens out the variation in tissue thickness encountered in the axial projection of the calcaneus[55] (Fig 4-40).

Oblique Projection of the Lower End of the Fibula

An additional view of the lower leg helps to demonstrate an incomplete oblique fracture of the lower end of the fibula. This projection separates

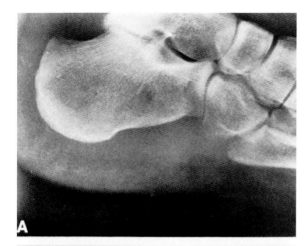

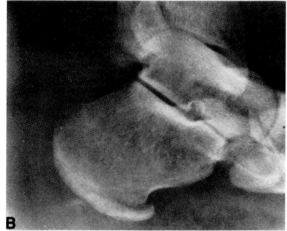

FIGURE 4–39   Talocalcaneal Joint

(A) Conventional lateral radiograph of the foot. Dual-tube angulation technique demonstrates the relationship of the talus to the calcaneus while compromising adjacent anatomy. Note the fracture of the inferior portion of the calcaneus, demonstrated by chance on the dual-tube angle projection designed primarily to demonstrate the talocalcaneal joint. (Courtesy Cullinan AM: *Producing Quality Radiographs*. Philadelphia, JB Lippincott Co, 1987.)

the lower end of the fibula from the tibia and calcaneus. The patient is placed on the side of the injured ankle. The cassette is elevated on a foam wedge to an angle of 30 to 35 degrees. The leg is placed on the cassette with the foot at a right angle to the lower leg to avoid overlapping the lower end of the fibula on the calcaneus. The toes should be pushed upward as far as possible.

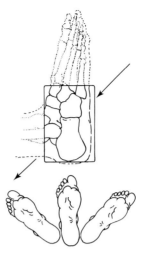

FIGURE 4–40   Axial Oblique Projection of the Calcaneus

The conventional AP axial view of the calcaneus uses a 45 degree cephalad angle. Top, With this position, there is a significant difference in the thickness of the part from the talocalcaneal joint to the soft tissues at the posterior aspect of the heel. Bottom, After the axial projection is made, internal and external 45 degree obliques can be used to help balance structural differences.

The x-ray tube is angled 30 degrees anteriorly, toward the toes, with the CR entering the ankle at the level of the internal malleolus at the posterior aspect of the ankle.[70]

Stress Imaging of the Ankle

Inversion trauma to the ankle may necessitate stress evaluation. An inversion force is applied to the lateral dorsal part of the foot with the knee slightly flexed. This maneuver, known as the talar-tilt angle, produces separation of the articular surfaces of the tibia and talus, with the talar-tilt angle opening laterally on the AP view.[71]

As an alternative, with the heel fixed, a force is applied to the anterior aspect of the distal tibia, which causes an anterior and inferior dislocation of the talus relative to the tibia.[71]

C A U T I O N : Stress maneuvers should be performed only under the direction of a physician.

Imaging of the Ankle Through a Cast

If centering points are difficult to determine through a cast, placing the patient's other leg adjacent to the cast can help to locate the external

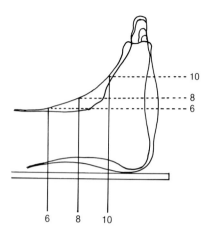

FIGURE 4–41   Extremities in Casts

Note the configuration of the foot and leg indicated by the dotted lines. Measurements taken just above the ankle joint would show 6 cm adjacent to the joint, 8 cm above the ankle joint, and 10 cm at the instep of the foot. Because of the variations in the thicknesses of plaster used in casts, obtaining actual measurements may be difficult. It may be necessary to use a grid or Bucky and 80 kVp or more to demonstrate the tibia and fibula, as well as the ankle mortise. (Courtsey Cullinan AM: *Producing Quality Radiographs*. Philadelphia, JB Lippincott Co, 1987.)

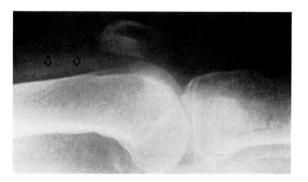

FIGURE 4–42   Horizontal Beam Lateral View of the Knee

A fat–blood fluid level caused by communication between the medullary canal of the tibia and the joint space (arrows) is shown. (Courtesy Keats T: *Emergency Radiology*. Chicago, Year Book Medical Publishers Inc, 1984.)

malleolus of the leg in the cast. The use of a high kVp (85 kVp or greater) technique with a grid or Bucky helps to image the ankle or foot within a dense cast.

A reinforced cast makes accurate measuring difficult (Fig 4-41).

Tibiofibular Joint Imaging

With the patient prone, the affected tibiofibular joint is centered to a cassette positioned over the midline of the table. The leg is rotated internally until the sagittal plane forms an angle of about 45 degrees with the horizontal plane. An additional 5 to 10 degrees of internal rotation places the leg in a position that approaches the lateral position. The CR is directed perpendicular to the long axis of the leg to enter through the tibiofibular joint. The proximal end of the fibula and the tibiofibular joint are well demonstrated.[72] This position is the same as that used for the posteromedial oblique projection of the knee joint.

An alternative is the anterolateral oblique projection. The patient is positioned supine with the knee joint supported on a foam sponge.[72]

Lateral Imaging of the Knee

There is some disagreement in the literature as to the value of the cross-table lateral as compared with a routine overhead lateral view to demonstrate knee-joint effusion. In the cross-table lateral view, Singer[73] states, when the patient's in the supine position, joint fluid is redistributed away from that portion of the suprapatella bursa measured for the fat-pad-separation sign to more dependent parts of the joint. A lateral view should be obtained with an overhead tube instead of a cross-table lateral study so that fluid will not gravitate over the femur, masking the effusion.[35]

Posttraumatic effusion of the knee can indicate intra-articular injuries, including ligament strains, ruptures, cartilage tears, and fractures. The fat pads are best demonstrated on the lateral radiograph with the joint in 30 degree flexion. Increased flexion may obliterate an effusion. Elastic support bands or tightly rolled-up pants legs can obliterate an effusion.[35]

Eisenberg[3] states that for the lateral view, when evaluating for possible knee effusion, the knee should not be placed in more than 15 degrees of flexion.

Horizontal Beam Lateral of the Knee

The cross-table lateral view of the knee can be used to demonstrate a fat–fluid level that implies an intra-articular fracture. A horizontal beam image may be required to demonstrate a fat–fluid level in a suprapatella bursa, indicating a fracture with extrusion of marrow fat into the fluid of the bursa[27,35] (Fig 4-42).

Tunnel Projections of the Knee

The degree of cartilage loss in the medial or lateral femoral tibial compartments caused by osteoarthritis can be evaluated with the tunnel view of the knee. Weight-bearing AP projections may demonstrate some narrowing of the knee-joint space. According to Resnick,[74] conventional tunnel views provide significantly more information regarding the degree of chondral erosion in the medial or lateral femorotibial compartments. Both the AP and PA tunnel views can be used to demonstrate cartilage destruction.

> CAUTION: If the x-ray tube is only slightly off center to the grid lines, a high ratio grid can produce grid striping artifacts when used with the 40 degree (or greater) angulation needed for tunnel projections.

Three routine projections are commonly used for tunnel imaging of the knee[75] (Fig 4-43).

Modified Erect Tunnel Projections of the Knee. The knee may be examined in the erect position using either of two alternative tunnel projections.

With the cassette placed on an adjustable stool beside the x-ray table, the patient stands next to the stool, facing the table. The knee to be examined is flexed and the stool and cassette

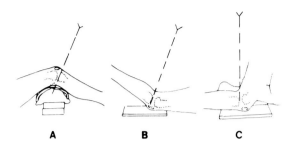

FIGURE 4–43 Conventional Tunnel Projections

(A) Beclere, (B) Camp-Coventry, and (C) Holmblad. (Courtesy Turner GW, Burns CP, Prevette RG Jr: Erect positions for "tunnel" views of the knee. *Radiol Technol* 1983;55:560-642.)

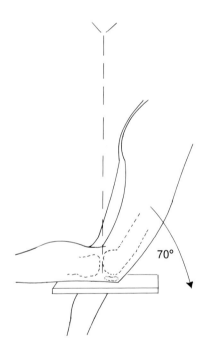

FIGURE 4–44 Erect Tunnel Projection of the Knee

(Courtesy Turner GW, Burns CB, Prevette RG Jr: Erect positions for "tunnel" views of the knee. *Radiol Technol* 1983;55:640-642.)

placed under the knee and centered to the apex of the patella. The patient leans forward after the stool has been adjusted for height, placing the hands on the table for balance. With the femur at an angle of 70 degrees, the CR is directed perpendicular to the film plane[75] (Fig 4-44).

In another modification, the patient is positioned erect against an upright Bucky and the knee is flexed by placing the foot on a low stool. The femur should be at an angle of 70 degrees to the film plane. The cassette is centered to the apex of the patella and the CR is directed horizontally[75] (Figs 4-45 and 4-46).

Intercondyloid Fossa Imaging (Oblique). With the knee positioned for the standard PA tunnel projection, the patient's body and thigh are rotated internally and externally 45 degrees for two separate oblique projections. Slight changes within the joint space, including loose bodies and compression of the tibial plateau, are well demonstrated with oblique tunnel projections.[55]

CAUTION: To minimize patient discomfort, it is necessary to support the lower leg when performing these projections.

Tangential Projection of the Patella

In conventional imaging of the patella, the patient may be either supine or prone. The knee is flexed approximately 90 degrees and the CR is directed to the patellofemoral joint.

In a modification to demonstrate subluxation of the patella (Hughston's method), the patient is prone and the knees are flexed to 55 degrees, with both feet resting on the x-ray collimator. Pathological subluxation usually occurs at 55 degrees of flexion since the greatest lateral force is applied to the patella at this point. The x-ray beam is directed 45 degrees cephalad and enters at the patellofemoral joint. Both knees are examined simultaneously.[76]

Stress Imaging of the Patella (Tangential Projection). If the previous maneuver does not demonstrate the degree of subluxation, the quad-stress maneuver may be considered. Again, with the knee flexed 55 degrees and the feet on the collimator, the patient is asked to extend the flexed knees against the resistance of the locked collimator. Tension of the quadriceps places a greater lateral stress on the patella and may show a definite lateral excursion.[76]

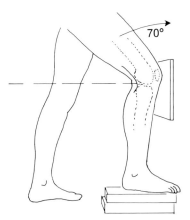

FIGURE 4-45 Erect Tunnel Projection of the Knee

(Courtesy Turner GW, Burns CB, Prevette RG Jr: Erect position for "tunnel" views of the knee. *Radiol Technol* 1983;55: 640-642.)

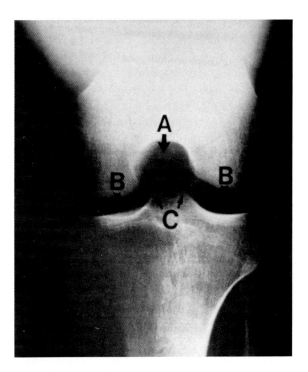

FIGURE 4-46 Tunnel View of the Knee

This image was obtained using the position and projection of the CR shown in Fig 4-45. The intercondyloid fossa (A), joint space (B), and tibial spines (C) are well demonstrated. (Courtesy Turner GW, Burns CB, Prevette RG Jr: Erect position for "tunnel" views of the knee. *Radiol Technol* 1983;55:640-642.)

CAUTION: As with all stress imaging, this maneuver should be carried out under the direction of or in the presence of a physician.

Oblique Projections of the Patella for Trauma

An oblique trauma radiograph demonstrates the patella free of the distal end of the femur. This projection is used when the AP and lateral images of the patella do not show an obvious fracture, but a patella injury is suspected. With the patient supine, the cassette is placed under the knee at its lateral aspect. The tube is positioned opposite to the knee, on the opposite side of the table, and angled 45 degrees. The CR enters the medial aspect of the patella being examined. The patella is seen elongated and magnified. The tibial plateau is also elongated along its horizontal plane.

Without moving the patient, a second cassette is positioned on the medial aspect of the knee and a 45 degree transtable oblique is made from the opposite side, with the CR entering the lateral aspect of the patella.

On the lateral oblique radiograph, the fibula is superimposed on the tibia, but is projected clear of the tibia on the medial oblique[77] (Figs 4-47 and 4-48).

Modification of Patellofemoral Projection. A unique tangential view of the patellofemoral joint (mountain view) has been used by orthopedic surgeons for many years. No special devices are required to give a better view of the articulating surfaces of the patellofemoral compartment than seen in the standard tangential (sunrise) view. Using a straight-back chair and a long-handled step stool, the patient is placed at the end of an x-ray table. The chair is positioned so that it leans at a 45 degree angle against the end of the x-ray table. The patient is then placed supine with the knees flexed 45 degrees over the table edge and supported by the back of the chair. The handle of the step stool is used along with the patient's ankles to support the cassette, which is perpendicular to the beam. A Velcro strap is

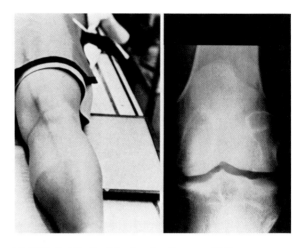

FIGURE 4–47 Positioning for Trauma Oblique Radiography of the Knee

Note that the CR enters the knee just inferior to the patella. Left, The cassette is positioned to allow for the 45 degree tube angle. Right, A bipartite patella is noted on the conventional AP image. (Courtesy Daffner RH, Tabas JH: Trauma oblique radiographs of the knee. *J Bone Joint Surg* 1987;69-A:568-570.)

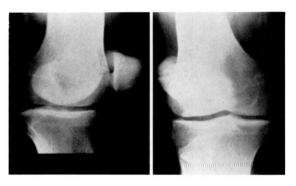

FIGURE 4–48 Trauma Oblique Radiograph of the Knee

Left, Medial oblique. Right, Lateral oblique. (Courtesy Daffner RH, Tabas JH: Trauma oblique radiographs of the knee. *J Bone Joint Surg* 1987;69-A:568-570.)

used to strap the calves of the legs together to prevent rotation. The CR is directed caudad 30 degrees from the horizontal. Both knees are exposed simultaneously.[78]

Imaging of the Femur

The neck of the femur should be visualized without foreshortening. With internal rotation (about 15 degrees), the lesser trochanter is not seen. To visualize the lesser trochanter in the AP position, the leg must be straight or rotated externally. An externally rotated leg shortens the neck of the femur radiographically. Often with a complete and separated fracture of the neck of the femur, the foot will be in lateral rotation. If the knee is included in the image, the patella should superimpose on the femur.

> CAUTION: In patients with known trauma, the leg should be rotated only on the advice of a physician, or the rotation maneuver should be omitted.

Axial Imaging of the Femur. The axial projection of the femur (frog lateral) presents a lateral view of the femur, but it does not change the position of the acetabulum.

> CAUTION: This position is contraindicated if a fracture is suspected. A cross-table axiolateral image, with the unaffected leg elevated, should be made.

Imaging of the Pelvis

The pelvis has four fat stripes that sometimes can be used to indicate trauma. See Chapter 3, Fig 3-5. Because of variations among people, and from side to side in the same person, the pelvic fat pads here are not as reliable an indicator of fracture as they are in other parts of the body.[35]

Shenton's line, an imaginary curvilinear line following the curve of the lower border of the superopubic ramus, serves as a comparison between sides and can be used to determine whether there are any alterations in the hip structure[4] (Fig 4-49). Careful positioning to avoid patient rotation maximizes this important diagnostic sign.

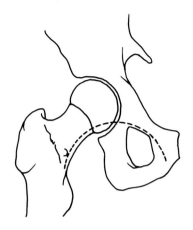

FIGURE 4-49   Shenton's Line

An imaginary curvilinear line formed by the inferior margin of the neck of the femur with the superior and medial margins of the obturator foramen. This continuous arc is used to compare one side of the pelvis with the other when a fracture is suspected.

> CAUTION: Patients often roll away from the injured area. Also, older patients with little pelvic fat sometimes will move intermittently during the examination.

The pelvis is a cup-shaped structure. In the AP view, the more posterior segments image in better focus than the anterior iliac wings. A small focal spot (0.6 mm or less) can reduce image blur (Fig 4-50).

Because of its curved nature, it is difficult to image the acetabulum. Complicated trauma to the acetabulum with adjacent soft-tissue injury may be better evaluated by CT.

Evaluation of Trauma to the Pelvis. Patients who fracture their pelvis are at high risk for additional injuries to the head, chest, abdomen, or extremities. Hemorrhage is an immediate threat to life. Lower genitourinary-tract injuries, such as a rupture of the urinary bladder or, in males, avulsion of the membranous urethra, should be suspected in patients with pelvic fractures.[79]

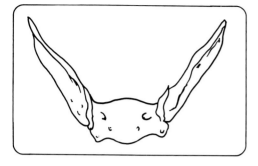

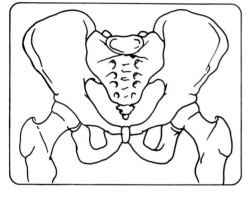

FIGURE 4–50 Pelvic Anatomy

Because of the relationships of anatomical structures within the body, different segments of anatomy image in better focus than others. Top, The pelvis is a cup-shaped structure. Bottom, Anterior anatomical segments when radiographed in the AP position enlarge significantly. The use of a small focal spot (0.6 mm or less) can reduce image blur.

> C A U T I O N : The placement of lead gonadal shielding should not compromise the examination.[7] See Chapter 3, Fig 3-2.

A subtle nondisplaced fracture of the femoral neck may be demonstrated in the supine position if the CR is directed 40 degrees cephalad. This angled projection, when used for patients with hip injuries, demonstrates a nondisplaced fracture of the femoral neck not otherwise seen on standard views. It eliminates the femoral neck foreshortening that may hide an undisplaced fracture on a routine AP projection. Flex-

ion of the unaffected hip or an oblique position is avoided by this technique. This projection can also be used as an alternative when fractures of the pubic rami are suspected.[80]

> N O T E : This projection is similar to the routine view used to evaluate the rectosigmoid barium-filled colon.[80]

Tomography is sometimes used to demonstrate subtle fractures of the pelvis and/or femur. Young et al[81] suggest the following views of the pelvis for fracture evaluation.

1. An AP view with the patient supine.
2. A pelvic inlet view with the patient supine and the x-ray beam directed 40 degrees caudad and entering at the umbilicus. The inlet view of the pelvis may demonstrate a subtle compression or the expansion of the pelvic ring seen in lateral or AP compression fractures. The coronal nature of pubic rami fractures that appear vertically oriented on the AP view may also be demonstrated.
3. A pelvic outlet view with the CR directed 60 degrees cephalad, to enter at the symphysis. The outlet view of the pelvis, although not diagnostic of any pelvic fracture, can provide an indication as to the amount of vertical displacement of the fracture fragments in cases of vertical shear.

During and following a hip pinning (nailing), radiographs must be made in the true AP and lateral positions to evaluate the fixation device (Fig 4-51). Whenever possible, the entire device must be included on both images.

Cross-Table Radiography of the Hip

It is difficult to align the x-ray beam to the center of the grid for cross-table lateral radiography of the hip. Placing the grid with its lines perpendicular rather than parallel to the tabletop helps to minimize grid cutoff[7] (Fig 4-52).

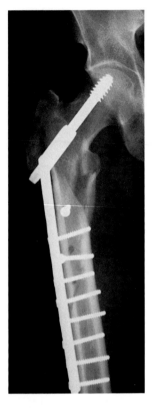

FIGURE 4–51 AP Hip and Femur, Following Hip Pinning

The entire length of the fixation device must be visualized. A hip pin is shown in position through the neck and head of the femur, mounted on an extension plate held in position by metallic screws. To provide stability, these screws bridge the femur from cortex to cortex. A lateral image should also include both ends of the fixation device. *Note:* If both ends of the fixation device cannot be demonstrated on a single image, a second image is required.

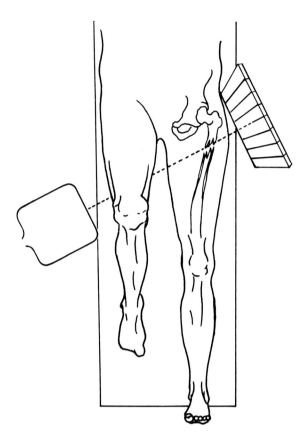

FIGURE 4–52 Grid-line Placement for Axiolateral Projection of the Hip

A grid cutoff is a common occurrence during axiolateral imaging of the hip. Since patients vary in size, it is unlikely that the center of a 10 in by 12 in grid cassette positioned parallel with the tabletop would be aligned with the hip of every patient being examined. By placing the grid cassette with the grid lines perpendicular to the tabletop or floor, the CR can be raised or lowered to coincide with the location of the hip being examined. *Note:* A similar positioning approach can be used with cross-table myelography. (Courtesy Cullinan AM: *Producing Quality Radiographs.* Philadelphia, JB Lippincott Co, 1987.)

C A U T I O N : Left or right misalignment of the x-ray beam to a perpendicularly positioned grid will result in a unilateral grid cutoff.

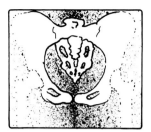
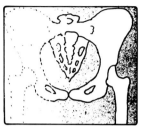

FIGURE 4–53 Relationship of the X-ray Tube to the Grid for Bedside Radiography

When an x-ray tube with a 72 in focal range is used erroneously at a 40 in FFD at the bedside, there is a loss of radiographic density bilaterally. Left, Up to 2 in segments of both lateral aspects of the pelvis appear to be underexposed. This also occurs when a high ratio grid, such as a 12:1 grid (40 in focal range) is used at a shortened FFD. Right, When the tube is positioned to one side of the grid, or if the grid is tilted beneath the patient, one side of the radiograph would seem to be adequately exposed while the other side would appear to be significantly underexposed. This illustration represents the positioning of the x-ray tube approximately 1.5 in off center to the right side of the pelvis. The higher the ratio grid, the greater is the image cutoff as the x-ray beam strikes the lead lines of the grid, which act as an almost solid lead barrier. The focused lines on the opposite side of the grid permit the passage of a higher percentage of the x-ray beam.

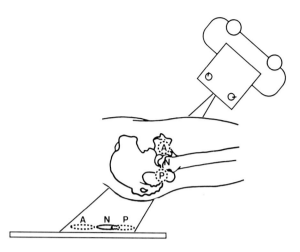

FIGURE 4–54 AP Angled Projection of the Pelvis

When evaluating the pelvis for congenital dislocation of the hips, it is difficult to demonstrate the relationship of the femoral head to the acetabulum. Following the conventional AP projection, a modified projection can be made with the CR directed to the symphysis pubis at a 45 degree cephalad angle. This angulation projects an anteriorly displaced femoral head above the acetabulum (A) and a posteriorly displaced head below the acetabulum (P). The normal position of the femoral head in the acetabulum is indicated (N). (Drawn from data of Martz CD, Taylor CC: The 45 degree angled roentgenographic study of the pelvis in congenital dislocation of the hip. *J Bone Joint Surg* 1954;36-A: 528-532.)

Imaging of the Pelvis at the Bedside

It is difficult to keep the x-ray cassette and grid in alignment with the CR to avoid grid cutoff during radiography of the pelvis at the bedside (Fig 4-53).

The FFD for the AP and lateral projections may also vary. The foot of the bed, if elevated, may shorten the FFD. Because of design limitations, many mobile units are not able to achieve an increased FFD in the overhead position. Depending on the location of the bed in the room, a significant increase or decrease in FFD may occur with the lateral projection.

Imaging of Congenital Hip Dislocation

If a congenital dislocation of the hip is suspected, a modified view of the hip joints made with the CR directed to the symphysis pubis at an angle of 45 degrees cephalad will project an anteriorly displaced femoral head above the acetabulum. A posteriorly displaced femoral head will project below the acetabulum[82] (Fig 4-54).

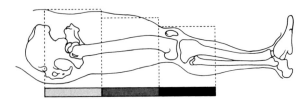

FIGURE 4-55 Absorption and Density Differences of the Leg

Body parts vary in thickness and mass density. A representative illustration from the acetabulum to the lower portion of the leg shows that when using simultaneous exposures, significant absorption density differences are seen among the hip, femur, and lower leg. With the hip appropriately exposed, the femur would be approximately 2X overexposed and the knee approximately 4X overexposed. These differences in absorption make it difficult to expose the entire leg for leg-length measurements or for femoral arteriography. A compensating filter (Fig 1-4) can be used to overcome this step-wedge–like effect and to balance tissue differences.

Tomographic Imaging of a Pelvis in a Cast

If a heavy plaster cast masks the bony detail of the hip, a thick section (zonogram) can be used to "remove" the cast and determine the relationship of the head of the femur to the acetabulum.[55]

Orthoradiographic Measurements of the Lower Extremities

It is relatively simple to evaluate differences in length between the lower extremities using a conventional x-ray unit. Unfortunately, however, there are significant differences in tissue thickness between the pelvis and the lower leg (Fig 4-55).

A single exposure from hips to ankles, made with a 14 in by 36 in cassette, is not recommended even at a 6 ft FFD, since the divergence of the x-ray beam produces considerable distortion of the proximal and distal portions of the image.

With the patient supine, using a single cassette (14 in by 17 in), bilateral simultaneous ser-

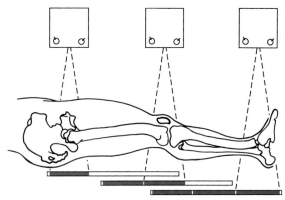

FIGURE 4-56 Leg-Length Measurements

A 14 in by 17 in cassette can be used with a Bell and Thompson ruler or similar measuring device simultaneously to expose both hips, knees, and ankle joints for leg-length measurement. The first exposure is made of the hips (left) with the bottom two thirds of the cassette masked with lead. The second exposure is made of the knees with appropriate cassette masking, and, finally, the third exposure is made of the ankles, while masking the upper two thirds of the cassette. Technical factors are adjusted between each exposure to make up for the differences in tissue absorption. See Fig 4-55.

ial Bucky exposures of hips, knees, and ankle joints can be made without moving the patient. A standard 40 in FFD is usually used and all data should be recorded so that it will be easier to duplicate the study, if necessary. Three individual serial exposures are made with lead dividers shielding the remaining two thirds of the cassette. A Bell and Thompson ruler or similar measuring device placed on the table is imaged along with the extremity[83] (Fig 4-56). Since this technique is used for measurement only, bony detail is not essential. High kilovoltage (85 kVp or greater) used with low mAs can produce excellent radiographs.

Six tightly collimated individual exposures of knees, hips, and ankle joints with a ruler in place can also be used for this procedure (Fig 4-57). It may be necessary to place the ruler beneath the soft tissue of the extremities if a high kVp technique is used.

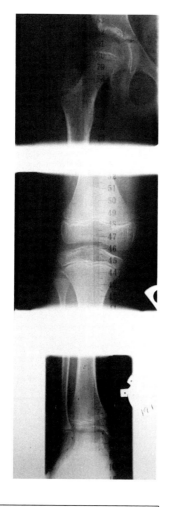

FIGURE 4–57   Leg-Length Measurement

Using the technique described in Fig 4-56, individual exposures of each hip, knee, and ankle (of the right and left legs) may also be made. The right leg is shown with three tightly collimated exposures. The measurement device is best seen behind the knee in this illustration. Since this procedure is used to determine leg length, and not to evaluate osseous abnormalities, a slightly underexposed image is acceptable. The use of a high kVp/low mAs technique helps to balance tissue density. If possible, the ruler should be placed beneath the soft tissue of the leg. (Courtesy Eastman Kodak Company, Rochester, NY.)

CAUTION: Since the extremities are not centered to the midline of the table and the patient cannot be moved between exposures, grid focus must be considered.

Slit Scanography to Measure Leg Length

A 14 in by 36 in cassette is used in combination with a motorized x-ray–tube column or crane that can continuously move a narrow aperture x-ray beam longitudinally down the x-ray table. A slit-beam diaphragm fitted to the x-ray tube or collimator with a 1/16 in aperture produces a slit-scan effect. Long exposure times (8 to 10 seconds) are used for slit scanography. Some modified units can be programmed to scan only over the hips, knees, and ankles.[84]

Because of the decrease in thickness from hips to ankles, the use of gradient intensifying screens has been suggested for measurement, with the fastest screens used over the hips, the midspeed screens over the knees, and the slowest screens over the ankles.

X-ray film that is 14 in by 36 in or larger is difficult to handle and store. Large sheets of fanfold film that can fit into conventional film folders are available commercially.

CAUTION: Changes in the beam intensity should occur at the tube. The use of compensatory filtration in the collimator minimizes radiation exposure to the patient.[55]

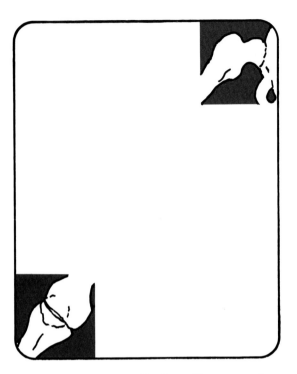

FIGURE 4–58 Preoperative Bone Measurement

The cassette is placed diagonally beneath the uninjured femur. The head of the femur and the knee are separately exposed, with the CR directed perpendicular to the joints. Actual measurements can be made from the hip to the knee joint to determine the length of the metallic rod needed for repair of the opposite leg.

Preoperative Bone Measurement

Internal fixation with a metallic rod is used to repair fractures of long bones such as the femur. See Chapter 3, Fig 3-3.

Prior to surgery, radiographs can be made of the noninjured long bone to obtain images free of traction devices, to avoid handling of the fractured femur, and to determine the length of the metallic rod needed for the operative procedure. A cassette is placed diagonally beneath the uninjured femur and the metallic fixation rod is placed adjacent to the long bone. A tightly collimated exposure is made of the head of the femur to include the upper end of the metal rod. A second tightly collimated exposure is then made. The CR must be directed through the joint being imaged to achieve an accurate measurement[85] (Fig 4-58).

CAUTION: The patient must not move as the tube is repositioned from over the hip and upper end of the rod to the knee and lower end of the rod.

CHAPTER FIVE

The Axial Skeleton: The Skull, Vertebral Column, and Bony Thorax

The axial skeleton is made up of the skull, vertebral column, and bony thorax (Fig 5-1).

THE SKULL

The emergence of CT and MRI imaging has led to a general decline in the use of conventional radiography of the skull. However, facilities without the newer technologies still must depend on traditional methods to image the skull, facial bones, mandible, sinuses, and mastoids, or transfer the patient to a facility where a CT or MRI examination can be performed.

ANATOMICAL / PATHOLOGICAL OBSERVATIONS

Trauma procedures account for the major part of conventional skull radiography. Trauma to the skull or facial bones is often accompanied by other serious injuries, such as an injury to the cervical spine. Maintaining vital signs and patient comfort requires basic patient-care skills.

An airway must be preserved and maintained, bleeding controlled, and shock treated before any radiographs are made. Swelling and skin discoloration can develop rapidly and obscure the nature of a fracture on physical examination.[27]

The departmental positioning routine must be modified if the radiographic examination threatens the condition or life of the patient. Even when it has been established that the patient is stable, the patient's movement should still be minimized. A variety of restraining devices, such as sandbags and soft collars, are available to restrict the movement of injured patients.

> C A U T I O N : A patient with a head injury should never be left unattended. A radiographer working alone in a trauma situation must be able to summon assistance.

Several years ago, a US Department of Health and Human Services publication[86] presented a comprehensive evaluation of the management of head trauma by plain-film skull radiography in which the benefits of posttrauma

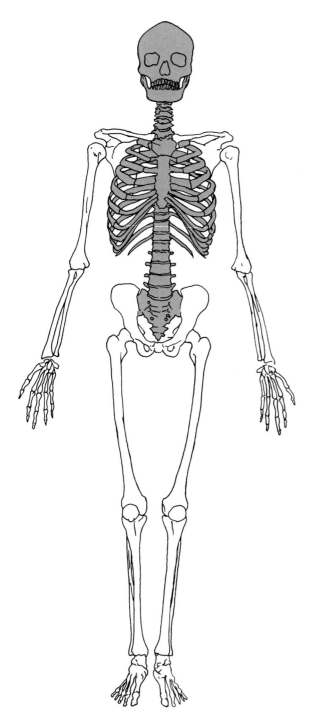

FIGURE 5–1 Axial Skeleton

The axial skeleton consists of the skull, vertebral column, and bony thorax. It is shown here in relationship to the full skeleton.

skull imaging were assessed. According to this publication, the number of skull fractures revealed by skull radiography for trauma has been found to range from 2% to 26.6%, with the larger values seen in the examination of children. When additional studies were made on both adults and children, no more than 5% of the skull x-ray examinations ordered for trauma demonstrated fractures. However, patients may suffer severe brain damage and/or bleeding even though their skull radiographs show no sign of fracture. Undiagnosed compound depressed fractures often lead to intracranial infection, which can result in death. Fractures that are clinically significant may not be apparent in standard views.[86]

Conversely, a skull fracture does not always indicate underlying brain damage. As early as 1913, it became obvious that skull radiographs, while of value in determining the extent of bone injury, were of limited help in the evaluation of brain injury or disease. Normal anatomical structures such as sutures and arterial or venous channels on the inner surface of the skull are often difficult to distinguish from fractures.[87,88] Vascular markings (channels) in the skull can simulate fractures; vessel grooves have white cortical margins whereas fractures do not.

Radiographic signs indicating significant head injuries include (1) a shift of the calcified pineal gland from the midline owing to an extradural or subdural hematoma, and (2) fluid levels in the sinuses or air in the subarachnoid spaces or ventricles.[89]

Because of conflicting advice regarding skull radiography following an apparently uncomplicated head injury, representatives of the Royal College of Radiologists (Great Britain) met with neurosurgeons in 1983 and passed joint recommendations to use the following criteria to determine the need for skull x-rays following head injury.

1. Loss of consciousness or appearance of amnesia at any time.
2. The presence of neurological symptoms or signs.
3. The discharge of cerebral spinal fluid or blood from the nose or ear.

4. Suspected penetrating injury or scalp bruising or swelling.
5. Alcoholic intoxication.
6. Difficulty in assessing the patient (eg, the young, epileptics).[90]

NOTE: Abusive behavior by a patient does not always indicate a misuse of drugs or alcohol; a neurological condition may exist. Additionally, the chronic substance-abuse patient could also have a serious injury, such as a fracture extending into an artery, representing a medical emergency.[86]

Facial contours, as well as skull types, influence cranial positioning. Asymmetry of the cranium or facial bones or deviation of the nasal bones from the median plane often complicates skull positioning. Skull types include dolichocephalic, the long narrow skull; mesocephalic, the average skull; and brachycephalic, the short, broad skull (Fig 5-2).

POSITIONING CONCEPTS

The complexities of skull positioning can be minimized if the similarities of the basic projections are noted and if there is an understanding of the entrance and exit points of the x-ray beam and the relationship of tube angulation to the position of the skull.

Many skull positions or projections are similar except for minor adjustments to the x-ray tube or the patient. If the projections are grouped into five basic categories, the radiographer will find it easier to recall base lines and planes when required to perform more complex skull examinations (Fig 5-3, page 104; Tables 5-1 through 5-5). A positioning atlas should be consulted if additional information is needed.[1-4]

A routine skull film series includes several basic projections.

• PA (no tube angle) (Fig 5-4, page 104; Table 5-1).

• PA (tube angle caudad) (Fig 5-4, Table 5-1). Many departments modify the PA (Caldwell) projection with variations in the x-ray tube angulation from 0 to 23 degrees to evaluate the

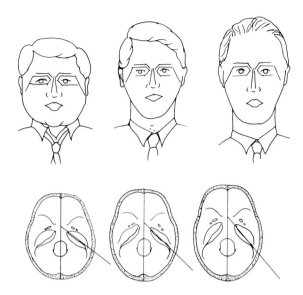

FIGURE 5–2 Skull Types

The type of skull, as well as the contours of the face, influences cranial positioning. The brachycephalic, short and broad skull (left); the mesocephalic, or the average-shaped skull (center); and the dolichocephalic, the long, narrow skull (right) represent typical skull shapes and facial contours. There is a slight change in the location of the petrous ridges in relationship to the median plane among these skull types. In the mesocephalic skull (center), the angle formed by the median plane and the petrous ridges is approximately 47 degrees. In the brachycephalic type, the angle is approximately 54 degrees (right), and in the dolichocephalic type, it is about 40 degrees (left). When examining the petrous ridges, it may be necessary to make minor changes in the positioning of the skull and/or the angulation of the x-ray tube or the patient's head to overcome these differences.

sphenoidal fissures, the petrous ridges, the internal auditory meatus, and so on (Figs 5-4 through 5-6, Table 5-1). Modified PA oblique projections include the Hough,[91] Stenver, and Rhese methods (Fig 5-7, page 104; Table 5-1).

• AP semiaxial (tube angled caudad) Towne (Fig 5-8, page 104; Table 5-2). In the AP projection, a variety of caudad tube angles may be used to project the dorsum sella into the foramen magnum (Fig 5-9, page 104). On the angled AP view, since the orbital structures are projected caudally, a calcified pineal gland may be seen.

(Text continues on page 109)

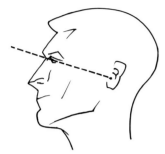

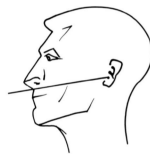

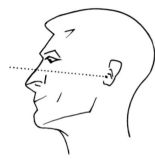

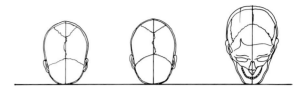

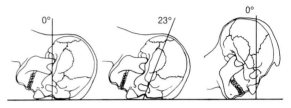

FIGURE 5-3
Surface Lines of the Skull

(A) In the lateral aspect, the various surface lines of the skull are shown. The orbitomeatal (dashed line), the infraorbitolmeatal (dotted line), and the acanthiomeatal (solid line) lines are used to determine the placement of the skull for specific positions. (B) In the frontal aspect, the median plane (a), the supraorbital line (b), and the interpupillary line (c) are used as positioning reference points. See Chapter 2, Fig 2-13.

FIGURE 5-4   Variations on the Basic PA Projection

This illustration shows modifications of the PA projection. Left bottom, In a standard PA projection, the nose and forehead are on the tabletop and the CR is perpendicular to the detector. Center bottom, In a typical caudad tube angle projection, such as the Caldwell, the head is in the PA position, but the tube is angled 23 degrees to evaluate the sphenoidal fissures, the petrous ridges, and the internal auditory meatus. Right bottom, The parietocanthial (Waters) method is shown with no tube angle and with the CR directed perpendicular to the film plane. In this projection, the patient's head is pulled away from the film plane, with the skull balanced on the chin and the nose, slightly away from the tabletop. Top, The relationship of the median planes to the film planes is shown with no rotation of the skull.

A

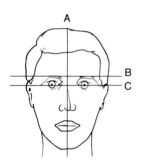

B

TABLE 5-1 Posteroanterior Projection (Caldwell)

Patient PA, prone or erect.
Median plane perpendicular to midline of tabletop or upright grid.
Head resting on forehead and nose.
Orbitomeatal line perpendicular to film plane.
CR directed 15 degrees caudad to exit through the nasion.
Modifications of Basic PA Projection
Center and collimate to area of interest and/or film.

To Demonstrate	Adjust
Frontal bone	CR perpendicular to the film
Superior orbital fissure	Direct CR 20 to 25 degrees caudad to exit through the orbits
Rotundum foramina	Direct CR 20 to 30 degrees caudad to exit through the nasion
Nasal bones	Seen on Caldwell
Sinuses (frontal/ethmoid)	Seen on Caldwell
Sinuses (fluid level)	Patient erect; CR must be horizontal to the floor
Sella turcica	CR directed 10 degrees cephalad to exit at glabella
Orbits	CR directed 20 to 25 degrees caudad to exit at nasion
Optic canal (Rhese)	The median plane and tabletop or upright Bucky grid form an angle of 53 degrees. Rotate head 37 degrees from the true PA position and rest on nose and chin. Adjust head so that the acanthiomeatal line of the opposite orbit is perpendicular to the film plane and tabletop. Direct CR perpendicular to the film plane to enter through the back of the skull and exit through the affected orbit (adjacent to the tabletop or upright grid). Each side is imaged separately. See Optic foramen, AP projection
Sphenoid strut (Hough)	Infraorbitomeatal line perpendicular to the film plane. Head is rotated so that the median plane is 20 degrees toward the side being examined. Direct CR 7 degrees caudad to exit through the center of the orbit. Each side is imaged separately
Temporal bone (Stenvers)	Rest head on nose, forehead, and zygoma
Note: The Stenvers method presents a true PA view of the petrous portion of the temporal bone.	Adjust head so that the infraorbitomeatal line is parallel with the transverse axis of the film plane and forms a 45 degree angle with the film plane and tabletop or upright grid. CR directed 12 degrees cephalad to enter at a point 1 in anterior to the external auditory meatus of the side closer to the film. Each side is imaged separately

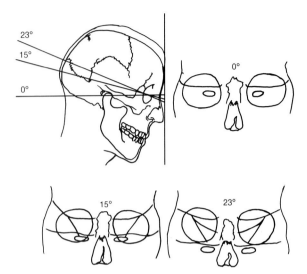

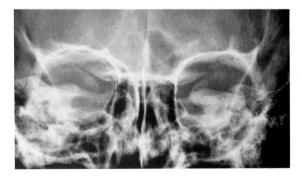

FIGURE 5-5   Modifications of the PA (Caldwell) Projection

The PA skull, in the erect position with three tube projections: 0 degrees, 15 degrees, and 23 degrees. In a schematic of the orbital areas (top left) with no tube angle (top right), the petrous ridges are almost superimposed on the superior orbital ridges. The sphenoidal fissures are not demonstrated. With the 15 degree caudad tube angle (bottom left), a modified Caldwell projection, the petrous ridges shift inferiorly, almost to the level of infraorbital ridges. The internal auditory meatus can be seen. The sphenoidal fissures are elongated in a bat-wing configuration. In the conventional 23 degree caudad projection (bottom right), there is elongation of the sphenoidal fissures and the petrous ridges shift below the infraorbital ridges.

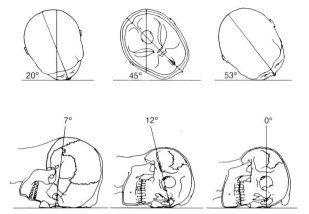

FIGURE 5-7   Modifications of the PA Projection (Hough, Stenvers, and Rhese)

Very slight tube angulations and/or changes in patient rotation produce different views of the skull. For example, with the patient rotated so that the median plane is placed 20 degrees toward the side being examined and the CR directed 7 degrees caudad (bottom left), the sphenoid strut will be demonstrated in a parieto-orbital projection known as the Hough method. With the patient positioned with the median plane at a 45 degree oblique angle to the film plane (top center) and the CR directed 12 degrees cephalad (bottom center), the petrous ridge is demonstrated in the projection known as the Stenvers method. A modified PA projection with the median plane at an angle of 53 degrees to the film plane (top right) and the CR directed perpendicular (bottom right) will demonstrate the optic canal in cross section in the lower outer quadrant of the orbit. This is known as the Rhese method.

FIGURE 5-6   Caldwell View

Radiograph made using 15 degree caudad tube angle. Note the excellent demonstration of the sphenoidal fissures. The petrous ridges and the internal auditory meatus are well visualized in the center of the orbits.

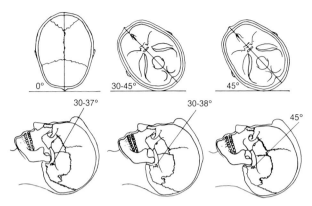

FIGURE 5-8 Modifications of the AP Projection (Grashey, Owen, and Mayer)

A true AP perpendicular beam study is not shown. A typical Grashey or Towne projection directs the CR through the foramen magnum at a 37 degree caudad tube angle to the infraorbitolmeatal line. A modification of this projection directs the CR at a caudad angle of 30 degrees to the orbitomeatal line (left). As the CR is directed toward the feet, the dorsum sella is projected downward into the foramen magnum. See Fig 5-9. The 45 degree semiaxial projection is not a routine projection, but is shown along with a 45 degree rotation of the skull (right) to illustrate that the Mayer projection is simply an exaggerated Towne projection, in a 45 degree oblique position with the chin depressed. A modification of the Owen projection utilizing a 30 to 38 degree caudad angulation with a 30 to 45 degree oblique rotation of the skull (center) is also used to image the mastoid structures.

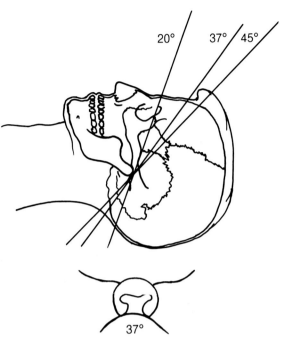

FIGURE 5-9 Semiaxial AP Projections, with Various Degrees of Caudad Projection of the CR

Directing the CR 37 degrees caudad gives a good representation of the dorsum sella within the foramen magnum with good visualization of both posterior clinoid processes. A lesser angle (20 degrees) will superimpose the superior portion of the dorsum sella on the occipital bone. A greater angle (45 degrees) will project the dorsum sella below the inferior margin of the foramen magnum. Depending on patient habitus or condition, the desired angulation can be achieved by combining tube tilt and part tilt angles. The orbitomeatal line or the infraorbitolmeatal lines should be adjusted perpendicular to the film plane, depending on the angulation used.

TABLE 5–2 Semiaxial (Towne) Projection

Patient AP, supine or erect.
Flex neck to place orbitomeatal line perpendicular to film plane.
Median plane perpendicular to midline of tabletop or upright grid.
Top of film placed at top of skull.
CR directed 30 degrees caudad to enter about 2 in above glabella and exit through foramen magnum.

> N O T E : If infraorbitomeatal line is used perpen-
> dicular to the film plane, an adjustment must be
> made to direct the CR 37 degrees caudad.

Modifications of Basic AP (Semiaxial) Projection
Center and collimate to area of interest and/or film.

To Demonstrate	Adjust
Jugular foramen, foramen magnum	CR directed 40 to 60 degrees caudad
Posterior cranial vault	CR directed perpendicular to enter midway between the frontal eminences
Zygomatic arch	Orbitomeatal line perpendicular to the film. Median plane is perpendicular to the midline of the table or upright grid. CR directed 30 degrees caudad to enter at glabella
Mandible	CR directed 30 degrees caudad to enter midway between the temporomandibular joints at a point about 3 in above the nasion
Mastoids (Mayer)	Head adjusted so that the median plane forms an angle of 45 degrees with the film plane, tabletop, or upright grid, thus placing the infraorbital line parallel with the transverse axis of the film plane. The side closest to the tabletop is the side to be examined. CR directed 45 degrees caudad to exit through the dependent external auditory meatus. Each side is imaged separately

TABLE 5–2 *continued*

NOTE: A short or thick-necked patient or a patient with severe kyphosis may find it difficult to depress the chin adequately in the AP supine position. With most patients, it is easy to overcompensate and depress the chin too far. Overcompensation often occurs with the Mayer method because of the oblique rotation of the skull.

To Demonstrate	Adjust
Petrous ridges (Arcelin— Reverse Stenvers)	Head rotated so that the median plane forms an angle of 45 degrees when rotated away from the side being examined and forms a 45 degree angle with the film plane and tabletop or upright grid. Infraorbitomeatal line is parallel to transverse axis of film plane. Direct CR 10 to 12 degrees caudad to enter at a point 1 in anterior and 1 in superior to the external auditory meatus of the elevated side (the side being examined). Each side is imaged separately
Optic canal (Rhese)	See Optic canal PA. Head rotated 37 degrees from the AP position so that the median plane forms an angle of 53 degrees with the film plane and the tabletop. The acanthiomeatal line of the unaffected orbit is perpendicular to the film plane. Center the cassette to the uppermost orbit. CR directed perpendicular to the middle of the cassette to enter the uppermost orbit in its lower outer quadrant. Center cassette to the CR. Each side is imaged separately

TABLE 5–3 Lateral Projection

Patient PA, supine or erect.
Head lateral.
Median plane parallel (horizontal) to film plane and midline of tabletop or upright grid.
Interpupillary line perpendicular to film plane and tabletop or upright grid.
Infraorbital line parallel to transverse axis of tabletop or upright grid and film plane.
CR directed perpendicular to film to enter 1 to 2 in above and in front of the external auditory meatus.
Modifications of Basic Lateral Projection
Center and collimate to area of interest and/or film.

To Demonstrate	Adjust
Sella turcica	Direct CR to enter about 1 in above and in front of the external auditory meatus
Sinuses	Direct CR to enter outer canthus of eye
Facial bones	Direct CR to pass through the prominence of the zygoma (malar bone)
Nasal bones	Direct CR to pass through the bridge of the nose at a point 3/4 in distal to the nasion
Zygomatic arches	CR enters and exits through the prominence of the zygomatic arches
Temporomandibular joint	Open- and closed-mouth images are taken separately of each side. The side of interest is closest to tabletop. CR directed 15 degrees caudad to enter at the upper parietal region and exit at temporomandibular joint closest to the film
Mastoids (Henschen)	CR directed 15 degrees caudad through the external auditory meatus closest to the tabletop or upright grid
Mastoids (Schuller)	CR directed 25 degrees caudad through the external auditory meatus adjacent to the tabletop or upright grid
Mastoids (Lysholm/Runstrom II)	CR directed 35 degrees caudad through the external auditory meatus adjacent to the tabletop or upright grid. Exposure is made with the mouth open
Mastoids (Law)*	Images of each side are taken separately. Head rotated so that the face forms a 15 degree angle with the tabletop or upright grid. CR directed 15 degrees caudad to enter about 1 in posterior and 2 in above the uppermost external auditory meatus

*Note: The original Law method utilized a nongrid dual tube angle technique—25 degree caudad and 20 degree anterior angulation.[1] A modification of the Law method is essential for grid techniques to avoid angling against a grid.

TABLE 5-4 Parietoacanthial Projection (Waters)

Patient prone or erect.
Head resting on chin.
Median plane perpendicular to film plane and midline of tabletop or upright grid.
Orbitomeatal line adjusted to form an angle of 37 degrees with film plane.
CR directed perpendicular to film plane to enter at the posterosagital suture and
   exit at the acanthion.
Center cassette to CR.
Modifications of Basic Parietoacanthial Projection
Center and collimate to center of interest and/or film.

To Demonstrate	Adjust
Orbital floors and margins (Modified Waters)	Adjust orbitomeatal line to form an angle of 55 degrees with the film plane
Sinuses	Seen on Waters view
Sphenoid sinuses	Have patient open mouth and position as for conventional Waters

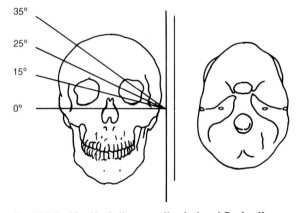

FIGURE 5-10 Variations on the Lateral Projection (Henchen, Schuller, and Lysholm)

Left, The skull in the erect, true lateral position (no tube angle) with caudad tube angulations of 15, 25, and 35 degrees. The 15 degree angulation (Henchen method) can be used to image the mastoid and petrous areas. The 25 degree angulation (Schuller method) is often used to image temporomandibular articulation. The Lysholm (Runstrom II) method uses a 35 degree caudad angulation to demonstrate the mastoid cells, antrum, external auditory meatus, and related structures. This illustration shows that positioning for these three unique lateral projections requires only minor changes in tube angulation. Right, The transverse-section schematic shows the external and the internal meatus of both petrous ridges represented as small ovals. The x-ray beam enters the top of the head, passes through the internal meatus of the petrous ridge, and exits through the external meatus.

- Both laterals (Fig 5-10, Table 5-3). A minor variation in tube angle in the lateral position is all that is often needed to achieve complex views with the skull in the lateral position.

NOTE: Leaman[92] evaluated 88 sets of bilateral skull x-rays, each demonstrating an unequivocal skull fracture. When only one lateral view of the skull was shown to radiologists for interpretation, only two of the fractures were not seen.

- Parietoacanthial (Waters) (Fig 5-4, Table 5-4). The Waters method traditionally is performed in the PA position with a nonangled tube technique. Significant soft-tissue swelling may hinder evaluation of the maxillary sinuses. The soft tissues of the upper lip and related structures often superimpose over the lower portion of the maxillary sinuses, septum, and turbinates. Even in the erect position with a horizontal beam technique, a small amount of fluid in one of the inferior recesses of the maxillary sinuses can be missed. With the mouth open, in the Waters method, the sphenoidal sinus can be visualized.

In a modification of the standard Waters view, the patient is requested to tuck the tightly compressed lips and adjacent cheek areas into the oral cavity during the x-ray exposure. This simple compression technique may eliminate

TABLE 5–5 Submentovertex (Base) Projection

Patient supine or seated with neck hyperextended and head resting on vertex of the skull.
Infraorbitomeatal line parallel to film plane.
Median plane perpendicular to film and midline of tabletop or upright grid.
CR directed perpendicular to infraorbitomeatal line to enter median plane between the angles of the mandible and exit at vertex of the skull.

> N O T E : If patient cannot assume the position to get the infraorbitomeatal line parallel to the film plane, direct the CR until it is perpendicular to the infraorbitomeatal line and center the cassette to the CR.

Modifications of Basic Submentovertex Projection
Center and collimate to area of interest and/or film.

To Demonstrate	Adjust
Mandible	Direct CR to enter median plane between the angles of the mandible and to exit at vertex of skull
Sinuses	Direct CR to enter median plane between both angles of the lower jaw and to exit at the vertex of the skull
Zygomatic arches	Direct CR to enter midway between the zygomatic arches and to exit at vertex of the skull
Zygomatic arch (axial oblique)	Rotate head 20 degrees toward the side being examined. CR directed tangential to the parietal eminence and body of the mandible. Each side is imaged separately
Temporal bone petrous portion (Taylor)	Adjust head so that the supraorbitomeatal line is parallel with the film plane or upright grid. Direct CR at an angle of 15 to 20 degrees to enter the median plane of the throat at a point 1 in above the external auditory meatus

the need for a repeat examination or tomography[93] (Fig 5-11).

> N O T E : Horizontal beam imaging is needed to demonstrate fluid levels within the skull.

- Submentovertex (base) (Fig 5-12, Table 5-5).

DISEASES OR CONDITIONS REQUIRING SPECIAL CONSIDERATION

Intercranial Calcifications

Skull or brain pathology can be seen on plain-film radiography if a tumor contains calcifications, causes bony erosion or growth, or results in an enlarged sella turcica or the shift of a calcified pineal gland.[94] Increased intracranial pres-

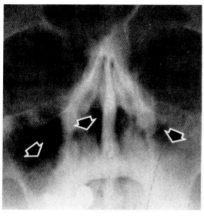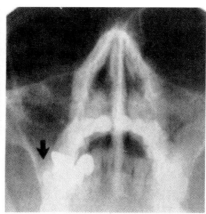

FIGURE 5–11 Modification of the Waters Method

In the conventional Waters projection, there is superimposition of the lips and adjacent soft-tissue structures over the lower portion of the maxillary sinuses, septum, and turbinates (left, arrows). A modification of the Waters method is known as the "no lip" Waters view. The patient is positioned as for the Waters projection, but is asked tightly to tuck and compress the lips and adjacent cheek areas into the oral cavity during the x-ray exposure. This maneuver avoids superimposition of the soft tissues of the upper lip and adjacent areas over the maxillary sinuses, septum, and turbinates. The no-lip Waters view demonstrates a small amount of fluid or mucosal thickening on the right side (arrow) and mucosal thickening in the left maxillary antrum (right). (Courtesy Dixit JK: The "no lip" Waters view. *AJR* 1989; 151 : 839-840.)

sure may change the size, shape, and mineralization of the sella turcica[95] (Fig 5-13).

The pineal gland is usually 3 to 5 mm in its greatest diameter, but can be as large as 10 to 12 mm, and it contains sufficient calcification for its detection on skull radiographs in 33% to 76% of patients. The frequency of visualization increases with age.[96] Accurate positioning provides the radiologist with the information needed for measurement and may lead to more sophisticated imaging studies, such as CT or MRI.

CAUTION: Rotation of the skull during positioning can give the illusion of a pineal shift.

CAUTION: Dirt, tightly woven hair, or screen artifacts can simulate intracranial calcifications.

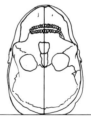
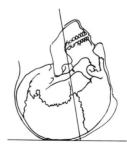
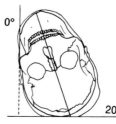

0°

20°

FIGURE 5–12 Variations on the Base Projection

In the base projection, the CR should be perpendicular to the infraorbitomeatal line, which optimally should be parallel to the film plane (top and center). This is difficult to achieve with most patients, particularly in the recumbent position. The base projection is also useful to demonstrate bilateral zygomatic arches. A 20 degree rotation of the skull is used to radiograph a single zygomatic arch (bottom). This projection is particularly helpful in the demonstration of a depression of this structure.

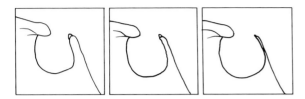

FIGURE 5-13 The Sella Turcica

The size, shape, and degree of mineralization of the sella turcica may change with increased intracranial pressure or other disease. Left, Representative illustration of a normal sella turcica. Center, Widening and deepening of the pituitary fossa, with some thinning of the dorsum sella. Right, Further enlargement, with thinning of the dorsum sella.

Trauma

The location of a skull fracture is of major concern since, if a fracture crosses an artery, an arterial bleed may result. The presence of a fracture increases the chance of a hematoma by 164- to 400-fold.[97] A fracture through the mastoid air cells or sinuses may communicate with an infected area, possibly resulting in encephalitis or meningitis.[96] In 1913, Stewart and Luckett[88] independently reported on the same patient who had suffered a fracture through the frontal sinuses and had developed pneumoencephalus. Such findings had not been reported or described previously.

Less than 3% of all skull fractures are associated with intracranial air, however, trauma represents the most frequent cause of pneumoencephalus, accounting for approximately 75% of all cases; about 8% of fractures of the paranasal sinuses produce pneumoencephalus. Approximately 3% to 4% of all skull fractures involve significant depression of bony fragments. Bony fragments that have been dislodged more than 0.5 cm are likely to impinge on the cerebrum.[96]

C A U T I O N : Trauma to the eyes, nose, and mandible is frequently accompanied by fracture, significant facial edema, and/or possible cervical spine injury.

Major types of skull fractures include[97]:

1. Linear fracture of the skull vault (Fig 5-14).
2. Basal fracture.

N O T E : Air–fluid levels in the sphenoid sinus or clouding of the mastoid air cells are often the only radiographic findings suggesting a basilar skull fracture (Fig 5-15).

3. Suture fracture.
4. Compound fracture of the skull vault.
5. Depressed fracture of the skull vault.[27]

N O T E : A tangential or silhouette projection may be required to demonstrate a depressed skull fracture (Fig 5-16).

If an oblique position of the skull, tangential to the fracture, is indicated, it may be helpful to place a small lead "0" marker on the scalp at the point of trauma. If the "0" is projected and depicted as a "1" in the image, the interpreter can be certain that a tangential projection has been achieved.[96]

C A U T I O N : In the presence of a skull fracture or a soft-tissue injury, head clamps, if applied too aggressively, can worsen the situation. Head clamps should be used as a positioning aid and not as a restraining device. They should center the skull to the cassette to avoid rotation in the frontal position and to guarantee a true lateral position.

Head-holding devices with small, round sponges at the ends of a C-arm are often used in tight contact with the skull. In the presence of a skull fracture, depression of bone fragments can occur[98] (Fig 5-17, page 114). If a skull-restraining device is needed, head-holding devices with larger spongy surfaces that come into contact with the skull are safer.

Skull radiography to evaluate trauma requires consideration of facial injury and/or of

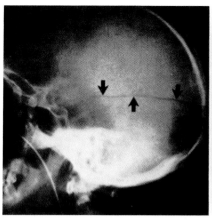
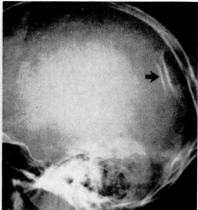

FIGURE 5-14 Skull Fractures

Fractures should be described in terms of their extent, their location, the depth of depressed fragments, and their relationship to major vessels. Lateral radiographs of the skull demonstrate two major types of fracture—linear (left, arrows) and depressed (right, arrow). (Courtesy Quencer RM: Neuroimaging and head injuries: Where we've been—where we're going. *AJR* 1988; 150: 13-18.)

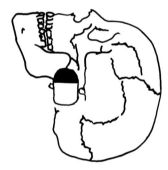

FIGURE 5-15 Lateral Skull to Demonstrate Air-Fluid Level in Sphenoid Sinus

A fluid level in the sinus could be exudate from sinusitis, blood, or cerebral spinal fluid. An air-fluid level in the sphenoid sinus often occurs with a fracture at the base of the skull. It is represented here by a black-white interface, with the black indicating air in the superior portion of the sphenoid sinus and the white representing fluid in the dependent portion of the sinus cavity. Clouding of the mastoid air cells often accompanies a basilar skull fracture. In the presence of a suspected fracture, this is an important diagnostic sign.

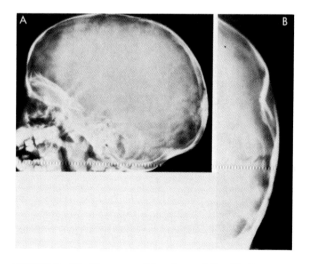

FIGURE 5-16 Depressed Fracture of the Skull

Left, A conventional lateral skull film of a child subjected to head trauma does not demonstrate a fracture. Right, A tangential or silhouette projection taken with the CR positioned through the site of injury shows a depressed skull fracture. (Courtesy Keats T: *Emergency Radiology.* Chicago, Year Book Medical Publishers Inc, 1984.)

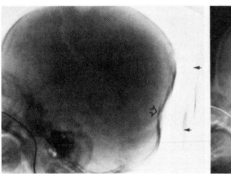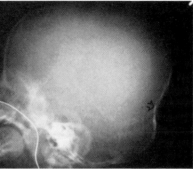

FIGURE 5–17   Potential Hazards of Using Head Clamps for Skull Radiography

A negative reproduction of a right lateral radiograph shows a significant depression of the posterior parietal and occipital bones with some overlap (open arrows). The border of the head holder's sponge (closed arrows) is less depressed than the adjacent cranium. In a positive reproduction, the iatrogenic nature of the depression is not immediately apparent unless the radiologist is aware that head clamps were used. (Courtesy Rosenblum J, Yousefzadeh DK, Ramilo JL: Skull radiography in infants: Potential hazards of the use of head clamps. *Radiology* 1986;161:367-368.)

the presence of free air within the skull. Air or gas may also appear within the brain or its covering after surgery.

A trauma series includes:

1. Cross-table, brow-up, lateral view using a horizontal beam technique (Fig 5-15, Table 5-3).
2. AP (no tube angle) (Table 5-2).
3. Caldwell (Fig 5-4, Table 5-1).
4. Towne/Grashey (Fig 5-8, Table 5-2).

A typical facial-bone series includes:

1. Caldwell or modified Caldwell (Figs 5-4 and 5-5, Table 5-1).
2. AP semiaxial angled projection (Figs 5-8 and 5-9, Table 5-2).
3. Lateral (Fig 5-10, Table 5-3).
4. Parietoacanthial (Waters) (Fig 5-4, Table 5-4).

SUPPLEMENTARY IMAGING OF THE SKULL AND FACIAL BONES

The Maxilla and Mandible

Occlusal films are often used for intraoral or extraoral images of the maxilla and mandible. Fractures of the palatine and alveolar process of the superior maxilla and body of the mandible

can be visualized using occlusal film. An occlusal film may demonstrate the symphysis menti, which is obscured by the cervical vertebrae on the PA view of the mandible.

> C A U T I O N : The decision to use an occlusal film for an intraoral superoinferior projection must be carefully weighed since the x-ray source is close to the lens of the eyes. As dental x-ray equipment is not available in many radiology departments, the use of a standard radiographic tube for occlusal radiography requires extremely tight beam collimation or the addition of an extension cone to minimize radiation to the lens of the eyes, the thyroid, and the sternum.

Sometimes, because of the trauma associated with a facial injury, attention is paid only to the severely traumatized area. When one side of the mandible is injured by a direct force, there is a tendency to fracture the opposing side.[27] For example, a fracture of the left ramus or body of the mandible with displacement is almost always accompanied by a fracture in or near the condylar neck of the right side. The opposite side must be imaged (Fig 5-18).

If the patient can assume either lateral position, both sides of the mandible can be evaluated

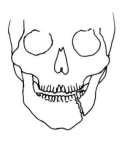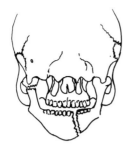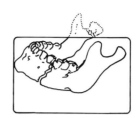

FIGURE 5–18 Mandibular Imaging

Injuries to the face often are associated with significant swelling, making it difficult to position a patient properly. In the PA mandible (left), a fracture is shown on the left side. A dotted segment, representing the condyle and condylar neck, is also shown (center). If a fracture existed in this area, it would not be seen in the PA projection. The semiaxial (Towne) projection projects the mandible downward (center). Note that both fractures can be seen in this elongated view. In the axiolateral mandible view (right), the left side of the mandible is well visualized, with the fracture seen extending into the teeth. *Note:* The fracture line, represented by the dotted lines on the right side of the mandible, is projected off of the image. In a conventional axiolateral, the head and condylar neck are often superimposed on the anterior structures of the cervical spine.

with conventional tomography. The uninjured side of the mandible can be placed against the tabletop and a 2 to 3 cm section made to evaluate the condyle and ramus. The tomographic fulcrum is then adjusted to the level of the injured side of the mandible (about 15 cm) and an additional section made.

The mandibular condyle is equally difficult to see in the lateral view. If the patient can safely project the mandible forward in relationship to the maxilla, this jutting effect will help to demonstrate the condylar head and neck (Fig 5-19) If the patient is unable to perform this maneuver, a positioning modification can help to visualize the condyles in the axiolateral position. With the patient's head turned an additional 15 degrees from the axiolateral projection, toward the x-ray tube, the ramus and condylar head and neck will not superimpose on the anterior cervical vertebrae.

> CAUTION: Since the body of the mandible will be foreshortened with this position, a conventional axiolateral projection is also required.

The Temporomandibular Joint

The temporomandibular joint, situated in a radiodense area of the skull, has a free range of movement, with a gliding movement between the articular surfaces. It is difficult to visualize the condylar necks of the mandible with the head in the PA position and the forehead against a grid cassette or Bucky table. On the standard PA view, the condyles, the coronoid processes, and the upper portion of the rami bilaterally may superimpose on the petrous bones, mastoid processes, and zygomas. If the patient's mouth can be safely opened to its maximum, the condylar portions of the mandible will be visualized (Fig 5-19).

Transcranial laterals with the mouth open and closed are the positions most frequently used to demonstrate the temporomandibular joints (Figs 5-10 and 5-20). Conventional tomographic techniques are often used to evaluate the temporomandibular joint in the open- and closed-mouth positions (Fig 5-21).

Supplementary views include the Towne (Fig 5-8), submentovertex projection (Fig 5-12), and panoramic radiographs (Fig 5-22).

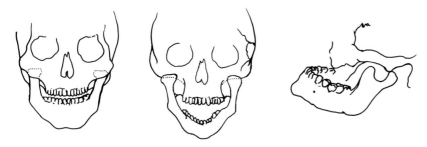

FIGURE 5-19   Modified Projection of the Mandible

If it has been determined that the patient does not have an obvious fracture of the mandible, some modification of the routine projections may be attempted in order to demonstrate the condylar portion of the mandible. Left, In the PA projection, the necks and heads of the condyles are not shown. Center, If the patient is instructed to open the mouth, the mandible will move forward on the condylar eminence and the necks and heads of the condyles will be seen. Right, If the patient is positioned as for a conventional axiolateral mandible and then asked to jut the teeth of the lower jaw foward, placing the lower teeth anterior to the upper teeth, the mandible will move forward.

C A U T I O N :   These maneuvers help to demonstrate the entire mandible; however, they should not be attempted in the presence of a suspected fracture.

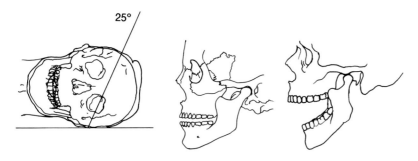

FIGURE 5-20   Temporomandibular Joint

Left, A representation of the temporomandibular joint with the patient in the lateral position and the CR directed caudad 25 degrees to exit at the joint being examined. Center, The mandibular condyle is shown in the joint space with the mouth closed. Right, When the mouth is opened, the mandibular condyle slides forward, out of the joint space.

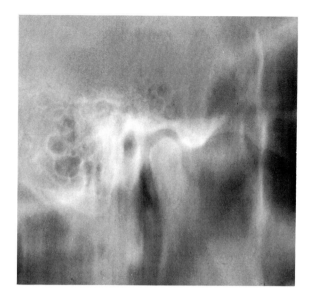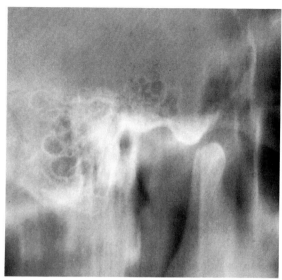

FIGURE 5–21 Tomography of the Temporomandibular Joints

Linear tomography of the temporomandibular joints in the (A) closed- and (B) open-mouth positions. Note the linear striations in the image as a result of artifacts associated with linear tomography.

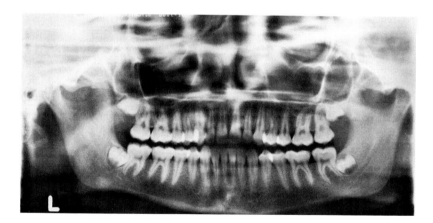

FIGURE 5–22 Pantomographic Study

Pantomographic units use a slit-scan tomographic motion with the x-ray tube and the cassette moving in opposite directions to each other. The maxilla and mandible can be seen from one temporomandibular joint to the other. Note the horizontal parasitical streaks (top of image) caused by the horizontal linear movement of the tomographic unit. (Courtesy Eastman Kodak Company, Rochester, NY.)

The Salivary Ducts

The axiolateral mandibular projections can be used to examine patients with salivary-duct occlusion or those with calculi in the submandibular duct and gland.

The use of an oblique AP open-mouth projection may serve to visualize mandibular calculi not seen on a routine AP image. With the patient in the AP position and the mouth opened, the head is rotated laterally toward the affected side. The median plane forms an angle of 30 degrees with the vertical plane[99] (Fig 5-23).

Calculi in the parotid gland can be visualized by a tangential projection. With the mouth closed and the head turned slightly toward the side being examined, the patient is requested to puff out the cheeks with air. This maneuver projects the parotid duct from the teeth and mandible. A soft-tissue technique is required.

The Zygomatic Arch

The Waters and Towne methods are recommended for visualization of the zygomatic arch (Fig 5-8). The zygomatic arch is elongated by caudad tube angulation (Towne) or hyperextension of the patient's head (Waters).

A conventional submentovertex projection will also demonstrate the zygomatic arches (Figs 5-12 and 5-24). A slight oblique axial submentovertex projection is useful to demonstrate a depressed fracture of a zygomatic arch (Fig 5-12).

The Paranasal Sinuses

A sinus series can be used to demonstrate acute inflammatory or allergic thickening of the mucosal membranes of the sinuses, air–fluid levels within the sinuses, or evidence of bony destruction. A routine sinus series includes:

1. PA (Caldwell) projection (Fig 5-4, Table 5-1).
2. Parietoacanthial (Waters) projection (Fig 5-4, Table 5-4).
3. Lateral projection (Fig 5-10, Table 5-3).
4. Base (submentovertex) (Fig 5-12, Table 5-5).

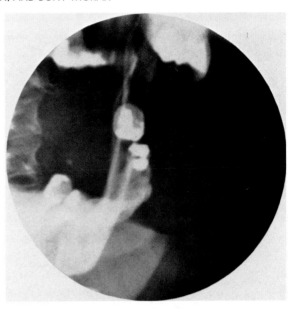

FIGURE 5-23 Submandibular Calculi

An oblique AP open-mouth position, with the head slightly rotated toward the side being examined, can demonstrate submandibular calculi. A single stone is seen in this image. This image is easy to overexpose. (Courtesy Eastman Kodak Company, Rochester, NY.)

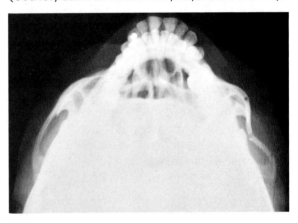

FIGURE 5-24 Modifications of the Submentovertex Projection (zygomatic arches)

An underexposed base projection can be used to demonstrate both zygomatic arches. The left zygomatic arch is fractured in two places and is depressed. Sometimes an oblique submentovertex projection must be used to lift a depressed zygomatic arch from the surrounding facial structures. The skull is positioned as for a standard submentovertex projection, and then the head is turned to an oblique position. (Courtesy Eastman Kodak Company, Rochester, NY.)

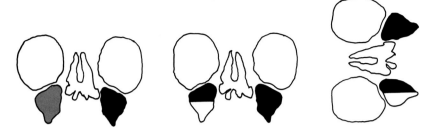

FIGURE 5-25   Free Fluid in the Sinuses

Representative Waters views are shown in this illustration. Left, A recumbent Waters view demonstrates what appears to be aerated sinuses bilaterally. Center, When the patient is seated erect, an air–fluid level is seen in the right maxillary antrum. Right, When the patient is positioned in the decubitus position, right side down, the air–fluid level can be seen owing to the use of a horizontal beam.

The erect position is preferred for demonstrating air–fluid levels. However, when examining a patient in the erect position, a caudad or cephalad tube angle can obscure an air–fluid level.

CAUTION: Fluid in the sinuses can cling to the walls of the sinus cavities and, depending on its viscosity, sometimes will slowly change its position. Allow enough time for the fluid to change position before the exposure is made (Fig 5-25).

The Orbits

A fracture of the inferior orbit can cause orbital fat and the inferior rectus muscle to herniate downward. Blowout fractures are produced when trauma is directed to the eyeball. The impact can force the eye backward into the cone-shaped orbital apex, causing a rapid increase in orbital pressure with recoil in the globe. The paper-thin bony margins of the orbital floor (the roof of the maxillary antrum) and the medial wall of the orbit fracture easily.[96] Extraocular muscles may be trapped in these fractures, which can result in a temporary impairment of eye movement. Soft-tissue density seen in the maxillary sinuses could be blood, fat, or mucosal edema.[100] Conventional tomography is helpful in evaluating an injury of this type.

A slightly modified shallow Waters position can also be used to evaluate the orbits. If a stereo technique is used, even when there is no intent to view these images stereoscopically, considerable information can be gained. For example, with the patient in a conventional or shallow Waters position, three separate views are made: (1) with no tube angle, (2) with the tube angled 5 degrees caudad, and (3) with the tube angled 5 degrees cephalad.

A fracture in the floor of the orbit is usually seen on one of these views. It is always difficult to make a slight adjustment to the position of the patient's skull when repeating an examination. With this technique, adjustments are made prior to exposure.

Additional radiographs are almost never needed, since the 5–0–5 degree tube angulation technique produces three slightly different Waters views (Fig 5-26). The 5 degree caudal/0 degree images constitute a stereo pair; the 0 degree/5 degree cephalad images are also a stereo pair. The 5 degree caudad and cephalad images can be viewed stereoscopically, as well. Patient cooperation is required since any motion will negate the stereo effect.

The Nasal Bones

The parietoacanthial (Waters) or intraoral projections demonstrate lateral or medial displacement of bony fragments of the nose. An occlusal

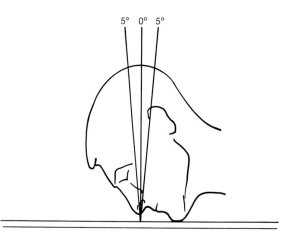

FIGURE 5-26 Modified Projection of the Orbits

The use of a modified projection (shallow Waters) in conjunction with a stereo technique helps in the evaluation of the orbits. A Waters projection is shown with tube angulations of 5 degrees caudad, 0 degrees, and 5 degrees cephalad. It is important that the patient not move between exposures. The three resultant images are modifications of the basic Waters projection. Any two views, if placed in a stereo viewer, would offer a three-dimensional representation of the orbital areas.

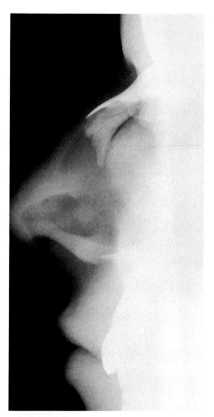

FIGURE 5-27 Lateral Nose Radiograph

A soft-tissue technique similar to that used for a finger is needed to visualize the nasal bones laterally. The anterior nasal spine (maxilla) is well demonstrated. No other osseous structures are seen with this technique.

film held in place by the teeth can be used for a superoinferior projection. High speed mammographic single emulsion screen-film systems (5 in by 7 in or 8 in by 10 in) can be substituted for the occlusal film to minimize dosage to the eyes while producing excellent detail of the nasal bones. The cassette should be covered with a plastic wrap. The corner of the cassette is gently placed in the mouth, with the patient holding the cassette to support its weight.

The lateral view shows the nasal bone and soft tissues of the nose (Fig 5-27). A compensatory filter helps to balance the wide variation in radiographic density in the lateral position.

A Foreign Body In the Eye

There are approximately 30 methods, or modifications of existing methods, for precise localization of an opaque foreign body in the eye. Tech-

niques popular in the United States include the Sweets method and the Pfeiffer modification of the Comberg method.[1]

To determine the location of a foreign body in the eye requires movement of the eye and two separate exposures on the same x-ray film. If it is within the eyeball, movement between the two exposures will demonstrate the foreign body in both positions.

With the patient in the lateral position and looking up and down for two separate images, it is often possible to localize an opaque foreign body in the eye. Since the muscles move with the eyeball, a foreign body lodged in a muscle or located in the eyeball also moves (Fig 5-28). A for-

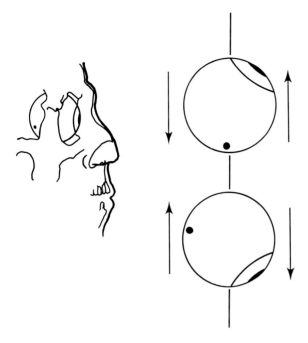

FIGURE 5-28 Foreign Body in the Eye

Conventional radiographs can be made to determine whether a foreign body is within the eye or is in an adjacent structure. Left, With the patient in the lateral position, a foreign body seen as a black dot appears in the posterior aspect of the eyeball. Top right, When the patient looks up, a foreign body in the eyeball will swing downward. Bottom right, When the patient looks down, the foreign body moves upward. The reverse would occur with a foreign body located anteriorly. If the foreign body is outside of the eyeball, it will not change position as the eye moves.

eign body external to the eyeball will not move with eye movement.

A shallow Waters method—two separate exposures made on two separate cassettes and the patient looking up and down or from left to right—can also be used to demonstrate the movement of a foreign body in the eyeball.

For many years, nonscreen or direct exposure studies of the eyes were made with cardboard film holders. Dosage to the lens of the eyes can be significantly reduced with the use of screen-film systems. Screen-film imaging is acceptable if the screens are cleaned with the screen cleaner and under the conditions recommended by the manufacturer of the screens.

If the surface of the eye is to be seen free of superimposed bone, occlusal films may be used for lateral or superoinferior projections.[1]

The Mastoid Portion of the Temporal Bone

A conventional imaging series of the mastoid portion of the temporal bones includes:

1. Semiaxial projection (Towne) (Fig 5-8, Table 5-2).
2. Semiaxial oblique projection (Mayers) (Fig 5-8, Table 5-2).
3. PA projection (modified Caldwell) (Fig 5-4, Table 5-1).
4. PA oblique projection (Stenvers) (Fig 5-7, Table 5-1).

With radiography of the temporal bones, the ears should be taped forward, away from the mastoid cells. The entrance point of the CR can be marked on the adhesive tape so that, if needed, corrections or adjustments in positioning can be made easily.

> C A U T I O N : The tape should not be placed over the mastoid-cell areas.

Conventional tomography or CT of the petrous area is often required to evaluate the minute structures of the middle and inner ear. When available, CT is the preferred imaging method. Linear or pluridirectional conventional tomographic units can be used for plesiotomographic studies (1 mm sections). If an older, conventional tomographic unit cannot be adjusted to 1 mm settings, a "book" cassette holding four closely matched pairs of intensifying screens may be used with a conventional Bucky. The exact 1.0 mm spacing of the pairs of intensifying screens in the "plesiocassette" guarantees equidistant spacing for four simultaneously exposed tomographic images. If a book cassette is not available, four individual cassettes can be used with three 1.0 mm thick aluminum spacers.

The lowest level needed in the four-section study must be determined. For example, when starting with a 10 cm section in the PA or AP position, three sheets of aluminum, each 1.0 mm thick, are required for the plesiosectional study. The initial 10 cm section is made with the first cassette. A sheet of aluminum, exactly the size of the cassette, is then inserted into the Bucky tray and a second cassette is placed on top of the aluminum sheet. This elevates the second cassette exactly 1.0 mm from the position of the first cassette. The fulcrum level remains at 10 cm but because of the aluminum spacer, a 10.1 cm level is achieved. A third section is made with a third cassette and two sheets of aluminum for a 10.2 cm level, and a fourth section, using three sheets of aluminum and a fourth cassette, produces a 10.3 cm image. The four tomographic sections—10.0, 10.1, 10.2, and 10.3 cm—are all made with the fixed fulcrum level of 10.0 cm.

> CAUTION: Identical cassettes must be used for all four exposures. Differences in the thickness of the cassettes or variations in methods of screen mounting can negate the 1.0 mm spacing effect of the aluminum sheeting.[69]

The Soft Tissues of the Scalp

Tangential (silhouette) views with the head in an oblique position can help to evaluate elevation of the scalp caused by soft-tissue or bony lesions, a depressed skull fracture, or foreign bodies within the scalp[101,102] (Fig 5-29).

STEREO RADIOGRAPHY

To avoid grid cutoff, stereo skull techniques require tube angulation in the direction of the lines of the grid rather than tube shifts to the right or left, against the grid. See Chapter 1, Fig 1-13. For example, with a modified Caldwell projection, the patient is placed in the PA position, the tube is angled 10 degrees caudad, and an exposure is made. A second image is then made with the tube angled 15 degrees caudad to produce a stereo pair.

For the AP Towne–Grashey projection, the tube is usually angled caudal 30 degrees or

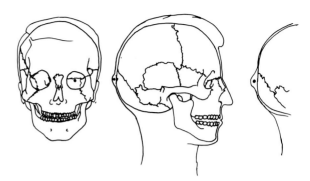

FIGURE 5-29 Soft-tissue Demonstration of the Scalp

Left, A dense foreign body is seen as a black dot in the left orbit in a frontal view. Center, The foreign body may or may not be visualized in the posterior aspect of the skull owing to scalp burnout with typical exposure factors. Right, A tangential or silhouette radiograph made through the area of concern using a soft-tissue technique will project the foreign body away from the skull and show its relationship to the bone or soft tissues of the skull. (Drawn from Brandt C: A shot in the dark: Foreign body localization. *Radiography* 1987;53:26-27.)

greater. A shift of 5 degrees on either side of the original caudad angulation results in stereo images. For example, a 35 degree caudad angulation requires a 40 degree angle for the second exposure to produce a stereo pair; a 30 degree tube angulation could also be used with a 35 degree angulation for a stereo pair.

For the lateral and submentovertex projections, shifts of 3 degrees caudad and 3 degrees cephalad from the originally centered beam (a total shift of 6 degrees) produce a stereo effect (Fig 5-30).

> CAUTION: Shifting across the skull would result in grid cutoff, as well as a distortion in all PA / AP projections similar to that seen with rotation of the skull.

> CAUTION: Stereo skull images made with tube angle shifting must be placed sideways in a stereo viewer for a three-dimensional effect (Fig 5-30).

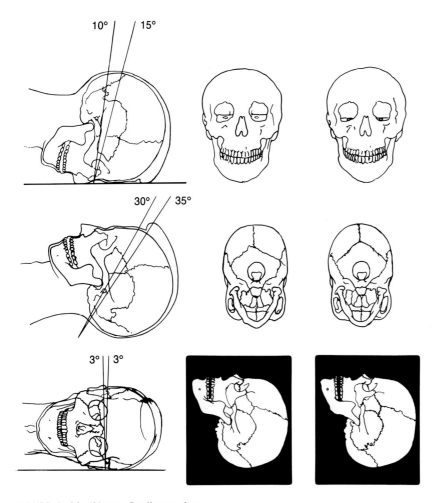

FIGURE 5–30 Stereo Radiography

Stereo radiography of the skull can be accomplished in several positions. In the PA position, (top left), the CR is directed caudad 10 and 15 degrees to make up a stereo pair (top center and top right). Top center, the 10 degree caudad tube tilt places the petrous ridges approximately in the center of the orbits. Top right, The petrous ridges are seen lower in the orbits when the 15 degree caudad tube angulation is used. Left center, In the AP position, semiaxial projection, the CR is directed caudad 30 and 35 degrees. Center, The dorsum sella is projected into the foramen magnum. Center right, The 35 degree caudad projection places the dorsum sella even lower in the foramen magnum. Bottom left, In the lateral position, the x-ray tube is angled 3 degrees caudad and 3 degrees cephalad. When viewed, these images must be placed sideways in the viewer as shown here (bottom center and bottom right). Each pair of images, when viewed in a stereoscopic viewer, will produce a three-dimensional effect. It is important that the x-ray tube be shifted in the direction of the grid lines to avoid grid cutoff.

ISOCENTRIC RADIOGRAPHY

Isocentric radiography requires three reference planes and coordinates to image the skull with the patient in a fixed supine position. In order to perform isocentric radiography of the skull, (1) the ceiling mount and (2) the x-ray tube must be able to rotate around the patient's head with (3) the CR always passing through the midpoint (the intersection of the horizontal and vertical axis), 80 to 90 cm from the focal spot.[103]

TECHNICAL CONSIDERATIONS

Image Blur

Poor image geometry can result in the blurring out of a fracture (Fig 5-31). Whenever possible, the site of a fracture should be in intimate contact with the image detector. For example, if a patient has a fracture of the right temporal region, the fracture will be more sharply defined

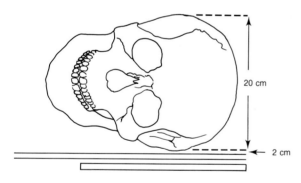

FIGURE 5–31 Image Geometry

With multiple injuries, it is not always possible to position a patient for both lateral skull radiographs. An increased OFD combined with a large focal spot can cause the side of the skull furthest from the detector to image out of focus. In the lateral position, the down side of the patient's skull is almost in contact with the cassette (approximately 2 cm). The upper side can be 15 to 20 cm away from the detector. When combined with the tabletop/Bucky-tray distance, an increased OFD of 30 cm or greater is possible for the structures furthest away from the tabletop. The use of a small focal spot (0.6 mm or less) helps to minimize image blur.

on the right lateral view. The opposing view made with the fracture site away from the detector results in a less sharply defined, seemingly wider, fracture. Unfortunately, the fracture may completely "disappear," depending on the size of the focal spot, the OFD, the focal object distance, the tabletop/Bucky-tray relationship, or the screen-film combination used. See Chapter 1, Fig 1-4.

When used at its maximum milliampere setting, a small focal spot may also produce image blur owing to focal spot "blooming." A high milliampere value combined with a short exposure time may necessitate the selection of a large focal spot, which should be avoided if possible.

When patient habitus or deformity forces an increase in the angulation of the x-ray tube, the parallax effect of dual emulsion film is accentuated. To minimize parallax, the skull should be elevated on a 10 to 15 degree radiolucent, artifact-free sponge, and the tube adjusted to achieve the desired projection. This elevation of the patient's head increases the OFD, but when used with a 0.6 mm or smaller focal spot, it is better than further distorting the radiographic anatomy by an exaggerated tube angle. See Chapter 2, Fig 2-14.

Cathode–anode placement can also affect resolution. See Chapter 1, Fig 1-6. Patient and equipment motions are major contributors to image blur.

Fixed-Kilovoltage Technique

Most adult skulls are similar in size and composition as compared with the abdomen or the thorax where, depending on body habitus, wide variations in size and absorption exist.

When a fixed mAs/variable kVp technique is used, kilovoltage is lowered as centimeter measurements decrease. For example, a technique that requires 70 kVp for a PA skull might require only 60 kVp for the lateral image. However, in the lateral position, the superimposed petrous ridges could be underpenetrated at the lower kilovoltage value, resulting in a shorter scale of contrast. At 70 kVp for both the PA and lateral projections, but using one half the mAs for the lateral, an image with adequate penetration and contrast is produced.

The fixed- (moderate to high) kilovoltage technique offers several technical benefits:

1. Uniform screen-film response. When using rare-earth screens, the fixed kVp setting helps to overcome kVp dependency. See Chapter 1.
2. Increased exposure latitude.
3. Better penetration of dense bony structures.

Lesions of the cranium can be focal or widespread or osteoblastic or osteolytic, which may influence the selection of technical factors.

Filtration

Proper exposure of the skull in the lateral position will result in overexposed images of the sinuses and facial bones. Compensatory filters are available for cephalometric procedures that help to visualize the osseous structures of the anterior facial bones, sinuses, and soft tissues. An underpart filter can be of value in preserving the soft-tissue structures of the face in the lateral position.[9] A sliding adjustable aluminum filter at the exit of the collimator accomplishes the same effect while reducing dosage to the part under study.[10]

Intensifying Screens

The demonstration of minor osseous changes or minute calcifications in the skull may require a detail screen-film combination. Single or double emulsion mammographic screen-film systems can produce exceptional bony detail.

CAUTION: The need for increased osseous detail must be weighed against the potential increase in dosage to the eyes, thyroid, and sternum. Using a higher speed screen-film combination, if possible, and optimizing the image chain with the use of a small focal spot may be the appropriate imaging choice.

Scatter Control

Until the mid-1940s, many skull and facial bone examinations were made without a grid or Bucky because of limited generator output and slow speed screen-film options. These nongrid techniques permitted greater freedom for angulation of the x-ray tube and/or cassette. When used with grids, dual tube angle projections result in grid cutoff.

A high mA, short exposure time image may show grid lines if the grid is "captured" in motion during a Bucky exposure. A primary beam leak with associated undercutting of the image degrades the image of the scalp and adjacent soft tissues of the facial bones. See Chapter 1, Fig 1-11.

Radiation Protection

When evaluating the cranium, the possibility of a cataractogenic dose to the cornea must be considered. The eyes of the patient in the AP position receive a higher entrance dose as compared with the exit dose in the PA position.[104] The use of the PA position, whenever possible, combined with high speed, rare earth screen-film systems, lowers radiation dosage to the lens of the eyes since primary radiation enters the posterior skull rather than the eyes and remnant radiation exits through the lens of the eyes.

Radiation dosage to the eyes is significantly increased with conventional tomography (Table 5-6). However, lead shields, if placed over the lens of the eyes to reduce dosage during tomography, may mask a fracture of the orbit.

TABLE 5–6 Radiation Exposure to Lens of Eye for 12 Radiographic Exposures During Intracranial Tomography*†

Projection	
AP	17.60 R
PA	0.90 R
Exposure reduction	95%

*50 mA, 6 seconds, 70 kVp, 45 in source-to-image distance, 3.2 mm half-value layer, trispiral tomographic motion; exposure includes backscatter.
†Courtesy Frank ED, Stears JG, Gray JE, et al: The use of the posteroanterior projection: A method of reducing x-ray exposure to specific radiosensitive organs. *Radiol Technol* 1983; 54: 343-347.

CAUTION: If the AP position must be used for tomography, patients should be asked to keep their eyes closed during the x-ray exposure so as not involuntarily to follow the tomographic tube motion.

Use of the ID Blocker as a Reference Point

An ID blocker in each cassette shields a segment of unexposed film for recording patient data and related information. By establishing a positioning routine and using identical cassettes from the same manufacturer, one can usually identify the side and/or position of the patient's skull by the location of the blocker on the image.

CAUTION: A different make or type of cassette may have a different position for the ID blocker. An inverted Kodak X-Omatic cassette changes ID blocker orientation. See Chapter 1, Fig 1-14.

The lead letter R or L should also be placed in the same position each time for specific views. The use of copper-backed markers minimizes burnout of the lead letters by the unattenuated primary beam.

THE VERTEBRAL COLUMN

In the adult, the vertebral column, situated in the median plane of the posterior trunk, consists of 7 cervical, 12 thoracic, and 5 lumbar vertebrae and an ankylosed sacrum and coccyx. The bony spine supports and protects the spinal cord.

ANATOMICAL / PATHOLOGICAL OBSERVATIONS

The vertebral column normally curves in both a convex and a concave manner. The cervical and lumbar regions form a convex curve, a bend with a ventral convexity (lordosis). The thoracic and sacrococcygeal segments form a concave curve. The sacrum and coccyx normally have a slight downward tilt. An exaggeration of the normal posterior curve is known as kyphosis. Scoliosis is a deviation of the spine from the median plane.

The most common use of conventional radiography of the vertebral column is to demonstrate fractures of the vertebral bodies, spinous or transverse processes, and extension–flexion injuries. Other indications for radiography of the spine would include ruling out protrusion or herniation of the intervertebral disks or bony destruction from primary or metastatic tumors or evaluating spinal curvature.

POSITIONING CONCEPTS

A variety of positioning aids may be used to support the spine during radiography.

CAUTION: Support devices, including folded sheets or pillows, must be free of such contaminants as iodine or barium to avoid artifacts.

Basic positioning of the various segments of the spinal column can be found in Tables 5-7 through 5-9. The lateral spine is presented in Table 5-7 since this projection should be the first image made on a trauma patient.[105]

Imaging of the Cervical Spine

Routine projections of the cervical spine include lateral (Table 5-7), AP (Table 5-8), AP open mouth (Table 5-8), and both obliques (Table 5-9). Descriptions of trauma projections are given under "Supplementary Imaging of the Spine." The protocol for examining trauma patients can be found under "Conditions or Diseases Meriting Special Consideration."

Demonstration of the Anterior Arch of C-1. A supplementary image of the cervical spine can be used when hyperextension of the neck must be avoided. In a modified basal projection, a small cushion is placed under the shoulder of a supine patient. The neck is slightly extended. The CR is directed 10 degrees superior to the line perpen-

(Text continues on page 131)

TABLE 5-7 The Lateral Vertebral Column

Area	Position of Patient	Projection of Central Ray	Demonstrates (View)
Cervical	Patient lateral, recumbent or erect; the coronal plane passing through mastoid tip parallel to tabletop or upright cassette holder; median plane of head parallel to film plane	CR directed perpendicular to film plane, tabletop, or upright grid device to enter at level of C-4 (just above the thyroid cartilage)	Lateral apophyseal joints; vertebral bodies; articular pillars; spinous processes
Thoracic	Patient lateral recumbent; midaxillary line centered to midline of tabletop	CR directed perpendicular to film plane tabletop or upright grid device, to enter 3 in below sternal angle (at level of T-6)	Lateral intervertebral foramina; vertebral bodies and intervertebral spaces; spinous processes
Lumbar	See Thoracic position	CR directed perpendicular to film plane, enters at L-4	See Thoracic view; junction of L-5/S-1
L-5/S-1	Patient recumbent lateral; center the plane lying 1.5 in posterior to the midaxillary line to the midline of tabletop	CR directed perpendicular to film plane, enters at point midway between crest of the ilium (L-4) and anterior superior iliac spines (ASIS; L-2)	Junction of L-5/S-1
Sacrum	Patient recumbent, lateral; the coronal plane 2 in anterior to sacrum centered to midline of table	CR directed perpendicular to film plane, to enter at midportion of sacrum	Sacrum
Coccyx	Patient recumbent lateral; align coccyx to midline of table	CR directed perpendicular to film plane, to enter at coccyx (just below top of greater trochanters)	Coccyx

TABLE 5-8   The AP Vertebral Column

Area	Position of Patient/Part	Projection of Central Ray	Demonstrates (View)
Cervical	Patient supine or AP erect; chin elevated to place the occlusal plane and the mastoid tips in the same transverse plane, perpendicular to film plane; median plane of body and head centered to midline of tabletop or upright cassette holder	CR directed 15 to 20 degrees cephalad to enter at level of C-4, increase the cephalad angulation if patient cannot elevate the chin	Vertebral bodies; spinous processes; interpediculate spaces; intervertebral spaces
Cervical (open mouth)	See Cervical position	CR directed perpendicular to film plane	Atlas; axis; C-1/C-2 articulations

NOTE: The lower edge of the upper incisors and base of skull should be superimposed sightly above the level of C-1. If the odontoid is obscured by the incisors, the chin is not elevated enough. Overelevation of the chin will cause obscuring of the odontoid process by the base of the skull. A space between the central incisors sometimes produces a vertical radiolucent line, which gives the illusion of a fracture of the odontoid process.

Area	Position of Patient/Part	Projection of Central Ray	Demonstrates (View)
Thoracic	Patient supine; median plane centered to midline of table	CR directed perpendicular to film plane to enter at level of T-6	Vertebral bodies; pedicles, spinous and transverse processes; intervertebral disk spaces
Lumbar	See Thoracic position	CR directed perpendicular to film plane, to enter at level of L-4	See Thoracic view
L-5/S-1	See Thoracic position	CR directed cephalad 30 degrees for males, 35 degrees for females, to enter midline at level midway between iliac crests (L-4) and anterior superior iliac spines (ASIS, S-2)	Junction of L-5/S-1; sacroiliac joints
Sacrum	See Thoracic position	CR directed cephalad 15 degrees, to enter median plane about 2 in above the level of the symphysis pubis	Sacrum; sacroiliac joints
Coccyx	See Thoracic position	CR directed 10 degrees caudad to enter median plane about 2 in above symphysis pubis	Coccyx

TABLE 5-9 The Oblique Vertebral Column

Area	Position of Part/Patient	Projection of Central Ray	Demonstrates (View)
Cervical	Supine or erect; 45 degrees oblique		
	LPO	AP projection; CR directed 15 degrees cephalad to enter at C-4	Intervertebral foramina, right; vertebral bodies; pedicles; disk spaces
	RPO	AP projection; CR directed 15 degrees cephalad to enter at C-4	Intervertebral foramina, left; vertebral bodies; pedicles; intervertebral disk spaces
Cervical	Prone or erect; 45 degrees oblique		
	RAO	PA projection; CR directed 15 degree caudad to enter at C-4	Intervertebral foramina, right; vertebral bodies; pedicles; disk spaces
	LAO	PA projection; CR directed 15 degrees caudad to enter at C-4	Intervertebral foramina, left; vertebral bodies; pedicles; disk spaces
Thoracic	Patient supine; 70 degrees oblique from plane of table		
	LPO	AP projection; CR directed perpendicular to film plane, enters to right of the median plane at level of sixth thoracic vertebra	Apophyseal joints, right; vertebral bodies; disk spaces
	RPO	AP projection; CR directed perpendicular to film plane to enter to left of the median plane at level of sixth thoracic vertebra	Apophyseal joints, left; vertebral bodies; disk spaces
Thoracic	Patient prone; 70 degrees oblique from plane of table		
	RAO	PA projection; CR directed perpendicular to film plane to enter to left of the median plane at level of the sixth thoracic verterbra	See LPO view
	LAO	PA projection; CR directed perpendicular to film plane, to enter to right of the median plane at level of sixth thoracic vertebra	See RPO view

(continued)

TABLE 5-9 *continued*

Area	Position of Part/Patient	Projection of Central Ray	Demonstrates (View)
Lumbar	Patient supine; 30 to 45 degrees oblique toward side being examined; align sagittal plane passing 2 in medial to elevated ASIS to midline of table		
	LPO	AP projection; CR directed perpendicular to film plane to enter to right of the median plane at the level of the third lumbar vertebra	Apophyseal joints, left; vertebral bodies; disk spaces
	RPO	AP projection; CR directed perpendicular to film plane, to enter to left of the median plane at the level of the third lumbar vertebra	Apophyseal joints, right; vertebral bodies; disk spaces
Lumbar	Patient prone; see Supine position		
	LAO	PA projection; CR directed perpendicular to film plane, to enter 2 in lateral to the spinous process of the elevated side at the level of third lumbar vertebra	See RPO view
	RAO	See LAO position	See LPO view
Sacroiliac joints	Patient supine; 25 degrees oblique from plane of tabletop		
	Median plane slightly to right of midline of table LPO	AP projection; CR directed perpendicular to film plane, to enter at point 1 in medial to and at level of elevated anterior superior iliac spine (ASIS)	Sacroiliac joint, right side
	Median plane slightly to left of midline of table RPO	See LPO projection	Sacroiliac joint, left side

(continued)

TABLE 5-9 *continued*

Area	Position of Part/Patient	Projection of Central Ray	Demonstrates (View)
Sacroiliac joints	Patient prone; 25 degrees oblique from plane of tabletop		
	Median plane slightly to right of midline of table LAO	PA projection; CR directed perpendicular to film plane, to enter dependent posterior inferior iliac spine about 1 in below spinous process of L-5	See RPO view
	Median plane slightly to left of midline of table RAO	See LAO projection	See LPO view

Note: LPO/RPO positions = AP oblique projections; LAO/RAO positions = PA oblique projections; LPO view = RAO view; RPO view = LAO view.

dicular from the orbitomeatal line. It is directed to enter at a level 2.5 cm below the external auditory meatus (Figs 5-32 and 5-33). Radiographs are made with the slightly elevated head in the neutral position, rotated 30 degrees to the left and 30 degrees to the right, using a non-Bucky technique.[106]

Imaging of Cervical Intervertebral Foramina and Articulating Processes

The cervical oblique demonstrates the intervertebral foramina and the pedicles closest to the cassette.[1] A simple positioning maneuver, the jutting of the jaw forward, helps to visualize the anterior segments of the cervical spine in the oblique positions (Fig 5-34). In a nontraumatized patient, the head may be turned in a true lateral position for the oblique study.[4]

A method to demonstrate the laminae and articular processes of the upper cervical vertebrae requires a slight extension of the supine patient's head with the mouth opened wide. The CR is directed 35 degrees caudad to enter at the third cervical vertebra. With the head rotated 10 degrees to the side, the mandible is removed from the area of interest.[107]

Modifications of the Standard Pillar Projection

Woodford[108] suggests that to demonstrate the articular masses using the "pillar" view, the patient should be supine with the CR directed 35 degrees caudad to enter the midcervical region. Two separate exposures are made, with the chin rotated first to one side and then to the other, to demonstrate the contralateral masses.

With the neck in a neutral position, the articular facets can be demonstrated with the x-ray beam centered laterally at the C-4 posterior arch and angulated axial-oblique (dorsal and slightly caudad). With the cassette flat on the table on the side opposite the x-ray beam, there is a magnification (elongation) of the apophyseal joint spaces and their facetal boundaries. Adjacent bony detail and cortical margins are enhanced. Posterior arch elements, including the pillar bodies, are distorted and blurred (Figs 5-35 and 5-36). A nonmobile patient who cannot rotate the head or hyperextend the neck benefits from this projection, which avoids superimposition of the facial bones on the upper cervical vertebrae.[109]

Yochum[29] suggests that to demonstrate the articular processes and apophyseal joints, both

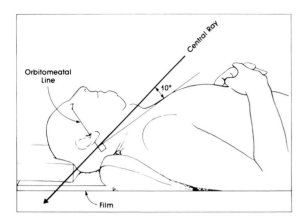

FIGURE 5–32 Modified Basal View of Neck to Demonstrate Fractures of the Anterior Arch of C-1

The head is in a neutral position and is rotated 30 degrees to either side using a tabletop technique. (Courtesy England AC III, Shippel AH, Ray MJ: A simple view for demonstration of fractures of the anterior arch of C-1. *AJR* 1985; 144: 763-764.)

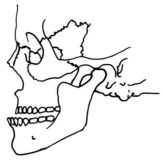

FIGURE 5–34 Jutting Mechanism to Demonstrate Forward Movement of the Jaw to Visualize the Anterior Structures of the Cervical Spine in the Oblique Position.

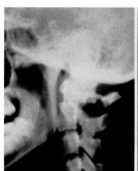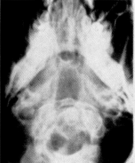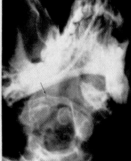

FIGURE 5–33 Lateral View of the Cervical Spine Compared with the Modified Basal View

Left, A lateral view of two fractures of the posterior arch of C-1. Center, A modified basal view with the head in a neutral position. Fracture of anterior arch of C-1 on right. Right, Modified basal view with the head rotated 30 degrees to the left more clearly demonstrates a fracture of the anterior arch of C-1 on the right (arrow). (Courtesy England AC III, Shippel AH, Ray MJ: A simple view for demonstration of fractures of the anterior arch of C-1. *AJR* 1985; 144: 763-764.)

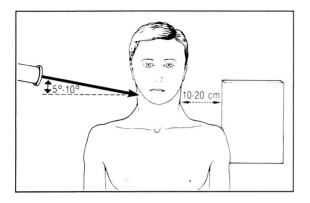
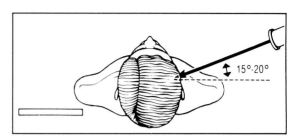

FIGURE 5–35   Frontal Dimension for Positioning for Magnified Axial-Oblique Projection of Cervical Facets (Left); Axial Dimension of Positioning (Right)

(Courtesy Tihansky DP, Augustine G: Magnified axial-oblique projection of cervical articular facets. *Radiol Technol* 1987;58:426-430.)

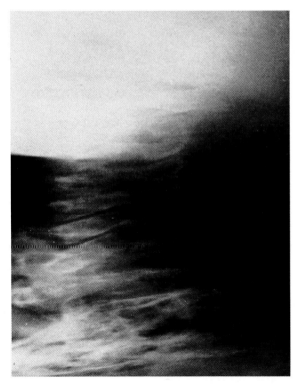

FIGURE 5–36   Magnified Axial-Oblique Radiograph of the Cervical Articular Facets

(Courtesy Tihansky DP, Augustine G: Magnified axial-oblique projection of cervical articular facets. *Radiol Technol* 1987;58:426-430.)

sides of the patient must be exposed for comparison. The patient is positioned PA with a 35 degree cephalad tube tilt. The head is rotated 45 degrees away from the side of interest. The CR is directed to enter C-5, 1 in lateral to the midline on the side of interest. This view can also be obtained in the AP position with a caudad tube tilt. Fractures of the articular pillars are frequently seen only on these special projections.

Imaging of Unilateral Facet Dislocation of the Cervical Spine

The patient, in the supine position, is rotated to a 22.5 degree angle. A foam-rubber sponge helps to stabilize the patient. A cassette is placed against the shoulder, perpendicular to the tabletop. The CR, parallel to the tabletop, is directed perpendicular to the film plane (Fig 5-37). The resultant 22.5 degree lateral oblique image, which resembles a lateral radiograph, is used to demonstrate dislocated facet joints.[108]

> N O T E : Tight beam collimation is required with nongrid exposures. If a grid cassette is used, the grid lines must be positioned perpendicular to the tabletop or floor to avoid grid cutoff.

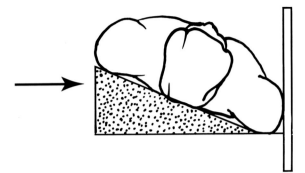

FIGURE 5-37 Positioning for the Cervical Facets

(Redrawn from Woodford MJ: Radiography of the acute cervical spine. *Radiography* 1987;53:3-8.)

Imaging of the Cervical Thoracic Junction

Visualizing the C-6, C-7 interspace is vital in examining the cervical spine, particularly with trauma patients.[110] Early diagnosis of a cervical spine injury is required to optimize treatment and prognosis (Figs 5-38 and 5-39).

The vertebral arch projection is used to demonstrate the posterior elements of the cervical and upper three or four thoracic vertebrae, the articular processes and their facets, the laminae, and the spinous processes. The patient is placed supine with the head hyperextended. The CR is directed 20 to 30 degrees caudad to enter the seventh cervical vertebra. The CR should coincide with the plane of the articular facets. A greater tube angle is required if the cervical curve is accentuated, and a lesser angle if the curve is diminished.[1]

The cervicothoracic lateral position, often referred to as the "swimmer's" position, is used to demonstrate lower cervical and upper thoracic vertebral alignment. A horizontal beam technique can be used with a grid cassette or upright Bucky if it is not possible to position the patient erect for the lateral cervicothoracic examination. The patient's arm adjacent to the image detector should be pulled upward and the arm nearer to the x-ray tube pulled downward.

In a modification of this projection, the patient is brought to attention in military fashion

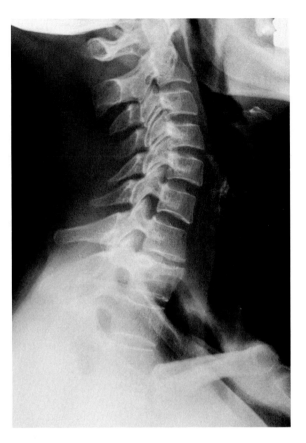

FIGURE 5-38 Lateral Cervical Spine to Include Upper Thoracic Vertebrae

It is imperative when evaluating the cervical spine for injury that the cervicothoracic junction be imaged. See Fig 5-39. (Courtesy Eastman Kodak Company, Rochester, NY.)

(head erect, shoulders back) in the right (or left) lateral position. The right shoulder is then shifted forward while the left shoulder remains back. This maneuver significantly diminishes the thickness of the part under study. The CR is directed perpendicular to T-2/T-3 to enter the body anterior to the left shoulder (closest to the x-ray tube) and exit through the right shoulder[55] (Fig 5-40).

Imaging of the Thoracic Spine

Basic projections to image the thoracic spine include the AP and lateral (Tables 5-7 and 5-8). Breathing techniques (up to 10 second expo-

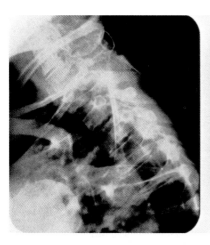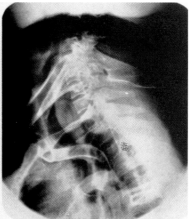

FIGURE 5-39 Upper Thoracic Vertebrae

Left, For an elderly man who is unable to raise his shoulders, a 5 degree caudad angulation helps to lift the shoulders off of the area of interest. Right, The upper thoracic vertebrae of a patient with a short neck and extremely stiff shoulders are imaged with a 5 degree caudad angulation. (Courtesy Eastman Kodak Company, Rochester, NY.)

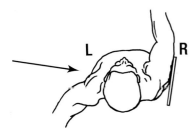

FIGURE 5-40 Modification of Cervicothoracic Lateral Position

This modification of the cervicothoracic lateral position helps to balance density between the lower cervical and upper thoracic regions. A high kVp (latitude) technique also helps to balance tissue density between the thinner cervical and the thicker thoracic areas.

sures) are often recommended for lateral thoracic-spine studies (Fig 5-41), but the mA station settings on modern x-ray equipment are often not low enough for such techniques to be used. Thus, depending on the speed of the screen-film system in use, a 10 mA or 20 mA station may have to be added to the x-ray unit in order to utilize breathing methods. Restraining devices are essential to immobilize patients and restrict their motion during prolonged exposures.

> C A U T I O N : Because shallow breathing does not fully depress the diaphragm, the lower thoracic vertebrae are often not imaged with the breathing lateral technique (Fig 5-41).

Imaging of the Lumbar Spine

Basic views include AP, lateral, and lateral lumbosacral spot (Tables 5-7 and 5-8). Oblique images of the lumbar spine are often made following the AP supine radiograph. If oblique projections are required, it may be easier to place

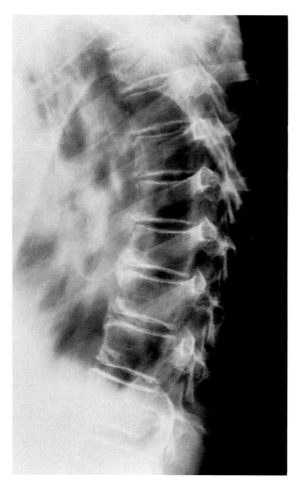

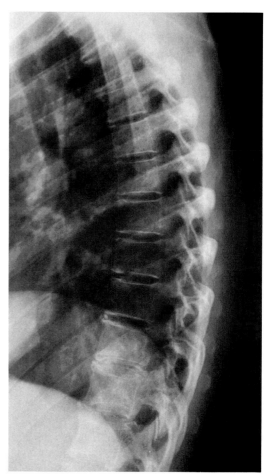

A B

FIGURE 5–41 Breathing Versus Conventional Lateral Thoracic Spine Technique

The thoracic spine is difficult to image in the lateral position because of superimposed ribs and pulmonary structures. (A) If the patient breathes rhythmically during an extended exposure of 5 seconds or longer at a low mA setting, the pulmonary vasculature can be blurred out. (B) With a conventional lateral image, an exposure made at deep inspiration with maximal downward excursion of the diaphragm demonstrates significantly more vertebrae than does the breathing lateral technique. Unfortunately, the pulmonary vasculature is superimposed on the thoracic spine.

the patient in the LPO or RPO position from the lateral position than to adjust the patient from the AP supine position.

In 1980, Rhea[111] suggested that the oblique view was an unnecessary component of the adult lumbar-spine examination. While the pars and facet joints are best seen on oblique views, evaluation of 200 consecutive lumbar examinations in adults resulted in a change in radiographic inter-

pretation in only four cases when oblique views were used. In the interests of reducing radiation exposure and costs, Rhea feels that the oblique view should be used for further evaluation if symptoms persist. A questionable abnormality in the standard three-view examination would also justify the use of oblique views. When compared with the AP and lateral studies in both males and females, the gonadal dose with oblique views is found to be increased by approximately 100%.

Imaging of the Sacroiliac Joints

A modified view of the sacroiliac joints can be used to image erosive changes too subtle to be imaged with CT.

With the patient supine and the hips and knees flexed, if possible, the CR is directed 23 degrees cephalad. A complementary image may be made with the patient prone and the CR directed 15 degrees caudad. This cost-effective method provides a more accurate evaluation of the sacroiliac joint 85% of the time than does the conventional AP view of the pelvis.[112]

CONDITIONS OR DISEASES MERITING SPECIAL TECHNICAL CONSIDERATION

Trauma

Conventional radiography is the primary imaging tool for evaluation of the cervical spine following trauma.

Even though spinal injuries are an everyday occurrence in trauma facilities, it is always an unsettling experience for radiographers to be confronted with these patients. A cervical spine injury must be anticipated when a patient sustains an injury above the level of the clavicle. While the cross-table lateral view of the cervical spine is important, it may not always demonstrate a fracture. Standard AP and open-mouth odontoid views help fully to assess the cervical spine.[113]

Even if a patient does not seem to have lost neurological function, supine horizontal beam lateral projections must be considered. The trauma patient should be kept supine throughout survey procedures. The radiographer should immobilize the patient's neck and head with sandbags or a soft collar to avoid further injury.

Sometimes only a limited examination of the cervical spine is possible because of the patient's condition. If no abnormalities are found on the survey examination, a complete study may be requested. After the survey radiographs

have been reviewed by a physician, permission should be obtained to turn the patient's head for supplementary projections.

> N O T E : Anterior displacement or jutting of the mandible further forward helps to avoid superimposition of the mandible on the cervical spine (Fig 5-34).

Yelton[114] recommends three basic rules for carrying out a cervical spine protocol in the emergency room:

1. The number of exposures should be limited to the minimum necessary for accurate diagnosis.
2. Manipulation of the patient should be minimal and extreme caution exercised if movement is required.
3. The examination should be easy to perform in the emergency-room setting.

> C A U T I O N : When cervical spine injuries are encountered, a physician should be alerted to be on standby to help in determining the appropriate number of images required for diagnosis.

Yelton[114] suggests that the supine position be used without manipulation of the patient and recommends the following basic sequence for emergency procedures.

1. Lateral projection of the entire cervical spine with a horizontal beam.

> N O T E : The lateral projection made using a 72 in FFD overcomes the increased OFD of the cervical spine relative to the cassette.

Horizontal beam projections should be reviewed by a physician before other images are made. If a specially equipped emergency room is not available, a mobile x-ray unit can provide positioning flexibility.

2. Supplemental lateral projection with traction if the initial lateral horizontal beam radiograph does not demonstrate seven cervical vertebrae.

> N O T E : With supine patients, someone is often asked to assist by applying traction to the arms to maximize the number of vertebrae seen in the lateral view. Tight beam collimation is necessary and lead gloves and a lead apron must be provided for this assistant.

3. Supplemental bilateral obliques in the AP projection. If seven cervical vertebrae are not visualized on the traction lateral, supplementary oblique AP projections are suggested. A 10 in by 12 in cassette is gently placed under the patient's shoulder. Yelton recommends that the CR be directed horizontally at a 45 degree angle to the midsagittal plane and 5 to 7 degrees caudad.

4. Routine AP 20 degree cephalad angulation projection. After evaluation of the survey images, when possible, the patient is transferred to the x-ray table for this projection. The head is extended so that the occlusal plane and the mastoid tips lie in the same transverse plane. The CR directed to the fifth cervical vertebra delineates the vertebral bodies and disk interspaces. This view may show a fracture of the transverse processes of C-7, which might not be seen on a straight AP projection because of the superimposition of the first rib.

5. An AP projection with a 20 degree caudad angulation with the CR directed to the fifth cervical vertebra. This projection demonstrates the articular facets and neural arches.

6. Routine AP projection of the upper cervical spine (open-mouth odontoid). This projection demonstrates the atlas and axis articulations.

7. Supplemental AP tomograms of the cervical spine, if indicated.

> N O T E : Linear parasitical striations of the incisors or nasal bones are seen with linear tomography. These striations can be eliminated if the tube/cassette traverses the incisors rather than moving in the direction of the incisors. Patient condition permitting, a slight tilt of the head away from the midline, left or right, helps to avoid streaking of the incisors or nasal bones during linear tomography.[69] See Chapter 1.

The autotomographic technique (AP moving-mandible procedure, also known as the chewing or wagging-jaw method) is sometimes used to image the cervical vertebrae (Fig 5-42). Autotomography, similar to linear tomography, produces parasitical streaks on the image since the incisors do not completely blur out because they are moving in the direction of the motion. If the patient does not have lower teeth, the blurring techniques usually produce good results.

Flexion and Extension Lateral Imaging. If the conventional radiographs do not demonstrate clinically suspected injury, flexion and extension views are sometimes made.

> C A U T I O N : The patient must move unassisted for flexion and extension views. These maneuvers should never be performed with someone moving the patient's head.[27]

If needed, flexion and extension views of the cervical spine can be made with the body rigid and supported and the patient seated. In the flexion position, the lower jaw can be jutted forward to minimize superimposition of the ramus of the mandible over the cervical spine (Fig 5-34). A similar maneuver is used for the lateral oblique projection of the mandible. See Fig 5-19.

Cervical spine fractures are not always isolated. Associated anomalies arise with as many as 67% of obvious injuries. A fracture seen on a routine radiographic series may require further investigation, such as with conventional tomography or CT.[27]

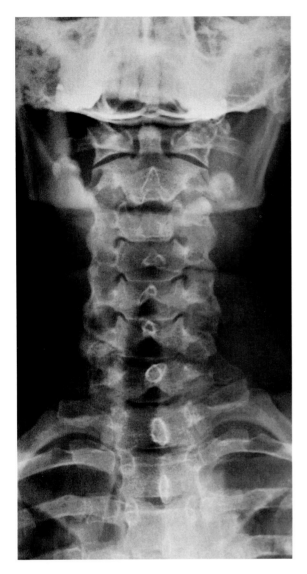

FIGURE 5-42 AP Wagging-Jaw Cervical Spine

An extended exposure combined with motion of the jaw blurs out the mandible so that all seven cervical vertebrae can be seen in the AP projection. Since linear striations are not seen, it is possible that this patient did not have lower teeth. (Courtesy Eastman Kodak Company, Rochester, NY.)

Imaging of the Thoracolumbar Region. Fractures of the thoracolumbar region account for about one third of all spinal injuries. Whenever possible, this area should be included when evaluating the lumbar vertebrae for trauma.[115]

A cross-table lateral lumbar image should include the lower thoracic vertebrae, at least to T-10, in case pain from a lower thoracic injury is referred to the lumbar or sacral area, thereby mimicking lumbar pathology. Conversely, patients with thoracic pain may have a lumbar spine injury.

Scoliosis

Scoliosis is a deviation of the spine to one side or the other from the median plane. Postural or pathological causes produce this rotating or twisting curvature, of the vertebral column, which is well documented in medical history. In Hippocrates' time, a bizarre method of treating scoliosis and other spine deformities, called "succession," involved tying the patient's ankles to a rung of a ladder and carrying the patient and ladder to the highest point of a building or other structure. The patient was then dropped vertically, head first, so that the ladder landed squarely on end.[116]

The positions required for scoliotic examinations vary with departmental routines and physician preferences. A typical routine includes an erect AP, an erect lateral, AP bending—left and right, and lateral—flexion and extension.

When examining the scoliotic spine radiographically in the lateral position, the direction of the lateral curvature determines whether a right or a left lateral position is used. The curvature should turn toward the cassette, thereby minimizing the OFD. The x-ray beam should enter the concave vertebral column. This allows the divergent x-ray beam to pass through and separate the projected vertebral interspaces.

Minimizing radiation dosage to the breast and bone marrow during the treatment and follow-up of scoliosis is a major concern. A study to evaluate the potential danger of low-dose fractionated exposures during early breast development was conducted between 1935 and 1965 on

TABLE 5–10 Comparison of Radiation Exposure to Thyroid, Sternum, and Breasts During Scoliosis Radiography*†

	Thyroid	Sternum	Breasts
Projection			
AP	0.100 R	0.160 R	0.344 R
PA	0.005 R	0.009 R	0.029 R
Exposure reduction	95%	94%	92%

*800 mA, 0.10 second, 83 kVp, 3.2 mm half-value layer, and 72 in source-to-image distance; exposures were measured at the skin surface and include backscatter.
†Courtesy Frank ED, Steatrs JG, Gray JE, et al: The use of the posteroanterior projection: A method of reducing x-ray exposure to specific radiosensitive organs. *Radiol Technol* 1983;54:343-347.

1,030 young women with scoliosis. The average age at diagnosis was 12.3 years; x-ray exposures were made over an 8.7 year period. Data were developed that resulted in the reporting of 11 cases of breast cancer, compared with six anticipated cases. Frequent exposure to low-level diagnostic radiation during childhood or adolescence may increase the risk of breast cancer.[117]

Osseous detail of the vertebral column is not a prerequisite for scoliotic evaluation. An image made with relatively high kVp, a low mAs value, and a high speed screen-film system will produce an outline of the vertebral column that is adequate for scoliotic measurements.

Attempts to reduce breast exposure during a scoliotic examination should include the following considerations.

- High speed screen-film imaging. Such systems (up to 1,200 speed), combined with aggressive shielding, greatly reduce dosage. However, for some physicians, high speed systems (800 and 1,200 speed) may exhibit too much quantum mottle for the initial evaluation, but should not be a problem with follow-up images.

- Breast shields. The female breast is sensitive to radiation, with patients between the ages of 10 and 19 at the greatest risk. One to four scoliotic examinations may be requested each year over a treatment period of three to four years, or until maturity[104,118] (Table 5-10). A shadow shield (Shadow Shield Inc, Cutten, Calif), to be attached to the collimator and placed in the path of the primary beam, has been available for many years to shield the gonads.

This device can also restrict dosage to the breasts during both lateral and frontal exposures and protect the bone marrow of the sternum in the lateral position. It is advisable to shield the sternum of male as well as female patients in the lateral position.

- PA versus AP projection. In 1988, organ dose and the quality of the radiographs associated with scoliotic examinations were evaluated. Dosages to the breasts, active bone marrow, and the thyroid, eyes, ovaries, and testes were measured using a pediatric anthropomorphic phantom in the AP and PA projections. While the dosimetry results with the phantom showed that the PA projection provided about a threefold reduction in breast dosage when compared with the AP view, the dose to the bone marrow doubled.[119] If breast shields are not available, the PA projection keeps unattenuated primary radiation from striking the breasts.

The vertebral column is further away from the cassette in the PA position, causing increased enlargement and image blur. Since evaluation of the vertebral alignment is the intent of the scoliotic examination, vertebral enlargement is not a problem. If there is concern about this increase in OFD, an increased FFD, up to 12 ft, can be used to overcome image magnification and image blur.

> CAUTION: The patient should always be reexamined in the same position (AP or PA) as in the initial examination.

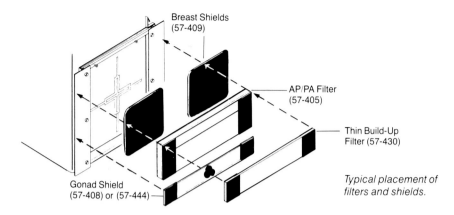

Breast Shields
(57-409)

AP/PA Filter
(57-405)

Thin Build-Up
Filter (57-430)

Gonad Shield
(57-408) or (57-444)

*Typical placement of
filters and shields.*

FIGURE 5–43   AP/PA Wedge Filter

A wedge (compensatory) filter should be used when performing full-spine examinations. Breast shields first are placed on the filter holder, and then the AP/PA wedge filter is placed on top of the breast shields. A gonadal shield is positioned below the AP/PA wedge filter. Built-up filters of this nature provide additional filtration in the cervical area, compensating for the added exposure that is required in the lumbar area. (Courtesy Nuclear Associates, Carle Place, NY.)

• Leaded acrylic compensatory filters. Compensatory filtration holds back much of the x-ray beam to the cervical area and as much as half of the exposure to the thoracic area, while permitting full exposure to the lumbar region. Since the compensatory filter selectively attenuates the x-ray beam, a similar radiographic density is achieved throughout the entire vertebral column (Figs 5-43 and 5-44).

> CAUTION: Compensatory filters made of metal will block the light from the collimator, making it impossible for the radiographer to see the field size. Lead acrylic filters permit the passage of the light beam, aiding in collimation.

Pathology in the Spinal Canal

Although CT can help to define soft-tissue masses, soft-tissue contrast is more clearly seen with MRI. Prior to the development of CT and MRI, the primary radiographic examination for suspected degenerative disk disease was myelography. The use of this invasive examination is fast declining, with the most common indication for myelography at present being the unavailability of MRI at a facility.[120]

Myelography examines the spinal canal and can be used to demonstrate neural tissues there. The first myelographic studies were made using air as a contrast medium. The subarachnoid space appeared as a decreased density on the radiograph. Oily-type iodinated materials were soon found to be of more value.[121] More recently, nonionic aqueous materials have replaced oil-based contrast agents (Fig 5-45).

> CAUTION: Most radiographs made during myelography are fluoroscopic spot films. The cross-table lateral myelogram requires careful alignment of the grid lines and the x-ray beam. If a grid cassette is placed on end with the grid lines perpendicular to the table, the upper portion of the cassette can usually be seen, thus making grid alignment easier.

A crosshatch grid will produce high contrast radiographs, but the CR must be directed to the center of both grids.

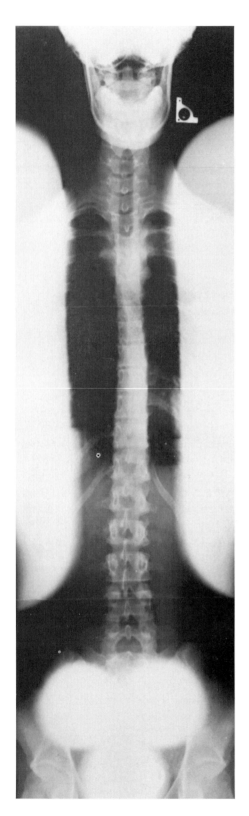

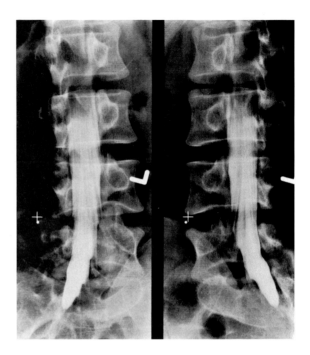

FIGURE 5-45 Lumbar Myelographic Study Using A Nonionic Contrast Medium

Fluoroscopic spot film made with a 0.6 mm focal spot. (Courtesy Eastman Kodak Company, Rochester, NY.)

FIGURE 5-44 Full-Spine Scoliosis Examination

A CLEAR Pb AP filter can be used to balance radiographic density throughout the spinal column. Note the positioning of the gonadal and breast shields. (Courtesy Nuclear Associates, Carle Place, NY.)

TECHNICAL CONSIDERATIONS

Image Blur

Positioning of the part and its relationship to the image detector can influence image blur. For example, when the thoracic or lumbar spine is positioned laterally, there is an approximate 15 cm OFD. Image resolution is further degraded by the distance between the tabletop and the Bucky tray. This increase in OFD results in more than a 30% enlargement in the size of the vertebrae. See Chapter 1, Fig 1-4.

Shallow breathing techniques using low mA values and long exposure times can be used to blur out vascular markings overlying the vertebral bodies of the thoracic spine (Fig 5-41). Breathing techniques used for the lumbar region also help to blur gas shadows that could obscure the vertebral bodies or spinous processes.

> CAUTION: Breathing techniques are not recommended with survey images, since calcifications or other abdominal pathology may be obscured by breathing.

Placing the anode portion of the x-ray tube over the thinner body part takes advantage of the anode-heel effect. See Chapter 1, Figs 1-6 and 1-8. For example, in a study of the cervicothoracic area in the AP position, the anode should be positioned over the cervical area and the cathode over the thicker thoracic region. With steep-angle targets (12 degrees or less), the heel effect occurs over a smaller area and may be more obvious, particularly if the tube is positioned transverse to a body part of equal thickness, such as the pelvis or skull in the AP or PA position. Of equal importance is the difference in the projected focal spot size. The segment imaged on the anode side of the x-ray tube has the potential for increased sharpness when compared with the segment of the image on the cathode side. See Chapter 1, Fig 1-6.

Kilovoltage Selection

Osteolytic or osteoblastic conditions affect bone density and can have a significant influence on x-ray technique. For example, Paget's disease in its early stages can produce osteolytic changes; in later stages, it can cause the enlargement of bone, with a thickening of the cortex and significant trabecular pattern changes. See Chapter 3, Fig 3-8. Osteoblastic conditions require an increase in conventional technical factors, whereas osteolytic conditions require a decrease.

A reduction in calcium in an osseous structure attributable to either disuse or disease results in a reduction in subject contrast. It is often suggested that, when examining osteoporitic patients, the mAs be decreased about 15% to 25%. A better option would be to reduce kilovoltage to overcome inherent poor subject contrast. A high contrast film used with moderate to low kVp also helps to minimize poor subject contrast when examining patients with osteoporosis. Crossover control screen-film combinations combined with lower kilovoltage produce excellent short scale contrast images because approximately half of the crossover of light is eliminated within the cassette. See Chapter 1, Fig 1-19. Latitude films produce a longer scale of contrast and are of marginal value when used with osteoporitic patients.

Since the cervical spine is relatively thin as compared with the rest of the vertebral column, it is difficult to expose the full vertebral column uniformly with a single exposure.

The cervicothoracic junction can be well demonstrated at a 40 in FFD with tight beam collimation and a high kilovoltage technique similar to that used for chest radiography. The use of the higher kVp results in a latitude technique that helps to overcome the density differences between the cervical and thoracic regions. High kVp can produce a latitude "look" even when using a high contrast screen-film combination.

The thorax is easily overexposed because of the radiolucent nature of the adjacent lungs. Additional exposure is needed in the AP or PA position to demonstrate the thoracic spine situated within the aerated thorax and superimposed on the dense, blood-filled, mediastinal structures. The AP or PA thoracic-spine projection requires approximately the same exposure as the AP/PA projection of the lumbar spine. Exposure factors for the lateral thoracic spine approximate those needed for the AP/PA projection.

The upper thoracic vertebrae, however, can be difficult to demonstrate in the lateral position because of the muscular nature of the superimposed shoulders and the limited amount of lung tissue in the apical areas (Fig 5-40). It is easy to overexpose the lower thoracic vertebrae in the lateral position since the heart and mediastinal structures are situated anterior to the thoracic spine and there is increased aeration of the retrocardiac segments of the lungs (Fig 5-41).

Filtration

A sliding aluminum filter or lead acrylic filter at the collimator exit acts as a permanent overpart filter that can be used for a variety of compensatory filtering techniques (Figs 5-43 and 5-44). Also see Chapter 1, Fig 1-4. The use of a compensatory filter selectively allows more x-ray exposure to the upper thoracic vertebrae and less to the lower segment, helping to balance radiographic density.

Minken and Ahlgren[122] developed an easy-to-use cross-table myelographic filter technique to image the entire cervical spine and the C-6/T-2 region simultaneously with one exposure. With the patient prone, a plastic container (a barium enema bag) filled with a solution of 40 ml of Urografin/Renographin 45% contrast medium mixed with 2,500 ml of water was positioned against the patient's neck at the shoulder, "filtering" the x-ray beam to the cervical area.

Scatter Control

Most of the scatter undercutting an image results from unattenuated primary radiation striking the tabletop. A primary beam leak at the posterior aspect of the lateral spine can cause severe undercutting of the image. The use of a primary beam absorber, such as lead-rubber sheeting on the tabletop to minimize a primary beam leak, prevents undercutting of the spinous processes by scatter radiation. See Chapter 1, Fig 1-11.

> C A U T I O N : If horizontal beam lateral projections are made, the grid must be positioned with the lead lines centered to the CR to keep the grid in focus regardless of where top to bottom centering occurs. Any shift from left to right will cause a unilateral grid cutoff.

If a grid cassette is used for a tube angle projection, the cassette must be positioned with the grid lines parallel to the direction of the CR (Fig 5-46).

Two low ratio grids can be positioned at right angles to each other to form a crosshatch grid. The use of a crosshatch grid is helpful with a large patient when high kVp is required. A grid cassette positioned transverse in the Bucky tray will also produce a crosshatch effect. For example, if the Bucky mechanism contains a low ratio grid, a 6:1 ratio grid cassette positioned transversely with an 8:1 ratio Bucky grid results in the scatter cleanup capability of a 14:1 ratio grid. See Chapter 1, Fig 1-12.

> C A U T I O N : The CR must be centered to the center of both grids. Tube angle techniques are not possible with crosshatch grids. If the grid cassette contains a large amount of lead to minimize backscatter, an exit type automatic exposure device may not operate properly.

THE BONY THORAX

The bony thorax is the frame of the thoracic portion of the axial skeleton. It is composed of 12 pairs of ribs and the sternum and their cartilages.

ANATOMICAL/PATHOLOGICAL OBSERVATIONS

The first seven pairs of true (vertebrosternal) ribs are connected by costal cartilage directly to the sternum. Each of the eighth to tenth ribs (false or vertebrochondral) is connected by carti-

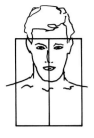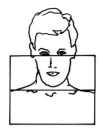

FIGURE 5–46   Grid Placement for Cross-table AP (oblique) Radiography

If it is necessary to angle the x-ray tube across the table, as in the magnified axial projection of the cervical articular facets (Figs 5-35 and 5-36), and if a grid is used for the study, the grid must be positioned as shown (left).

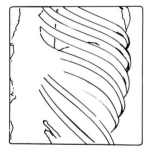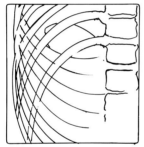

FIGURE 5–47   Tube Angulation for Radiography of the Ribs

Left, A tube angle of 20 to 30 degrees cephalad projects the ribs separately. Right, Angulation of the tube 30 degrees caudad projects the ribs onto each other. (Drawn from Pearson GR: Radiographic projection studies. *X-ray Technician* 1951;23:1-9.)

lage to the rib immediately above. The costal cartilage increases the length of the ribs, contributing to the elasticity of the thorax. The 11th and 12th ribs (false, floating, or vertebral) are not attached at their distal ends.

Portions of the ribs superimpose on the aerated lungs, the cardiac silhouette, or abdominal structures beneath the diaphragm, making radiographic visualization of the ribs difficult. Rib fractures may be as fine as a hairline and of little consequence, or they may exhibit serious displacement of fragments, causing hemothorax, pneumothorax, or subcutaneous emphysema.

POSITIONING CONCEPTS

Since the ribs curve in different planes, segments of the ribs must be visualized anteriorly, laterally, and posteriorly, as well as above and below the diaphragm. Sternal attachments and costovertebral articulations sometimes must be studied and may require special projections.

Perpendicular beam techniques are generally used. The hemithorax under study should be centered to the cassette. Oblique and angled projections may be used to avoid the overlapping of ribs and are recommended if the area of interest is in the axillary aspect of the thoracic cage. A cephalad tube tilt is used for AP and AP oblique positions, and a caudad tube tilt is used for PA and PA oblique positions. The degree of angulation, approximately 10 to 30 degrees, depends on patient habitus[123] (Fig 5-47).

The examination can be made in an erect or sitting position, if the patient can tolerate the procedure and if no other injuries are present. A metallic marker (lead B-B) is often used to identify a specific point of trauma.

> CAUTION: The lead shot marker should be removed upon completion of the examination. Patients have been known to leave markers in place for days. If not removed, the lead may become embedded in the chest wall, causing an inflammatory lesion.

If conventional AP, PA, or oblique projections do not demonstrate a rib fracture or lesion, the silhouette projection is recommended. See Chapter 2, Fig 2-8. Since the rib cage is a cylindrical structure, pathology in a rib can be best seen with the CR tangential to the pathology.[124]

TECHNICAL CONSIDERATIONS

Image Blur

The use of a small focal spot will minimize the image blur associated with an increased OFD, such as an anterior injury in a supine patient.

Kilovoltage Selection

In the early 1940s, low kilovolt/nongrid techniques using 40 to 55 kVp were recommended for radiography of the ribs above the diaphragm. The x-ray generators of that time were self-rectified or single phase, and these kilovoltage values, if correct, would have to be even lower if modern three-phase or constant-potential equipment were used. See Chapter 1, Fig 1-16.

If a grid were used, it usually was a 6:1 or 8:1 grid. Today, most Bucky grids are 12:1 ratio and produce excellent contrast at higher kVp levels.

> NOTE: Inspiration causes downward diaphragmatic excursion and demonstrates more of the upper rib cage. An expiration exposure, to visualize the ribs below the diaphragm, requires up to twice as much x-ray exposure as the above-diaphragm, full-inspiration technique. Exposure factors suitable for abdominal radiography, when combined with expiration, should adequately demonstrate the ribs below the diaphragm.

Screen-Film Technology

Contemporary x-ray techniques for radiography of above-the-diaphragm ribs utilize high ratio grids and moderate kVp values. The use of crossover control screen-film technology helps to produce abrupt black and white images. Rare earth intensifying screens combined with crossover control film permit the use of higher kilovoltages than do conventional screen-film combinations. A latitude film can be used to advantage when imaging the ribs (Fig 5-48).

> CAUTION: Rare earth screen-film combinations are kVp dependant and fall off in speed in the lower kilovolt ranges. See Chapter 1.

STERNUM

The sternum is connected to the first seven pairs of true ribs by costocartilage.

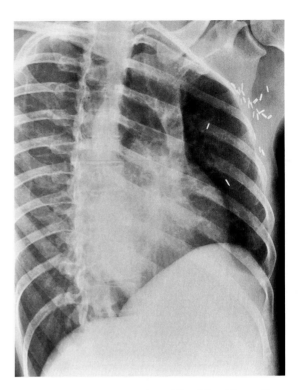

FIGURE 5-48 Radiography of the Ribs Above the Diaphragm Using Latitude Film

With a latitude x-ray film, abrupt black and white contrast is minimized. Note the excellent bony detail achieved without significant blackening of the lungs. (Courtesy Eastman Kodak Company, Rochester, NY.)

ANATOMICAL/PATHOLOGICAL CONSIDERATIONS

Fractures of the sternum are usually attributable to a direct violent force. Sometimes trauma in a specific area causes severe pain, masking other injuries such as a rib fracture, a punctured lung, or a pneumo- or hemothorax. See Chapter 7. Thoracic, abdominal, and head trauma must also be considered.[113]

POSITIONING CONCEPTS

Anterior structures of the chest, vessels, heart, and so on are considerably more radiodense than is the sternum. Superimposition of these

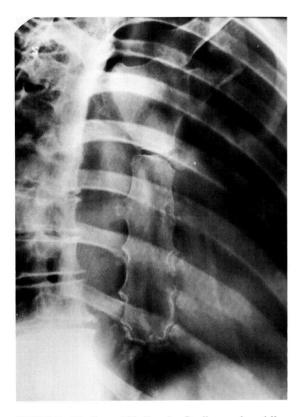

FIGURE 5–49 Use of Motion for Radiography of the Sternum

Superimposed pulmonary structures make it difficult to image the sternum. With the patient in the prone oblique position, an extended exposure time (5 seconds or greater) is used. The patient is asked to breathe rhythmically throughout the exposure. A low mA setting, combined with the long exposure, blurs out pulmonary vasculature.

structures on the ribs and the sternum may make it difficult to demonstrate the sternum in the AP or PA position.

It is interesting to review the literature concerning the development of special projections of the sternum. The use of the oblique position with a tube angle technique was reported in the literature as recently as 1988 in both American and British technical journals.[125,126] Actually, a similar projection was first developed in the early 1940s by Holly[127] to show the sternum free

of the thoracic spine, sternoclavicular articulations, and mediastinal structures. The patient is positioned prone, leaning across the long axis of the x-ray table. The position required for this projection may be difficult to assume and can only be used with ambulatory patients.

Garber[128] recommends angling the x-ray tube to the left side so that the sternum will be superimposed as completely as possible on the heart.

A patient with a small, asthenic chest requires a greater tube angle than does a larger patient with a well-developed chest in order to project the sternum away from the thoracic spine. Garber[128] recommends the following degrees of angulation at a 36 in distance (a 40 in FFD may be used): patient thickness of 20 cm, 19 degrees; of 25 cm, 15 degrees; and of 30 cm, 11 degrees.

Early sternum-demonstration techniques used a shortened FFD with the x-ray cone removed from the x-ray tube and the tube placed almost against the posterior thorax to blur out posterior structures. Since the sternum is against the cassette in this position, it remains in focus while the structures closer to the x-ray tube blur out. Large focal spots, often as great as 4 mm, contributed to image blur. This procedure is not recommended.

If a perpendicular beam is used, the degree of rotation of the patient can be determined by placing one hand on the sternum and the other on the thoracic vertebrae. The patient is then rotated until the vertebrae and sternum are no longer superimposed.[1,3]

The lateral view of the sternum is easy to obtain in either the recumbent or erect position. The hands should be clasped behind the back so that the shoulders are as far posterior as possible. Female breasts should be drawn laterally so that they do not superimpose on the sternum in the lateral position.

A conventional lateral chest radiograph often produces an excellent image of the lateral sternum.

Since many of these patients have a potential hemothorax or pneumothorax, a PA chest radiograph is often part of the positioning routine for evaluation of the sternum. See Chapter 7.

TECHNICAL CONSIDERATIONS

Motion may be used to help eliminate superimposed lung markings in the prone oblique position (Fig 5-49, page 147). The patient is instructed to breathe rhythmically during an extended exposure (5 seconds or greater) taken at a low mA setting. This shallow-breathing technique blurs out the pulmonary vasculature, as well as the ribs to a lesser degree. A similar technique is used to image the thoracic spine in the lateral position (Fig 5-41).

CAUTION: A patient in pain may find this breathing maneuver difficult to accomplish.

Scatter Control

The shape of the sternum in the lateral position follows the curvature of the chest and the typical collimated x-ray beam often results in a primary beam leak. Lead or other primary beam attenuating material should be placed on the x-ray table to absorb this radiation. The use of adjustable filters in the x-ray tube can also help to avoid this undercutting effect.[10] See Chapter 1, Fig 1-11.

CHAPTER SIX

The Abdomen: Plain-Film Imaging and Imaging of the Digestive and Genitourinary Systems

PLAIN-FILM IMAGING

A survey (scout) image of the abdomen, sometimes called a KUB (kidney, ureters, and bladder), often precedes radiography of the alimentary tract and the biliary, urinary, and reproductive systems. This study is performed to rule out congenital disorders, normal variants, and gross abnormalities before administering a contrast agent.

Other indications for conventional imaging of the abdomen include the evaluation of calcifications, gaseous patterns, masses, and organs for enlargement, duplication, or displacement and the presence of barium, opaque medication, or ingested foreign bodies.

The vascular and lymphatic networks found throughout the abdomen require special opacification techniques for their visualization.

ANATOMICAL AND PATHOLOGICAL OBSERVATIONS

Imaginary lines or planes divide the abdomen into nine regions (Fig 6-1, page 154). The ab-

dominopelvic cavity contains the stomach, the lower portion of the esophagus, the small and large intestines, the liver, the gallbladder, the spleen, the pancreas, the kidneys, the ureters, the bladder, and some reproductive organs. The peritoneum, a serous membrane, lines this cavity.

Adjacent structures of different densities provide subject contrast, which helps to identify normal anatomical and pathological conditions. Radiolucent fat produces subtle outlines of the psoas muscles, the liver, and the kidneys.[94]

A variety of names—such as peritoneal fat lines, properitoneal fat, retroperitoneal fat, and flank stripes—are used to describe the fat shadows that extend inferiorly from the lateral rib margins on both sides and gradually fade out over the iliac crests[27] (Fig 6-2, page 154).

Any gas seen outside of the bowel is diagnostically significant.

POSITIONING CONCEPTS

Basic positioning routines for abdominal procedures vary with departmental preference. Tables 6-1 through 6-4 summarize the routine projec-

TABLE 6-1 The AP/PA Abdomen

Area	Position of Patient/Part	Projection of Central Ray	Demonstrates (View)
Abdomen (Survey) AP	Patient supine or erect; median plane centered to midline of table or upright grid; no rotation of the body	CR directed perpendicular to film plane, to enter at the level of the iliac crests	Size and shape of liver; spleen and kidneys; abdominal masses or calcification; osseous structures of the pelvis, lower spine, and ribs
PA	Patient prone; see Abdomen AP position	See Abdomen AP projection	See Abdomen AP view
Colon (barium filled)	See Abdomen AP position	See Abdomen AP projection	Opacified colon
Small bowel (barium filled)	See Abdomen position; initial film in series should be centered above iliac crests to include duodenal bulb	See Abdomen projection	Opacified small bowel
Stomach (barium filled) AP	Patient supine; midportion of left half of abdomen centered to midline of the table	CR directed perpendicular to film plane, to enter at level of L-1	Opacified stomach and duodenum
PA	Patient prone; see Stomach AP position	See Stomach AP projection	See Stomach AP view
Oral cholecysto- graphy	Patient prone; right half of abdomen aligned to midline of tabletop	CR directed perpendicular to film plane to enter right side at level of ninth rib (varies with patient habitus	Opacified gallbladder
Excretory urography (contrast study)	See Abdomen position	See Abdomen projection	Opacified kidneys, ureters, and urinary bladder; osseous and soft-tissue structures of the abdomen

TABLE 6–2 The AP/PA Oblique Abdomen

Area	Position of Patient	Projection of Central Ray	Demonstrates (View)
Abdomen	Patient supine or prone in 45 to 70 degree RPO, LPO, or LAO, RAO position; degree of rotation depends on patient habitus	CR directed perpendicular to film plane	Soft-tissue structures of abdomen; lower spine; pelvis
Colon (barium filled)	See Abdomen position	See Abdomen	Opacified colon; splenic flexure; descending colon
	RPO	CR directed perpendicular to enter to the left of the median plane	
	LAO	CR directed perpendicular to enter to the right of the median plane	
	LPO	CR directed perpendicular to enter to the right of the median plane	Hepatic flexure; ascending colon; sigmoid colon
	RAO	CR directed perpendicular to enter to the left of the median plane	
Stomach (barium filled)			
PA	Patient prone in 40 to 70 degree RAO position; longitudinal plane midway between vertebrae and the anterior surface of the elevated side (left) coincides with the midline of the tabletop	CR directed perpendicular to film plane, to enter at about 1.5 in above lateral margin of lower ribs (L-2)	Opacified stomach; duodenum
AP	Patient supine in 40 to 70 degree LPO position; midportion of left side of abdomen aligned with midline of tabletop	See Stomach AP projection; CR directed perpendicular to film plane to enter 2.5 in below xiphoid (T-2)	See Stomach AP view

(continued)

TABLE 6–2 *continued*

Area	Position of Patient	Projection of Central Ray	Demonstrates (View)
Oral cholecysto-graphy	Patient prone in 15 to 40 degree LAO position	CR directed perpendicular to film plane, to enter midway between spinous process and right lateral margin of the body at the level of the gallbladder, as determined by the survey image	Opacified gallbladder
Excretory urography	Patient supine in 30 degree LPO or RPO position; longitudinal plane through vertebral column is parallel to midline of the tabletop	CR directed perpendicular to film plane, to enter at level of the iliac crests midway between median plane and lateral surface of elevated side	Opacified kidneys; ureters
	LPO		Right kidney in profile; proximal portion of right ureter may be superimposed on spine
	RPO		Left kidney in profile; proximal portion of left ureter may be superimposed on spine

TABLE 6–3 **Lateral Decubitus Abdomen**

Area	Position of Part/Patient	Projection of Central Ray	Demonstrates (View)
Abdomen (right or left)	Patient recumbent in lateral decubitus position, knees slightly flexed	CR directed horizontally and perpendicular to film to enter median plane of the body at the level of the iliac crests	Soft-tissue structures and gas-filled organs; pelvis; lower spine
AP	Dorsal surface of body close to edge of table and against cassette		
PA	Anterior surface of body close to edge of table and against cassette		

(continued)

TABLE 6–3 *continued*

Area	Position of Part/Patient	Projection of Central Ray	Demonstrates (View)
Colon (barium filled)	See Abdomen position	See Abdomen projection	Opacified colon
(double contrast)			Colon opacified with barium and air
Oral cholecystography	Patient in right lateral decubitus position; body raised to center gallbladder to 8 in by 10 in film	CR directed horizontally and perpendicular to the film plane to enter the right upper quadrant of the abdomen	Small gallstones heavier than bile seen only when accumulated in dependent gallbladder; stones lighter than bile seen only by stratification

TABLE 6–4 **The Lateral Abdomen**

Area	Position of Part/Patient	Projection of Central Ray	Demonstrates (View)
Abdomen	Patient recumbent, in lateral position (right or left); abdomen centered to midline of table; knees flexed; body not rotated	CR directed perpendicular to film plane, to enter at level of crest of the ilium	Soft-tissue structures of abdomen; lower vertebrae; antevertebral space occupied by aorta; intra-abdominal calcifications or tumor masses
Colon (barium filled)	See Abdomen position	See Abdomen projection	Opacified colon
Stomach (barium filled)	See Abdomen position	CR directed perpendicular to film plane, to enter midway between midaxillary line and anterior surface of the abdomen at the level of L-1	Opacified stomach; duodenal bulb; Duodenal loop
Oral cholecystography	Patient recumbent, in right lateral position; abdomen to midline of tabletop	CR directed perpendicular to film plane, to enter midway between the spinous processes and the anterior margin of the body	Opacified gallbladder

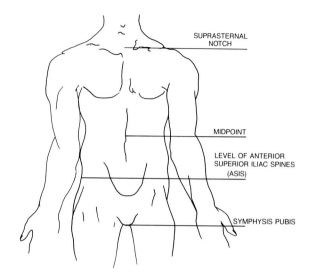

FIGURE 6–1(A) Surface Points of the Chest and Abdomen

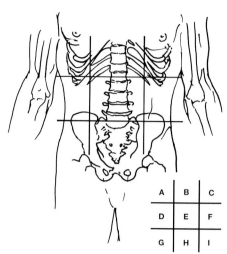

FIGURE 6–1(B) Regions of the Abdomen

(A) Right Hypochondriac
(B) Epigastric
(C) Left Hypochondriac
(D) Right Lumbar
(E) Umbilical
(F) Left Lumbar
(G) Right Inguinal
(H) Hypogastric
(I) Left Inguinal

tions presented to show that often only slight modifications are required to obtain similar views of adjacent areas.

Plain-film imaging of the abdomen usually begins with an AP supine image. Free intraperitoneal air will be demonstrated by horizontal beam radiography in 85% of the patients with a perforated viscus.[129] An upright chest image helps in the diagnosis of perforated hollow viscera. Free air, when present, pockets beneath the diaphragm within the abdomen, but takes time to rise to the highest point when the patient is placed in the upright position.

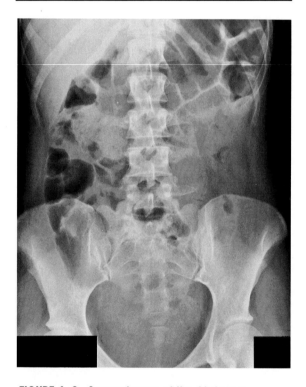

FIGURE 6–2 Survey Image of the Abdomen

There are significant radiolucent gas patterns throughout the intestines. Note the presence of radiolucent flank stripes from the lateral rib margins extending to the iliac crests bilaterally. (Courtesy Eastman Kodak Company, Rochester, NY.)

> C A U T I O N : When possible, the patient should be placed erect for a few minutes prior to the exposure to allow time for the air to rise and / or better to demonstrate air–fluid levels in the dilated bowel loops seen in many acute abdominal conditions. The upright position is often difficult to attain for an acutely ill patient.

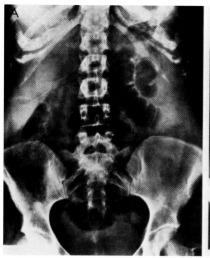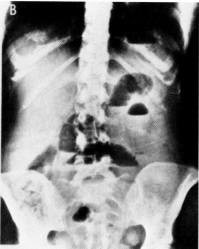

FIGURE 6–3 Supine versus Erect Abdomen

(A) A supine radiograph made to evaluate mechanical obstruction in small intestine shows a distended small bowel. (B) The upright radiograph (horizontal beam technique) shows dynamic air–fluid levels. (Courtesy Keats T: *Emergency Radiology.* Chicago, Year Book Medical Publishers Inc, 1984.)

With ambulatory patients or those transported to the x-ray department in a wheel-chair, the following sequence of exposures is recommended.

1. PA erect chest, if part of departmental routine. Pneumonia, atelectasis, or pleural fluid can often accompany acute abdominal disease.

> N O T E : High kVp / grid chest images help to visualize retrocardiac and retrodiaphragmatic disease.

2. Horizontal beam imaging of the abdomen. See Chapter 2, Fig 2-8. A horizontal beam image (erect or decubitus) should demonstrate dynamic air–fluid levels, a stepladder effect in the bowel (Fig 6-3).

   a. Upright abdomen to include the diaphragms, when indicated.

> C A U T I O N : If the patient is only partially elevated, a horizontal beam exposure will distort anatomy. Partial elevation of a patient because of patient condition requires that the x-ray beam be directed horizontally to demonstrate an air–fluid level within hollow viscera. Positioning the CR perpendicular to the patient and cassette allows a more accurate representation of the anatomy, but may miss an air–fluid level. See Chapter 2, Fig 2-5.

   b. Decubitus abdomen (horizontal beam)

   b-1. Lateral decubitus. When the patient cannot tolerate the erect position, a decubitus position is recommended. In the lateral decubitus position, patients lie on their side. The left lateral decubitus position (left side down, right side up) is used to demonstrate free air in the abdomen. If possible, patients should be placed on their left side for transport to radiology. The motion associated with transportation helps pocket any free air in the elevated portion of the abdomen. A nongrid chest technique with the cassette centered to include the right upper quadrant of the abdomen, diaphragm, and right lower lung will demonstrate free air superimposed on the gas-free liver. This lateral decubitus image can be made using a mobile unit if the patient is not able to undergo an abdominal imaging series (Fig 6-4). The condition of the patient limits the amount of time that the patient can tolerate the lateral decubitus position. A delay of ten minutes is suggested to allow the air to rise to the elevated side.

C A U T I O N : If the patient is placed in the right lateral decubitus position (right side down, left side up), free air may superimpose on the aerated splenic flexure of the colon or fundus of the stomach and may not be easily identified.

    b-2. Dorsal or ventral decubitus. The dorsal or ventral decubitus position may be employed for the examination of an immobile patient. See Chapter 2, Fig 2-8.

  c. Tangential. If it is not possible to obtain a horizontal beam radiograph (erect or lateral decubitus), a tangential horizontal beam image with the patient in the supine position may be used to demonstrate free air in the abdomen. See Chapter 2, Fig 2-8; Chapter 7, Fig 7-17.

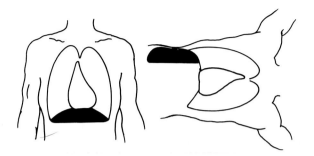

FIGURE 6–4 Lateral Decubitus Radiography for Free Air in the Abdomen

Left, An upright chest radiograph will often demonstrate free air beneath the diaphragm. Right, If the patient is positioned in the left lateral decubitus position, air will rise and superimpose on the gas-free lateral aspect of the liver.

    3. AP supine abdomen. An acute abdominal series to rule out free air or bowel obstruction should include a supine radiograph centered at the iliac crest, as well as an erect abdominal image and an upright PA chest study made with a 6 ft FFD.

Unless pathology in the posteroinferior lungs is suspected, the PA chest radiograph should adequately demonstrate the diaphragmatic areas. In an attempt to show the diaphragms on the upright abdomen, the lower portion of the abdomen may be cut off.

It is important to demonstrate the right iliac fossa to confirm an absence of gas or fecal shadows, commonly associated with acute appendicitis, Crohn's disease, and carcinoma of the cecum.[130] A gynecological mass may also account for the absence of gas or fecal material in the right iliac fossa.[131]

The erect image can also be used to diagnose an inguinal hernia, which may be present but is not seen in the supine image. The lower edge of the cassette should be positioned below the symphysis pubis to include the full obturator foramen, even though the diaphragms may not be included in this view (Fig 6-5). A decubitus position will not demonstrate a herniation.[131]

The diaphragm must be included in at least one erect view to demonstrate its relationship to

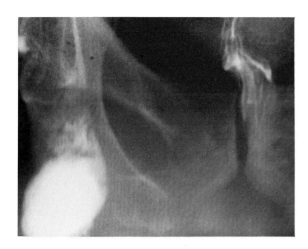

FIGURE 6–5   Segment of an Erect Abdominal Image

If an air-filled or barium-filled inguinal hernia is suspected and not seen in the supine image, the cassette must be positioned below the symphysis pubis to include the full obturator foramen. (Courtesy LO Martinez, Mount Sinai Medical Center, Miami, Fla.)

the lung fields. For the examination of large patients, it may necessary to place the cassette crosswise and make two separate exposures. A chest radiograph can be helpful in demonstrating a hiatal hernia.

CONDITIONS OR DISEASES MERITING SPECIAL CONSIDERATION

Bowel Obstruction

Blockage of the lumen of the large or small bowel results in a mechanical obstruction whereas decreased peristalsis in the small bowel produces a paralytic ileus. Both types of obstruction require supine and horizontal beam projections for optimal visualization.

If a gallstone obstructs the ileocecal valve, a small bowel obstruction may result. A stone may also erode through the wall of the gallbladder, creating a fistula to the small bowel. Since most gallstones are radiolucent, their visualization is difficult on plain radiographs.

Additional views can be helpful when an obstruction is suspected. Two supine abdomen radiographs made 15 minutes apart can be used to determine changes in the distribution of small-bowel loops. With the patient supine, a lateral projection of the anterior abdomen using a horizontal beam may help to evaluate air–fluid levels in an obese patient. See Chapter 2, Fig 2-8.

Intraperitoneal Air

Perforation of hollow viscera, as a result of disease or trauma may result in a pneumoperitoneum. Surgical intervention in the abdomen may also introduce air into the peritoneal cavity. When the patient is supine, the gas collects centrally beneath the abdominal wall and it is difficult to identify on the conventional supine radiograph.[89]

As little as 2 cc of intraperitoneal air can be seen if the patient is maintained in an upright position for 20 minutes prior to the making of a radiograph.[27] Since these patients are often in distress from intestinal perforation, this delay is not always possible.

CAUTION: Upright or decubitus images should be made on trauma patients with possible vertebral injury only if the spine has been evaluated and fracture ruled out.

Air in the Soft Tissues

Free air in the soft tissues can indicate puncture of an air-filled structure or an infection such as gas gangrene. See Chapter 3, Fig 3-11.

Ureteral Calculi

Nearly all urinary tract calculi are calcified. Plain films of the abdomen (AP and/or oblique) may show small calcific densities representing ureteral calculi or phleboliths. Rounded calcifications with central lucent holes or calcifications projected below the iliac spine are likely to be phleboliths. Irregularly shaped calcifications are likely to be ureteral calculi. Excretory urography is required for differentiation.[27]

Calcification in the kidneys sometimes can be masked by gas shadows. A prone radiograph may shift the gas away from the kidneys.

Accurate visualization of renal calculi with regard to changes in the size, number, or position of the stones is possible with conventional tomography of the kidneys. Tomographic sections made at intervals of 0.5 to 1 cm throughout the entire kidney can outline the renal size, contour, calcifications, and masses. This technique is particularly helpful if there is a previous history of reaction to contrast media. The size and number of stones can be more accurately determined with tomography than with ultrasonography.

Aneurysm

An outpouching or ballooning of a vessel wall can often be detected by the presence of calcification in the wall of an aneurysm. The pulsations of an abdominal aortic aneurysm may cause an erosion of the anterior segment of the adjacent lumbar vertebrae.

Fluid in the Abdomen

Ascites, an accumulation of serous fluid within the peritoneal cavity, changes the radiographic appearance of the survey image of the abdomen. Radiographically, organs within the abdomen lose their edges as fluid increases. Erect-position or other horizontal beam imaging can be used to demonstrate the fluid gravitating to the dependent portion of the abdomen.

Pregnancy

X-ray exposure of fertile females should be made only during the first ten days of the menstrual cycle (from the first day that menses begins). During the first trimester, x-radiation should be avoided unless the patient's condition requires a radiographic investigation. During the second and third trimesters, dosage should be limited as much as practical.

Ultrasound is the imaging modality of choice for evaluation of the abdomen for fetal measurements. Pelvimetry is rarely performed, and is used only if measurements of the bony pelvis of the gravid female are needed; it can provide an approximation of fetal age by visualizing the ossification patterns of the fetal bones. If a pelvimetry is needed, rare earth intensifying screen-film systems (up to 1,200 speed), combined with high kilovoltage, can greatly reduce x-radiation dosage (Fig 6-6).

Localization of Surgical Sponges

Surgical sponges contain radiopaque threads for easy identification by radiography (Fig 6-7). The density, size, shape, texture, and attenuation characteristics of the thread, as well as the quality of the x-ray equipment, film, and processing system, affect the detection of surgical swabs and sponges. Overlying surrounding tissue and bony structures of the body can obscure the radiopaque threads.[27,132]

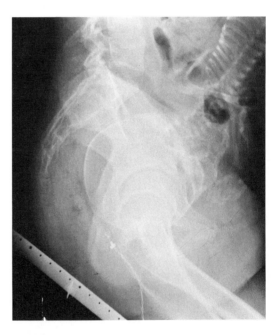

FIGURE 6-6 Pelvimetry

This image was made using a 1,200 speed screen-film system and high kilovoltage (110 kVp), significantly reducing radiation exposure. A Colcher-Sussman pelvimeter is in position for measurement purposes. (Courtesy Eastman Kodak Company, Rochester, NY.)

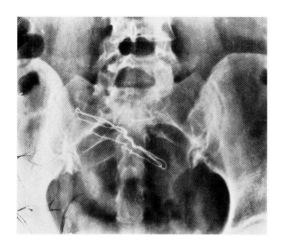

FIGURE 6-7 Localization of Surgical Sponges

An intra-abdominal surgical sponge is identified by the fine radiopaque threads used to make the sponge visible on x-ray. (Courtesy Keats T: *Emergency Radiology*. Chicago, Year Book Medical Publishers Inc, 1984.)

Localization of Foreign Bodies

Images for localizing foreign bodies must be made at right angles to each other. See Chapter 2, Fig 2-1.

Although foreign bodies generally pass easily through the alimentary canals of most patients, their ingestion does result in the deaths of some 2,000 children in the United States every year. The most common foreign bodies ingested by children are nuts and seeds (particularly peanuts) and lead-paint chips.[133]

Button-type alkaline batteries (used in cameras and watches) become time-release packets of lye. A small battery, if delayed in passage through the gastrointestinal (GI) tract, may leak its contents and result in an esophageal burn, perforation, or mercury poisoning.[133]

TECHNICAL CONSIDERATIONS

In the early years of radiography, all radiographs were "flat plates"—images made on thin sheets of glass with a single coating of emulsion. The scout or survey study of the abdomen was first known as a flat plate of the abdomen. In the 1920s, the glass plate was replaced by a cellulose-acetate base coated with dual emulsions. Today's film bases are made of plastic.

Image Blur

Exposures of the abdomen should be made at suspended respiration after complete exhalation. Forced exhalation may result in an increase in involuntary motion. If long exposure times are required, breathing or peristalsis may degrade the image.

The presence of overlying gas, drainage tubes, opaque sutures, or, occasionally, contrast media can influence the perception of radiographic detail.

Image blur increases as OFD is increased; for example, a surgical sponge lying anterior, near an incision, may be difficult to detect. The shortened FFD, common in some bedside- and operating-room studies of large patients, almost always results in imaging difficulties.

Kilovoltage Selection

An air-distended bowel produces a significant increase in the thickness of the abdomen. If technical factors are increased because of the air-distended abdomen, the image may be a greatly overexposed. Conversely, an abdomen distended by intra-abdominal fluid or blood necessitates an increase in exposure factors for adequate penetration.

High contrast images, made at moderate kVp, are needed to demonstrate calcific changes, such as flecks of calcium in arteries or veins or opaque gallstones or kidney stones.

Scatter Control

When it is necessary to include the abdomen from the symphysis pubis to above the diaphragm, a 48 in FFD can be used if this distance is within the focal range of the grid. See Chapter 1, Table 1-2.

Scatter from a primary beam leak can sometimes undercut the lateral aspects of an abdominal image, masking the flank stripes and adjacent anatomical structures. Tight beam collimation and the placement of lead sheeting on the tabletop can minimize image undercutting. See Chapter 1, Fig 1-11.

Radiographs to detect surgical swabs, sponges, or instruments are often made with low-power mobile equipment in the operating room or recovery area (Fig 6-7). Low ratio grids minimize grid focusing problems and help to overcome the limited output of some mobile equipment. Also, screen-film combinations of up to 1,200 speed can be used with mobile equipment at the bedside or in the operating room to augment limited output.

THE DIGESTIVE SYSTEM

The digestive system includes the alimentary canal, salivary glands, pancreas, liver, and biliary system. These organs help in the digestion and absorption of food and the elimination of waste. Peristalsis, an involuntary, progressive wavelike movement in the hollow alimentary canal, causes the contents of the hollow organs to be moved forward.

ANATOMICAL AND PATHOLOGICAL OBSERVATIONS

Contrast agents—air or gas (negative), water (isodense), barium, or aqueous iodine (positive) —are needed to evaluate the GI system radiographically.

The pharynx, shared with the respiratory and digestive systems, is the passageway for air from the nasal cavity to the larynx and for food from the mouth to the esophagus. It extends from the base of the skull to the level of C-6, where it becomes contiguous with the esophagus.

The esophagus extends from the pharynx to the stomach and carries food and liquids from the mouth to the stomach. It passes in front of the vertebral column through the upper portion of the mediastinum, slightly to the left of the midline. At the level of T-11, the esophagus opens into the cardiac orifice of the stomach. The stomach occupies the left upper quadrant of the abdomen and lies below the diaphragm to the right of the spleen, partially under the liver. The internal surface of the stomach is lined with a mucosal membrane that forms longitudinal folds (rugae).

The stomach contents empty by peristaltic activity, which normally takes place at the rate of about three peristaltic waves per minute. The movement is initiated in the body of the stomach and continues toward the pylorus. Peristalsis, moving food or contrast media rapidly from the mouth to the stomach, changes the outline and shape of the stomach. The small bowel originates at the duodenal bulb and terminates at the cecum. The duodenum, the first part of the small intestine, connects with the pylorus of the stomach and extends to the jejunum. The jejunum loops to the left upper quadrant of the abdomen, to terminate at the ileum, in the right upper quadrant. The ileum passes through the right and left lower quadrants and terminates at the ileocecal junction. Multiple small vascular projections of the mucous membrane (intestinal villi) extend into the lumen of the small bowel and aid in digestion by absorbing fluids and nutrients. These fingerlike mucosal villi (500 to 800 μm in length and 300 μm in thickness) cover the mucosal surface of the normal small bowel.[134] The large bowel, from the terminal ileum to the anus, is about 5 ft long. It includes the cecum, the ascending colon, the hepatic flexure, the transverse colon, the splenic flexure, the descending colon, the sigmoid, the rectum, and the anus.

POSITIONING CONCEPTS

Radiographic investigation of the GI system commonly consists of a combination of fluoroscopy and radiography. Fluoroscopy provides dynamic information, whereas radiographs (fluoroscopic spot films or Bucky follow-up images) furnish a permanent (static) record of the examination.

For positioning purposes, a simple schematic can be used to illustrate the GI tract in three dimensions[135] (Fig 6-8).

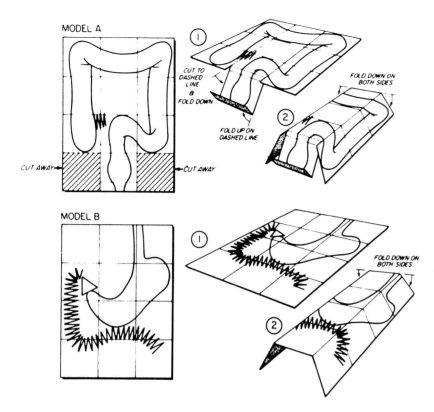

FIGURE 6–8   Schematic Models Made from Paper or Clear Film to Illustrate the Three-Dimensional GI Tract

This teaching aid can be used to help illustrate the effect of patient positioning on barium and air. Gas and barium change positions throughout the hollow viscera of the patient during a typical sequence of imaging. Since barium is heavy, it flows downward with gravity, while the gas rises. (Courtesy Munro TG: Brief communication: A simple model for teaching double-contrast examinations of the gastrointestinal tract. *J Can Assoc Radiol* 1989; 40: 162-163.)

Most upper GI studies begin with the patient in an erect position. This position helps to evaluate air–fluid levels in the alimentary tract. An esophageal study is usually performed as part of the upper GI study. During fluoroscopy, the esophagus can be viewed in the erect, horizontal, or Trendelenburg position. Fluoroscopic spot films are used with various combinations of breathing and positioning maneuvers.

GASTROINTESTINAL IMAGING

Barium sulfate (an insoluble substance), the contrast medium generally employed for examina-tion of the GI tract, is contraindicated in cases of GI-tract perforation.

> C A U T I O N :   Barium should not be administered in the presence of a suspected perforation.

If a perforation is suspected, a water-soluble ionic contrast agent should be utilized. This type of contrast is easily absorbed in the peritoneal cavity and excreted by the kidneys. Barium sul-fate, if spilled into the peritoneal cavity, could re-sult in a septic condition.

A water-soluble contrast material (iodine) administered orally will traverse the small intestines into the colon within two hours. The low viscosity of a water-soluble contrast medium makes it useful in evaluating an obscure or suspected intestinal perforation.[27]

Specific GI pathology may require a change in the preparation and consistency of the barium mixture. A thicker, pastelike barium mixture may be used for esophageal studies, along with a barium tablet to evaluate the transport of a solid bolus in the pharyngoesophagus and to determine the diameter of its lumen.[36]

After the ingestion of a barium mixture, the stomach is evaluated for contour, position, rugae, and peristaltic activity. Small amounts of barium manipulated over the surface of the mucosa during fluoroscopy demonstrate the mucosal relief pattern.

Because of the variations in the size and mobility of the stomach, it is difficult to give precise external localization points for positioning (Fig 6-8). It may be helpful to the radiographer if the fluoroscopist makes surface markings on the patient to aid in follow-up positioning.

Barium-filled segments of the small bowel have a distinctive appearance. The duodenal pattern is transverse and rigid. The jejunal mucosa appears delicate and feathery. The folds of the ileum resemble those of the duodenum.

The motility of the small bowel is quite rapid. Bowel function determines the transit time (up to six hours or longer) of the ingested barium meal. As the barium moves through the small intestines, full field images are made at specific intervals to evaluate motility and abnormalities within the small bowel. Sometimes follow-up images are made at 24, 48, or 72 hours following the ingestion of barium to check the progress of the barium meal.

The sequence and number of fluoroscopic spot film and follow-up overhead images needed for GI studies are determined by departmental preferences. Time-interval markers are needed on each image to document function on delayed studies.

Esophageal Imaging

Barium sulfate is usually used to outline the esophagus, commonly examined as part of an upper GI study. Short exposure times must be used during swallowing-function studies of the esophagus in the cervical area.

The RAO (35 to 40 degrees oblique) demonstrates the barium-filled esophagus between the vertebrae and the heart and aids in the study of the contour of the heart.

A barium-filled gelatin capsule may be used to evaluate esophageal obstruction or function in what seems to be a normal or equivocal barium esophagogram. Empty capsules, ranging from 1.5 to 10 mm in diameter and 15 to 25 mm in length (and available at any pharmacy), are flexible, inexpensive, and safe. Patient size and symptoms will determine the diameter of the capsule. After being swallowed, the barium-filled capsule retains its shape for about 10 to 15 seconds—long enough to evaluate an obstruction and for the capsule to dissolve and pass the site of obstruction.[136]

A drinking cup designed for double contrast esophagography includes a holder for barium, a feeding arrangement for air, and a feed valve that, in part, blocks the free discharge of barium from the cup. Continuous ingestion from this cup almost always results in successful double contrast imaging (after 5 to 10 seconds of ingestion). The patient drinks throughout the imaging while pinching the nose to increase the intake of air.[137]

Imaging of Foreign Bodies in the Esophagus. About two thirds of all foreign bodies can be demonstrated by radiography. Large bones, US coins, metallic objects, and drug packets can usually be seen. Fish bones, meat, and most other foods are more difficult to visualize. Small bones, foreign coins, peanuts, sunflower seeds, popcorn, plastic objects, and video-game tokens may or may not be seen, depending on their absorptive nature.[138]

Flat objects in the esophagus usually align in the coronal plane and are best seen in an AP view. In the trachea, flat objects are usually found in the sagittal plane. A lateral view best demonstrates a coin in the trachea.[138]

In the lateral view, the esophagus is seen between the vertebral bodies of the air-filled trachea, which helps to identify the position of a foreign body. See Chapter 7, Fig 7-27.

After plain-film evaluation, another method of establishing the presence of a foreign body in the esophagus is to have the patient swallow a cotton pledget (a small flat compress) drenched with barium. The ingested radiopaque cotton may be caught on the foreign body.[96]

CAUTION: Barium mixtures, particularly those with adhesive qualities, should not be used until conventional radiographs have been viewed to determine whether technical factors and positioning are adequate.

THE UPPER GI TRACT

Single Contrast Study

A single contrast study can be performed as a mucosal-relief study, as a complete filling study, or as a compression study. The complete filling or full-column study outlines the hollow viscera of the GI tract. A single contrast study made with high density barium may mask a lesion in a too-dense pool of barium. In the mucosal-relief study, the radiologist applies a small amount of barium to the mucosa. The compression study, made with moderate density barium, demonstrates tiny mucosal irregularities.[139]

Double Contrast Study

The double contrast study requires coating the inner surface of a hollow viscus with a thin coat of barium (positive contrast). Gas (a negative contrast) is used to distend the barium-coated stomach and/or bowel for better visualization of the mucosal lining (Fig 6-9).

On contact with fluid in the stomach, effervescent granules, tablets, or powders swallowed by the patient rapidly release as much as 300 to 400 mL of carbon dioxide on contact with the fluid in the stomach.[140] Other gases, such as carbon dioxide or gases released by carbonated beverages or gas-forming powders, may also be used.

Biphasic Study

A biphasic study employs both the single contrast, full-column technique and the double con-

trast technique to avoid the pitfalls of one or the other.

Many authors advocate a biphasic examination and use gas introduced by the bubbly-barium carbonated cocktail method (100% wt/vol, barium suspension) described by Op den Orth.[139] If the patient belches, commercially available effervescent powders may be used to produce additional gas.[139] The special bubbly-barium preparation is easily prepared with the assistance of a pharmacist.

Another barium formulation (96.8% wt/vol, sp gr 1.82), which can be prepared in the x-ray department, combines good mucosal coating properties in the double contrast phase with better penetration of the barium in the single-contrast study.[139-141]

For more specific information on barium preparations, a review by Op den Orth is suggested.[139] A comprehensive description of pa-

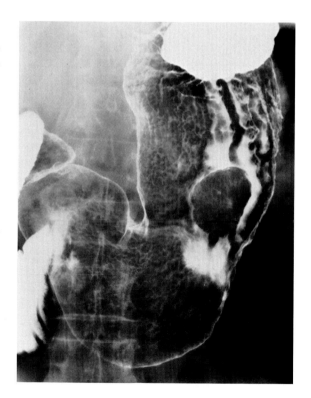

FIGURE 6–9 Double Contrast Study of the Stomach

(Courtesy Eastman Kodak Company, Rochester, NY.)

tient positioning for these studies is presented in an article by Levine and his colleagues.[140]

Hypotonic Duodenography

To perform hypotonic duodenography, an intestinal tube is passed via the mouth into the duodenum, which has been temporarily paralyzed by a drug (usually glucagon) given intravenously or intramuscularly prior to the examination. Glucagon diminishes gastric peristalsis and promotes relaxation of the lower esophageal sphincter and an increase in gastroesophogeal reflux.

During the atonic state, the duodenum can be distended to two to three times its normal size, pressing against and outlining the head of the pancreas. Either CT or ultrasonography, if available, will demonstrate the pancreas with less discomfort to the patient.

With delayed emptying, double contrast views can be obtained before the stomach is obscured by overlapping loops of the barium-filled duodenum or other segments of the small bowel.[1] Levin[140] describes double contrast imaging of the upper GI tract using an ingestion of effervescent granules and high density barium, after the injection of a hypotonic agent (glucagon).

The small bowel may also be studied radiographically by means of a small-bowel enema (enteroclysis). With this technique, an intestinal tube is advanced to the end of the duodenum (proximal jejunum) via the patient's mouth. Positive- (barium) and negative- (air) contrast agents are injected directly into the small bowel (Fig 6-10).

Imaging of the Small Bowel

The unique anatomy and remote location of the small bowel make it the most difficult segment of the alimentary tract to examine. There are more techniques for examining the small bowel than the combined total of upper-GI-tract and colon studies. A classic description of small-bowel radiography by Maglinte and his colleagues[142] is recommended for those who would like an update on improvements in barium imaging of the small bowel, who want to review guidelines

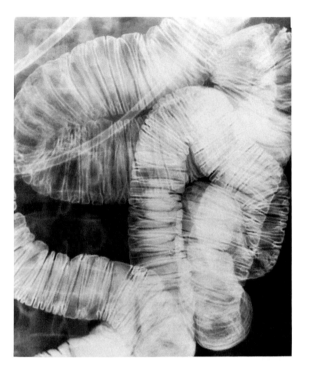

FIGURE 6–10 Small-Bowel Enema

(Courtesy Eastman Kodak Company, Rochester, NY.)

based on clinical indications for these studies, or who want an overview of the future direction of small-bowel radiography.[142]

THE LOWER GI TRACT

Proper preparation is essential for quality studies of the colon. Every department has a preferred preparation routine. If the patient has had a colostomy, ileostomy, or jejunostomy, the contrast agent may be administered through the stoma in the abdominal wall.

Single Contrast Study

The lower GI tract is examined by administering a barium sulfate enema for a full-column study.

Double Contrast Study

Double contrast enemas require a positive contrast agent (barium) and a negative contrast

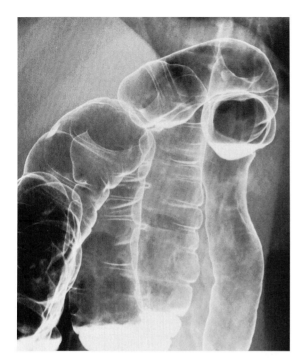

FIGURE 6–11 Fluoroscopic Spot Image, Double Contrast Barium Enema, Erect Position

(Courtesy Eastman Kodak Company, Rochester, NY.)

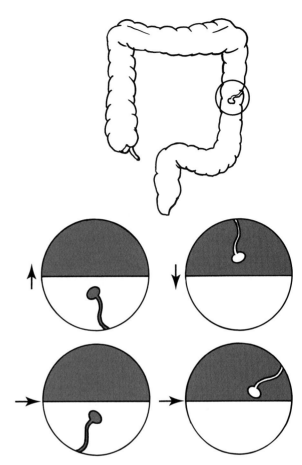

FIGURE 6–12 Effect of Positioning on a Polyp

Top, A polyp with a long, narrow stalk is shown on the wall of the descending colon. Bottom, Circular images demonstrate the polyp within the air-filled or barium-filled segments of the colon. In most situations, barium will coat the lining of the colon as well as the polyp. This illustration shows the polyp within the barium as a lucent shadow and within the air-filled colon as a structure lightly coated with barium.

agent (air), which distend the lumen and allow improved visualization of the mucosal lining, especially small polyps and intraluminal tumors (Fig 6-11).

An adenamatous polyp is a small sacular mass of tissue that arises from the wall of the colon and projects into the bowel lumen. Polyps may be sessile in nature, with a wide base, or they may be pedunculated, attached to the wall of the bowel by a long, narrow stalk. When surrounded by barium, a rounded filling defect is usually seen. When coated with barium, as in air contrast studies, sometimes the stalk is visible. Since barium is heavy, it flows downward, owing to gravity, and gas rises. By maneuvering the patient, the gas and barium are manipulated throughout the large bowel. Multiple views are helpful in the demonstration of polyps (Fig 6-12).

A compensatory filter used for decubitus air contrast imaging is employed to equalize radiographic density (Fig 6-13).

TECHNICAL CONSIDERATIONS

Image Blur

A small focal spot (0.6 mm) combined with a high ratio grid (10:1 ratio or greater) results in Bucky-quality fluoroscopic spot film images (Figs 6-11, 6-14, and 6-15). Bucky follow-up radiographs (10 in by 12 in or smaller) can often be eliminated owing to the Bucky-like quality of the

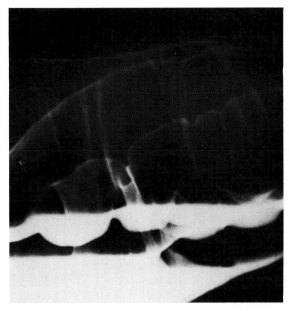

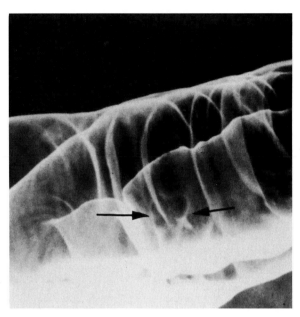

A

B

FIGURE 6-13 Compensatory Filter for Lateral Decubitus Radiography

Lateral decubitus images used with double contrast barium enemas exhibit extreme differences in film densities. Barium gravitates to the lower portions of the colon, while air rises to the top. (A) In a conventional decubitus view, the upright segment of the colon is overexposed. (B) A lateral decubitus compensation filter can help to balance tissue densities. A lesion is indicated by arrows in the filtered image. (Courtesy Nuclear Associates, Carle Place, NY.)

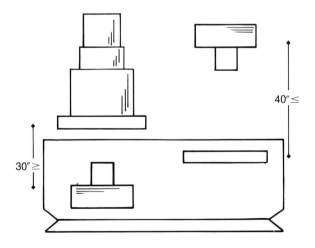

FIGURE 6-14 Comparison of Geometry with Fluoroscopic / Radiographic Equipment

Left, Fluoroscopic spot film images have a greater potential for increased image blur since these images are made using a shortened FFD, often 30 in or less. Right, Bucky radiographs are usually made using a 40 in or greater FFD. A 0.6mm focal spot should be used whenever possible for both under- and over-table imaging. This is particularly important with fluoroscopic spot films because of the reduced FFD. A 12:1 ratio grid is used in most Bucky tables. A lower ratio grid is often used with fluoroscopic spot films because of the tight beam collimation employed for four-on-one spot film imaging. See Fig 6-15. (Courtesy Eastman Kodak Company, Rochester, NY.)

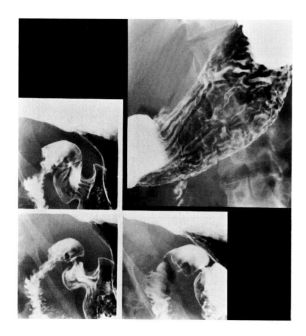

FIGURE 6-15 Fluoroscopic Spot Radiographs

This composite image is used to compare a full-field (8 in by 10 in) radiograph of the stomach (top right) and three segments of a four-on-one duodenal bulb series. A 0.6mm focal spot combined with a 12:1 ratio grid was used to generate the Bucky-like fluoroscopic images. (Courtesy Eastman Kodak Company, Rochester, NY.)

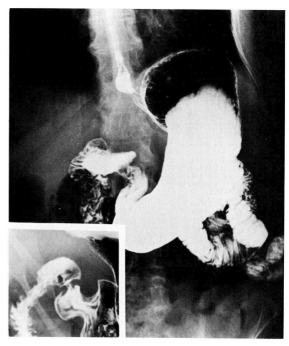

FIGURE 6-16   Comparison of Fluoroscopic Spot Film and Full Field Table Bucky Radiographs

The full field image of a barium-filled stomach is shown with a collimated four-on-one fluoroscopic spot film in the insert. The exposure time required for the collimated spot film is considerably longer than that required for the full field image since tight beam collimation necessitates an increase in exposure factors owing to the reduction of scatter radiation. The longer exposure time may result in image blur as a result of peristaltic activity. This stated difference in exposure length assumes that the same FFD and the same grid ratio were used. In reality, the spot film device uses a shortened FFD and lower ratio grid. (Courtesy Eastman Kodak Company, Rochester, NY.)

fluoroscopic spots. This technique significantly reduces radiation dosage to the patient. The elimination of some follow-up images is also cost-effective.[69]

Relatively short exposure times are required to overcome peristaltic activity or spasm of the alimentary tract. Image blur is often present on the tightly collimated fluoroscopic spot films since the tight beam collimation needed for this type of imaging results in prolonged exposure times. Full field radiographs of the same structures often exhibit less image blur since exposure times are shorter. Exposure times are also increased with deep oblique or lateral positions (Fig 6-16).

Although the under-table radiographic tube is in a fixed position, the fluoroscopic spot film device changes distance with the position or size of the patient (Fig 6-17).

Kilovoltage

Full-column barium examinations usually require a high kilovoltage technique to penetrate the barium-filled organs. High kVp helps to demonstrate a lesion or barium-filled crater through the barium. For example, an ulcer on the anterior or posterior surface of the stomach would be seen as an opacity superimposed on the barium.

Higher kVp techniques permit a reduction in mAs resulting in shorter exposure times and

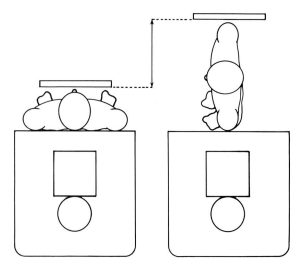

FIGURE 6–17 Fluoroscopic Spot Film Geometry

The FFD used for fluoroscopic spot film imaging is determined by the size and position of the patient. Image sharpness is influenced in part by the relationship of the part to the detector. Left, With the recumbent patient, the spot film tunnel is in contact with the patient. Right, When the patient is placed in the lateral position, anatomical structures on the down side of the patient will be magnified. The structures closest to the detector will be sharper and more accurate in size. A small focal spot will help to reduce image blur. (Courtesy Cullinan AM: *Producing Quality Radiographs.* Philadelphia, JB Lippincott Co, 1987.)

so minimizing patient- or organ-motion blur, lowering heat units, and reducing the potential for tube trauma.

Scatter

When a light flare from a primary beam leak is seen on the television monitor during fluoroscopy, the doctor repositions the image intensifier over the patient, reduces the collimator field size, or stops fluoroscoping. With conventional radiography, the radiographer does not have the advantage of seeing the effect of the primary beam leak, which will undercut the image (Fig 6-18). See Chapter 1, Fig 1-11.

Lower ratio grids are usually used in fluoroscopic spot film units to minimize grid cutoff and to reduce dosage to both the patient and the operator. See Chapter 1, Table 1-2. Because of

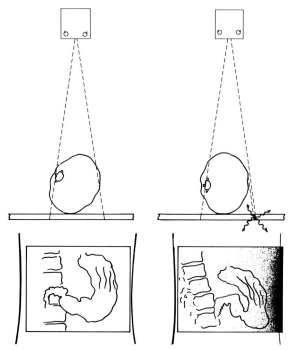

FIGURE 6–18 Primary Beam Leak

Left, An oblique position of a barium-filled stomach shows no primary beam leak. Right, In the lateral position, a primary beam leak permits unabsorbed x-radiation to strike the tabletop, thus emitting scatter in all directions, which undercuts the image, bottom. A piece of lead rubber, placed on the tabletop, or a tissue-equivalent filter helps to reduce image undercutting.

FOD variability, grid focus must be considered when using a fluoroscopic spot film tunnel (Fig 6-17).

> CAUTION: For a decubitus examination of the colon, the centering of the x-ray beam to the center of the patient (not to the center of the grid) results in a grid cutoff. The filterlike effect of unilateral grid cutoff resulting from miscentering of the grid will negate the advantage gained by using a decubitus compensatory filter.

Screen-Film Combinations

The National Council on Radiation Protection has estimated that more than 40% of the annual

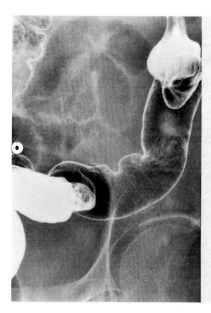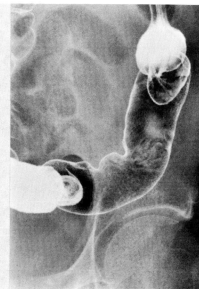

FIGURE 6-19 **High Speed Screen-Film Combinations for Fluoroscopic Spot Imaging**

A 400 speed screen-film image is shown (left) compared with a 1,200 speed image (right) taken on the same patient. The higher speed system permits the use of a smaller focal spot and a higher ratio grid, if needed. An up to threefold reduction in dosage is possible when a 400 speed system is replaced by a 1,200 speed system. (Courtesy Eastman Kodak Company, Rochester, NY.)

collective effective dose equivalent from medical x-ray examinations results from two fluoroscopic examinations—the upper GI study and the barium enema. The Center for Devices and Radiological Health is evaluating fluoroscopic equipment and examinations with regard to patient exposure to radiation.[143]

Chronic GI diseases such as Chron's disease or ulcerative colitis often require frequent follow-up studies. High speed screen-film combinations (up to 1,200 speed) reduce dosage to the patient, radiographer, and fluoroscopist during fluoroscopic spot film imaging (Fig 6-19).

> N O T E : There is no decrease in the amount of x-radiation used during the actual fluoroscopy.

Automatic Exposure Control

It is common practice to divide an 8 in by 10 in, 9.5 in by 9.5 in, or 10 in by 12 in cassette into four equal parts for tightly collimated views of the duodenal bulb and antrum of the stomach (Fig 6-15). Since less scatter radiation is produced, the AEC adjusts to a longer exposure time to maintain the preselected density. Longer exposures increase the production of heat units and, therefore, the potential for tube damage.

ACCESSORY ORGANS OF DIGESTION

The liver, gallbladder, biliary ductal system, and pancreas are accessory organs of digestion.

ANATOMICAL / PATHOLOGICAL OBSERVATIONS

The head of the pancreas, encircled by a loop of the duodenum, has always been a difficult area to demonstrate radiographically. Portions of the pancreas can be seen if calcifications are present. A survey study of the abdomen, including an upright or decubitus image, is the appropriate first step in the imaging workup of pancreatitis. Free air in the peritoneal space can indicate a perforated viscus, such as a perforated peptic ulcer, which may mimic the clinical signs of pancreatitis. The upper GI series is sometimes used to determine whether a mass in the head of the pancreas has affected the size of the duodenal loop or the position of the pyloric antrum.

On a conventional survey image of the abdomen, the liver may be partially outlined by air in the transverse colon and/or in the hepatic flexure. Blunt and penetrating trauma caused by accidents, stab or gunshot wounds, or hemorrhagic complications of a liver biopsy are common examples of liver injuries.

Bile, produced in the liver, is stored in the gallbladder until needed. Bile exits from the gallbladder via the cystic duct, which then carries it into the duodenum via the common duct. The common duct and the pancreatic duct usually join together in a common channel to form a papilla that is often called the ampulla of Vater.

Examination of the Gallbladder

Ultrasound is currently the preferred imaging modality for examination of the gallbladder.

Most gallstones are radiolucent and cannot be visualized on survey radiographs. Gallstones present in the gallbladder can occasionally be seen as faint calcifications in the right upper quadrant of the abdomen.

Gallbladder function can be determined by oral cholecystography. Iodinated contrast tablets or capsules, taken according to the manufacturer's recommendation, help to determine the concentration of bile and the emptying capabilities of the gallbladder.

If the gallbladder is not seen on the scout film, a 14 in by 17 in abdominal image should be

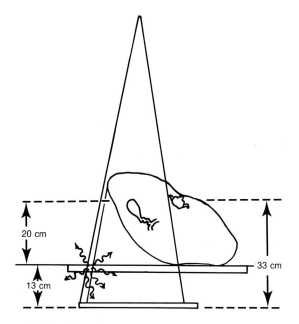

FIGURE 6–20   Gallbladder Imaging

A number of technical difficulties arise when attempting to evaluate the gallbladder, particularly in the oblique position. The gallbladder is a considerable distance (20 cm) from the tabletop. The tabletop/ Bucky-tray relationship (13 cm) adds to this distance and, therefore, to the potential for increased image blur. See Fig 1-4. In the oblique position, if a primary beam leak exists (see Fig 6-18), scatter may undercut the lateral aspect of the image.

taken. Depending on the size and position of the patient and the degree of respiration, the gallbladder can assume many positions. Sometimes a thin, elongated gallbladder will superimpose on the lumbar spine or pelvis. A left-sided gallbladder, while rare, can be ruled out with a full field image.

There are several reasons for the nonvisualization of the gallbladder:

1. The patient did not take the tablets or capsules as instructed.
2. The patient did not fast as instructed. Food would cause the contrast material to be expelled from the gallbladder.
3. Nausea or diarrhea may also prevent retention and absorption of the opaque material in the small bowel.

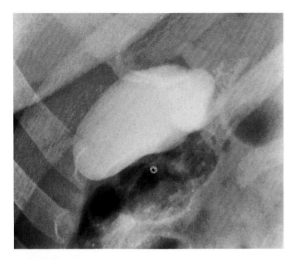

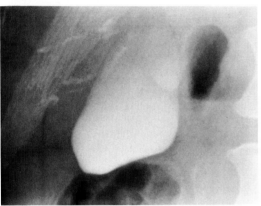

FIGURE 6-21 Fluoroscopic Spot Films versus Table Bucky Radiographs of the Gallbladder

A high ratio grid used with a small focal spot results in a fluoroscopic spot film image (top) similar in quality to a table Bucky study (bottom). (Courtesy Eastman Kodak Company, Rochester, NY.)

4. There was impaired liver function, blockage of the cystic duct, or disease of the gallbladder.
5. There were technical difficulties (Fig 6-20).

The routine study of the gallbladder includes a tightly collimated PA recumbent image of the right upper quadrant, an LAO of the right upper quadrant, and a horizontal beam PA image (erect or right lateral decubitus). The radiologist will often take upright fluoroscopic spots (Fig 6-21) to visualize the layering effect of stones. In exceptionally thin patients, the true lateral position helps to visualize the gallbladder, free of gas.

After the preliminary radiographs are checked, a meal consisting of fatty foods or a specially prepared fatty drink is given to promote emptying of the opacified bile from the gallbladder. The content of the fatty meal is determined by departmental preference. In approximately 20 to 30 minutes, an additional radiograph is made. Reduction in the size of the gallbladder is an indicator of gallbladder function. Small radiolucent stones may be better visualized on the postevacuation images since much of the iodinated bile is expelled from the gallbladder.

SUPPLEMENTARY IMAGING OF THE BILIARY SYSTEM

Endoscopic Retrograde Choledochopancreatography (ERCP)

In this technique, a fiber-optic endoscope is used to visualize the common bile and pancreatic ducts via the ampula of Vater. The object of this examination is to evaluate obstruction at the lower end of the biliary system, to locate suspected stones in postcholecystectomy patients, or to diagnose chronic pancreatitis. Stones can be extracted and tumors biopsied during an ERCP procedure.[144]

Percutaneous Transhepatic Cholangiography (PTC)

Patients with obstructive jaundice attributable to tumor or impacted stones may require a direct percutaneous needle puncture into an intrahepatic duct. External drainage of bile may be used to relieve jaundice and remove stones.[144]

N O T E : Since the contrast material used for ERCP and PTC studies is injected directly into the biliary ductal system, moderate to high kilovolt values may be necessary to penetrate dilated biliary structures.

Intravenous Cholangiography (IVC)

Ultrasound, the ERCP, and the PTC have rendered the IVC redundant. However, it is sometimes used if the gallbladder fails to visualize with an oral contrast medium or if the gallbladder has been removed.

When performing an IVC, stratification of bile or layering of the contrast material results from the difference between the specific gravity of the concentrated bile found in the gallbladder before the start of the IVC and that of the opacified lighter, new bile.

CAUTION: Radiolucent gallstones will not be seen if they level in nonopaque layers of bile, even with good visualization of the gallbladder.

The first IVC images are usually made 20 to 30 minutes after the injection. Delayed radiographs help to ensure mixing of the contrast material and bile to provide optimal visualization of the gallbladder.[145]

Since the intravenous contrast material must be imaged as it is being excreted, it is often poorly visualized. A better concentration of contrast material may be seen on a 24-hour delayed radiograph.

There is a significant failure rate with the relatively hazardous IVC study.[144]

Operative Cholangiography

Operative cholangiography is used during gallbladder surgery to determine the patency of the biliary ductal system and the presence or absence of residual calculi.

Oblique positions during operative cholangiography, after a direct injection of an opaque contrast agent, are obtained by asking the anesthesiologist to tilt the table slightly. Crosswise placement of the grid is necessary to avoid grid cutoff. This transverse positioning of the grid also allows the x-ray tube to be angled from the nonoperative side of the abdomen to image the right upper quadrant, without rotating the patient, keeping the x-ray tube to the opposite side and away from the surgical field[69] (Fig 6-22).

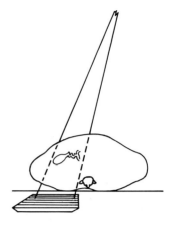

FIGURE 6–22 Operative Cholangiography

If an oblique radiograph of the biliary ductal system is needed during operative cholangiography, the grid or grid cassette should be placed in the transverse position. With the placement of the x-ray tube and grid as shown, the common duct is projected off of the vertebral column without rotating the patient. Since the x-ray unit is on the opposite side of the operating field, the possibility of contamination of the sterile field is minimized.

CAUTION: Air bubbles in the contrast material may mimic radiolucent calculi.

Postoperative Cholangiography

Postoperative cholangiography is employed after the removal of the gallbladder to demonstrate the patency of the biliary ductal system and to check for residual calculi. An opaque contrast agent is injected directly into the biliary system via a drainage tube inserted into the ductal system during surgery.

The improved technical quality of fluoroscopic spots may eliminate the need for overhead Bucky images (Fig 6-23).

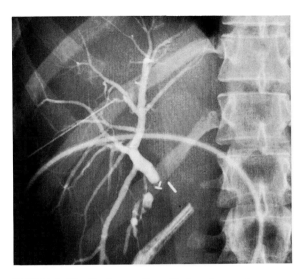

FIGURE 6–23 Postoperative Cholangiography

This fluoroscopic spot film was made using a 1,200 speed screen-film combination and a 0.6 mm focal spot. This technique may eliminate the need for some follow-up Bucky radiographs, avoiding a second injection of a contrast medium. The potential of introducing air bubbles into the biliary system is also minimized with a single injection. (Courtesy Eastman Kodak Company, Rochester, NY.)

The direct injection used for operative or postoperative cholangiography delivers undiluted contrast material into the biliary ductal system. It is common to see dilated biliary ducts holding large amounts of contrast material. Nonopaque biliary calculi can be obscured by a dense contrast agent. The use of moderate to high kilovoltage (85 kVp or greater) helps in the penetration of dense, opacified biliary ducts.

Conventional tomography used with low to moderate kVp, a high mAs value, and tight beam collimation can also help to produce higher contrast images. The use of a pluridirectional tomographic motion minimizes tomographic artifacts.

Scatter

It is difficult to center the patient, the grid, and the CR for decubitus images of the abdomen (Fig 6-24). Decubitus images require careful placement of the grid lines in relation to layered calculi.[69] In the erect position, a layering of stones could be masked if the grid were positioned parallel with the floor. In the upright position, a stationary or moving grid must be positioned so that the grid lines run perpendicular to the floor, opposite to the leveled calculi.[69]

C A U T I O N : Air bubbles in the contrast material may mimic radiolucent calculi.

C A U T I O N : Most fluoroscopy grids are mounted in the fluoroscopic tunnel so that when the unit is in the upright position, the grid lines are perpendicular to the floor. A layering effect is easily seen; however, a single gallstone, polyp, or small lesion within the opaque, filled gallbladder may "disappear" in a defective grid.

TECHNICAL CONSIDERATIONS

Kilovoltage Selection

A low to moderate kilovoltage should be used with any indirect routing of contrast material to an organ.

With an intravenous technique, there is a decrease in the density of the opaque medium since it has been diluted by bile or urine. For example, the IVC depends on liver function to deliver the contrast agent to the biliary structures. This results in very low subject contrast, requiring low-kilovoltage techniques to produce short-scale contrast images.

THE URINARY SYSTEM

The urinary tract includes the kidneys, ureters, and urinary bladder. These organs are studied radiographically to determine the presence of disease or trauma and to document urinary function.

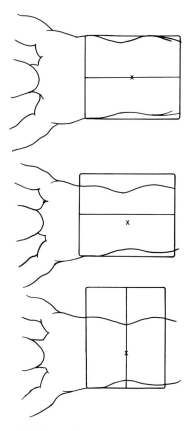

FIGURE 6–24 Grid Placement for Decubitus Radiography

The centering of a patient to a grid for lateral decubitus radiography requires careful centering of the CR to the center of the grid. Positioning the grid with the lines parallel with the tabletop assumes that all patients are exactly 14 in wide (top). Note that the center of the abdomen indicated by the "X" is approximately 1 to 1.5 in off center from the center of the grid. Centering to the center of the abdomen would result in grid cutoff in this image (center). If the grid is placed with the grid lines perpendicular to the x-ray table or floor, the CR can be directed to any point along the vertical line of the grid and still maintain grid focus (bottom). If the x-ray tube were moved left or right, however, unilateral grid cutoff would result.

ANATOMICAL / PATHOLOGICAL OBSERVATIONS

The kidneys, which are bean-shaped organs, lie in the retroperitoneal space. An adrenal gland caps the superior portion of each kidney. The kidneys filter the blood and excrete urine into the ureters, which carry the urine to the urinary bladder. Fat seen on a radiograph as an area of decreased density outlines much of the kidney during plain-film imaging. Renal dimensions can be determined by either plain-film radiography, conventional tomography, or intravenous urography. Radiopaque calculi in the kidneys, ureters, or bladder can often be demonstrated on a survey radiograph.

Blood may appear in the urine if there is injury to the renal collecting system, ureters, or bladder. In the presence of severe trauma to the kidney region, the lower ribs, the lumbar vertebrae, and the pelvis should also be evaluated for injury.

POSITIONING CONCEPTS

A survey radiograph is usually made to determine the cleanliness of the colon and/or the presence of calculi prior to the injection of a contrast agent. Patient-preparation routines to cleanse the colon of gas and fecal material vary from department to department.

Respiration and patient habitus and position may change the location of the kidneys. The kidneys move up and down approximately 1 in within the retroperitoneal space during respiration. In the erect position, depending on patient habitus, the kidneys can drop 2 in or more. In very thin patients, the kidneys may drop into the pelvic cavity.

The survey radiograph must be processed and viewed and appropriate adjustments made in technique before the injection of a contrast medium. If technical adjustments were made to the original survey image, it is good practice to review the second scout radiograph to be certain that the desired results were produced. Rapid automatic processing minimizes delay of the study.

Intravenous Urography (IVU)

An intravenous urogram (excretory urogram) visualizes the renal outlines, the collecting system, soft-tissue details, and psoas shadows. An IVU not only demonstrates static anatomy, but is also used to evaluate kidney function.

Prior to the injection of a contrast medium, preparation of the patient emotionally and the taking of a history to ascertain allergy are important. The type of contrast medium (ionic versus nonionic), the amount injected, the need for sensitivity testing, and the rate of injections should be determined by departmental policy.

Reactions to iodinated contrast media vary from patient to patient. Patients who suffer allergic reactions such as asthma, migraine headaches, or reactions to drugs or foods, particularly iodine compounds, are thought to be particularly sensitive. Symptoms may include hot flashes, urticaria, vomiting, pain in the arm and shoulder, itching, nasal congestion, lacrimation, salivation, a metallic taste, fainting, and spasm of the glottis.[146]

The contrast medium, needed to demonstrate the kidneys, ureters, and bladder, is removed from the blood via glomerular filtration and is excreted by the kidney. Visualization of the renal substance (nephrogram) depends on the amount of contrast medium reaching the kidneys within a given time. Visualization of the collecting system (pyelogram) depends on the ability of the kidneys to concentrate the urine.[89]

Life-threatening reactions include convulsions, cyanosis, shock, and cardiac arrest. Resuscitation equipment should include oxygen, a suction machine, a sphygmomanometer, a defibrillator, a cardiac monitor, and appropriate drugs.[147]

> CAUTION: To avoid delay in instituting cardiopulmonary resuscitation, electrical outlets must be easily accessible for the necessary equipment.

Just before starting the examination, the patient should be asked to void. A scout radiograph and scout tomogram, if part of the departmental routine, are made, processed, and reviewed. If necessary, technical or positioning errors are corrected at this time.

A basic examination of the excretory system includes:

1. AP survey image.
2. AP, LPO, and RPO projections following injection of opaque medium.
3. Postvoiding image of the urinary bladder.

To produce the best possible evaluation of the urinary tract, abdominal and ureteral compression are suggested. Gas within the colon overlying portions of the urinary tract sometimes can be displaced laterally by compression of an air-filled rubber bladder placed against the abdomen, below the kidneys. The compression device is attached to the table by a band that restricts patient motion, but limits oblique positioning.

Contraindications to compression include:

1. Known or suspected ureteral obstruction.
2. Possible ureteral stones.
3. Known or suspected abdominal mass.
4. Known or suspected aortic aneurysm.
5. Recent surgery.
6. Acute abdominal pain.
7. Trauma.

> CAUTION: To minimize the danger of metastasis in patients being evaluated for an intra-abdominal neoplasm, particularly infants and children, pressure on the abdomen by either prone positioning or the use of a compression band is not recommended.[148]

Oblique positioning is possible with the use of a compression device consisting of two small, inflatable rubber balloons held in place by sponge-rubber or plastic-foam blocks and a flexible cloth band that passes around the patient. The balloons are placed over the ureters, where they cross the promontory of the sacrum. Inflation of the balloons helps partially to occlude the ureters.[147]

A routine described by Hattery et al[147] includes a two-film technique for all but the smallest adults. The 14 in by 17 in lower film is positioned with the inferior margin of the symphysis pubis about 6 cm above the lower margin of the cassette. The x-ray tube is angled 10 degrees caudad. The 11 in by 14 in upper film is centered according to the patient's body habitus, with the film usually centered 2 to 4 cm above the umbilicus. The x-ray tube is angled 10 degrees cephalad. The entire renal and suprarenal areas and the diaphragm are included.

The contrast medium is injected and ureteral compression applied. Tomograms are made at levels 1 to 1.5 cm apart to include the full thickness of both kidneys. At eight minutes, the pelvis and calyces usually are well distended and can be imaged with and without compression. At ten minutes, on the decompression 14 in by 17 in radiograph, the ureters are generally well seen. Images exposed at approximately 20 minutes and a postvoiding radiograph best demonstrate the bladder. This filming sequence should provide adequate visualization of the kidneys, ureters, and bladder, with the renal parenchyma being well demonstrated on the tomograms. This routine does not utilize the oblique view as part of the standard examination, but only for problem solving in selected patients. It may be necessary to obtain a prone view to visualize the ureters adequately.[147]

Delayed radiographs can be used to help differentiate between inconstant filling defects such as clot and constant defects such as tumor.[36] Delayed radiographs also help to determine the function of a kidney associated with acute unilateral ureteral colic.

Ureteral obstruction sometimes can be demonstrated 40 minutes or longer after the injection of the contrast medium. In some cases, as long as 24 hours may be needed to detect the site and cause of an obstruction in the ureter.[147]

In the presence of blunt abdominal trauma, a "single shot" IVU may be taken. A single bolus of intravenous contrast material may be used to demonstrate gross renal abnormalities and help to determine whether both kidneys are present and functioning.[149]

Hypertension Series

Compression is not initially applied in patients being evaluated for arterial hypertension. Care-

fully timed radiographs taken two minutes and three minutes after injection demonstrate the time of appearance of the contrast medium in the renal collecting system. Some radiologists prefer "minute" sequence images obtained at 30 seconds and 1, 2, 3, 4, and 5 minutes after injection, with ureteral compression applied after the three-minute radiograph, followed by a standard urographic routine.[147]

Infusion Pyelography

An infusion pyelogram is particularly useful with poor renal function or when a patient cannot be dehydrated. For this technique, the patient is administered, by rapid intravenous infusion, a large amount of contrast medium with a volume of aqueous diluent. The amount of contrast medium and rate of infusion are influenced by the weight of the patient and are determined by the radiologist.[95] Opacification of the collecting system is not directly related to the speed of injection, but depends on the concentration of the contrast agent in the collecting system and distention. In healthy patients, parenchymal opacification is most intense during the first two minutes following injection. This opacification is a combination of "vascular" and "tubular" nephrograms.[147]

Retrograde Pyelography. The kidneys are studied by injecting a contrast medium via catheters inserted into the renal collecting system during cystoscopy. Sometimes, to opacify the entire ureter, the contrast medium is injected as the catheter is withdrawn.

Cystography

The contrast medium is injected into the bladder via a catheter to identify vesicoureteral reflux. A cystographic study consists of recumbent AP, left and right oblique positions. A postevacuation image is usually obtained in the recumbent AP position.

Although low to moderate kilovoltage values associated with urographic procedures demonstrate the outline of the bladder within the pelvis, a higher kilovoltage helps to show calculi or small tumors in the opacified bladder. Even a di-

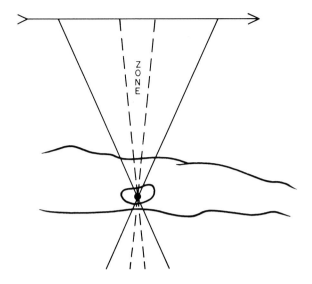

FIGURE 6–25 Extended Angle Tomography versus Zonography

Extended angle tomography, usually 40 degrees or greater, is represented by the solid lines. With increased amplitude, an increased exposure angle results and a thinner section is produced. With narrow angle tomography (zonography), represented by the dotted line, a thicker tomographic section is obtained. (Courtesy Cullinan AM: *Producing Quality Radiographs.* Philadelphia, JB Lippincott Co, 1987.)

luted contrast medium may be difficult to penetrate in a large, fully opacified bladder. Kilovoltage values in excess of 85 kVp may be required to penetrate a dilated opacified bladder.

Voiding Urethrogram

In the oblique position, while the patient is voiding, an exposure can be made to demonstrate the urethra. A moderate kVp technique is recommended to avoid overexposure of the urethra.

Retrograde Urethrography

If the urinary bladder cannot be filled with a contrast medium or the patient is unable to void when requested, a retrograde urethrogram may be indicated. A water-soluble contrast medium is injected via the urethral meatus to opacify the urethra. To obtain the image, the supine patient is rotated into a 45 degree oblique position, with the down leg flexed. Prior to injection, the penis is straightened.[95]

Tomography

Overlying bowel content and gas can obscure renal anatomy. Linear tomography may be achieved with exposure angles varying from 10 degrees (zonography) to a thin-section tomogram made with a 40 degree or greater arc (Fig 6-25). Tomograms should be made at the maximum intensity of the nephrographic phase.

A suggested routine includes:

1. A tomogram made at approximately the arm-to-kidney circulation time (generally 12 to 20 seconds). This time frame should allow demonstration of the vascular phase. Dense parenchymal opacification should be seen after the vascular phase has been reached (30 to 45 seconds). The cortex, corticomedullary junction, and medulla should be delineated.

2. A series of tomograms (one minute to four minutes after injection) are then made.[148]

TECHNICAL CONSIDERATIONS

Image Blur

A compression band can help to minimize involuntary motion, thereby reducing image blur.

There is approximately a 17% magnification factor in the radiographic size of the average adult normal kidneys because they are at a considerable distance from the detector.[95] Riggs[150] evaluated radiographic rooms in five hospitals and found that the tabletop/Bucky-tray distances varied from 6 to 13 cm. See Chapter 1, Fig 1-4. This finding explained an 8% "shrinkage" of the kidneys in comparative excretory urograms made in different rooms over a six-month period.[150]

CAUTION: Repeat evaluation of a patient for kidney size after transplant surgery requires that the same room be used to avoid varying degrees of magnification, which could signify a rejection of the transplanted kidney.

Kilovoltage Selection

While kilovoltage must be selected to suit the examination and/or patient size, the imaging system must also be considered. A low kilovoltage value used to produce high contrast radiographs may result in a falloff in screen speed with some rare earth screen-film systems. See Chapter 1.

CHAPTER **SEVEN**

The Respiratory System

The respiratory system includes the lungs, bronchi, trachea, larynx, pharynx, and nasal passages.

CHEST RADIOGRAPHY

The chest radiograph, the most frequently performed study, is also one of the most difficult to interpret. Changes in radiographic density occur as the result of pathology, different degrees of inspiration, or changes in radiographic technique. The amount of blood carried by the pulmonary vessels affects their visualization. Previous studies, if available, can help in the evaluation of subtle changes.

Duplication of radiographic densities in comparison radiographs and documentation of the time of the examination help in following the progression of a disease or the effect of treatment.

ANATOMICAL / PATHOLOGICAL OBSERVATIONS

The anatomical structures of the chest in close relationship to each other vary significantly in radiodensity and are visualized because of the natural contrast between adjacent structures. Radiographic density also changes with the amount of inspiration, the general health of the patient, or changes in radiographic technique and/or positioning.

The mediastinal space is bordered by the sternum anteriorly, the spine and ribs posteriorly, and the lungs bilaterally. The heart, blood vessels, thymus, esophagus, trachea, and bronchi lie within the mediastinal space.

A considerable portion of lung tissue does not image on the PA view, owing to the superimposition of mediastinal structures (Fig 7-1). The size and shape of the mediastinum can be affected by body habitus, scoliosis, sternal deformity, pregnancy, or different degrees of respiration.

Optimal radiographic demonstration of the outer edges of the lung fields, including the costophrenic angles, is essential. Short, horizontal septal lines, known as Kerley "B" lines, are often seen on the periphery of the lungs on the PA image. These lines extend laterally to the edge of the lungs. Kerley "A" lines, also seen on the PA image, are much thinner than adjacent blood vessels and radiate toward the hilar in the middle and upper zones.[89] It is important to demonstrate these interstitial patterns, which are imaged as faint lines.

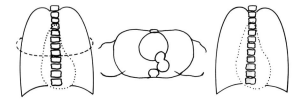

FIGURE 7-1   Lung Tissue Masked by the Mediastinum

Left, In the PA position, the cardiac silhouette is outlined. Major blood vessels and adjacent hilar structures are not shown in this illustration. A dotted transverse section represents the midthoracic area. Center, Note the amount of lung tissue behind the heart, anterior to the thoracic vertebrae on the right side of the chest. This area is difficult to demonstrate on PA or AP radiographs. Anatomical details such as vertebral bodies should be visible through the dense cardiac silhouette. Since the heart widens at its lower portion, the vertebral bodies and interspaces are more difficult to visualize. Aerated lung tissue behind the heart, adjacent to the soft-tissue structures (air–soft-tissue interface), should be faintly visible within the mediastinum. Since the air–soft-tissue interspace is visualized near the toe of the sensitometric curve, an extended latitude film will help to overcome the difference between the aerated lung and the dense mediastinum. Right, The shaded area, superimposed on the vertebral column, represents the aerated lung on the right side, abutted against soft tissues. A high kilovoltage / grid technique produces many shades of gray (long scale contrast), rather than abrupt blacks and whites, helping to demonstrate mediastinal information.

Most of the bronchial tree is invisible in a healthy patient. The thin walls of the bronchi are surrounded by aerated alveoli, making it difficult to identify air in the bronchi. Occasionally, the walls of some bronchi can be seen on end. If the alveoli are filled with fluid, the air in the bronchi contrasts with the fluid. This is known as an "air bronchogram," which represents air within an open airway surrounded by consolidated air spaces. A bronchogram is shown in Fig 7-2 to illustrate the extent of the bronchial tree.

The diaphragm may be seen at various levels within the thorax, and it moves significantly during full inspiration. For an average patient, full inspiration causes the diaphragm to move downward approximately 3 cm. The size of the liver limits the downward motion of the right hemidiaphragm. Other factors that affect the lo-

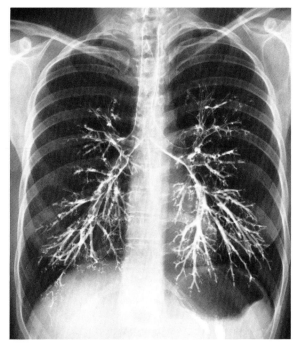

FIGURE 7-2   Visualization of the Bronchi by Use of an Opaque Contrast Medium

Except for the trachea and the right and left primary bronchi, the walls of the bronchi are very thin, and even when aerated, they are not normally seen by conventional chest radiography. For years, bronchography was used to study the bronchial tree, using an oily iodinated contrast material. Newer diagnostic techniques have all but eliminated this procedure. This image is shown to demonstrate the extent of the bronchial tree. An equally complex vascular system also forms a large part of the chest image. The major arteries are vaguely outlined, but would require angiography to be seen in their entirety. (Courtesy Eastman Kodak Company, Rochester, NY.)

cation of the diaphragm include patient habitus, positioning, and pregnancy.

The diaphragm separates the thoracic cavity from the abdomen. The upper surface of the diaphragm contrasts against the air-filled lungs; the lower surface requires air beneath the diaphragm to outline it. Occasionally, in the erect position, the air-filled fundus of the stomach abuts against the diaphragm, outlining the inferior surface of the diaphragm, as well as the superior wall of the fundus.

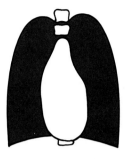 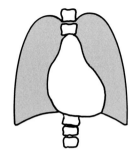

FIGURE 7–3   Inspiration Versus Expiration

Fully aerated lungs are required for routine radiography of the chest. The cardiothoracic ratio changes with varying degrees of inspiration or expiration. Left, On full inspiration, the diaphragm moves downward approximately 2 in and the heart narrows. Right, On full expiration, the diaphragm moves upward, widening the heart. Depending on the size of the heart and the position of the diaphragm, as much as 40% of the lungs can be superimposed on the mediastinum and diaphragm in the PA chest image. Any degree of expiration requires an increase in technical factors over the fully ventilated chest. Since most modern chest x-ray units use AECs, the exposure will be lengthened, depending on the degree of expiration. Although a satisfactory density is achieved on the radiograph, the cardiothoracic ratio may be significantly altered. When using manual techniques, changes in aeration of the lungs may produce various degrees of lung blackening on the image.

In the normal adult chest, the transverse diameter of the heart is usually less than half the internal diameter of the chest (cardiothoracic ratio). The cardiothoracic ratio changes with the degree of inspiration and patient positioning (Fig 7-3).

In addition to the heart, lungs, trachea, and bronchi, osseous and thoracic soft-tissue structures are demonstrated on chest images. An intrathoracic lesion touching a border of the heart, aorta, or diaphragm will obliterate that border on the chest radiograph, resulting in a "silhouette sign."[89]

Pulmonary lesions in the hilar region, anterior to the sternum, posterior to the heart, or behind the domes of the diaphragm, can sometimes be hidden in the PA projection. The entire bony cage should be visible on the radiograph.

Changes in the ribs constitute important findings for the radiologist.

A lump on the skin, braided hair, a prominent pectoral muscle, a mammary implant, or a nipple shadow superimposed on a chest radiograph may simulate a pulmonary nodule. Disposable nipple markers help to differentiate the nipple from a mass. When repeating an examination with nipple markers, a 5 to 10 degree PA oblique position helps to differentiate a small nodule from the nipple on the PA study. If the suspected lesion is a nipple, the mass and the marker superimpose. If a pulmonary mass exists, the marker and mass separate on the slightly oblique image. A small lead-shot nipple marker should not mask a pulmonary nodule.

> C A U T I O N :   If a single lead shot is taped directly to the nipple, the marker must be removed from the patient as soon as the examination is determined to be satisfactory. A metal marker allowed to remain taped in position may cause an inflammatory process.

POSITIONING CONCEPTS

Routine radiographs of the chest include the PA and lateral projections (Tables 7-1 and 7-2). Oblique radiographs help to evaluate changes in the cardiac silhouette (Table 7-3, page 184). Barium used to outline the esophagus delineates the cardiac shadow. Additionally, oblique projections are used to demonstrate the trachea and adjacent bronchi.

In 1943, Peter Kerley[20] suggested that radiographers fluoroscope the chest to learn how to position accurately for the oblique projection. Dr. Kerley's comment, unusual for the time, was, "There is, as you are aware, some vague opposition to radiographers' screening [fluoroscoping]. Let us hope that this medieval prejudice will soon be universally abandoned." Experience has helped radiographers to develop acceptable oblique positioning concepts without the use of fluoroscopy.

TABLE 7-1 The PA/AP Chest

Area	Position of Patient/Part	Projection of Central Ray	Demonstrates (View)
Chest (PA)	Patient erect in PA position; median plane of body perpendicular to film plane; dorsal surface of wrists placed on hips; shoulders rotated foward	CR directed perpendicular to film plane to enter at level of T-5/T-6	Bony thorax; cardiac shadow; lung fields
		CR directed perpendicular to film plane to enter at midsternum.	Heart
Chest (PA)	Patient prone; median plane of body perpendicular to midline of tabletop; head turned to one side; elbows flexed; hands on table beside head; no rotation of the body	See PA projection	See PA view
Chest (barium swallow)	See PA position	See PA projection	Esophagus
Chest (AP)	Patient erect in AP position or supine; median plane of body perpendicular to film plane; if possible, flex elbows, pronate hands, and place hands on hips	See PA projection	See PA view; cardiac shadow appears enlarged

Eisenberg and his collegues[151] reported on a prospective study to determine the optimum number of radiographic projections of the chest needed to evaluate applicants for Veterans Administration compensation. These studies were used to assess the extent of previous trauma or to determine the presence of a degenerative disease with a possible occupational relationship. Their study showed that 99% of the chest examinations (978 of 987) required only a single PA chest x-ray. In only nine (0.9%) of the 987 applications did a lateral or oblique view alter the radiographic diagnosis made using the single PA view. They estimated that at $5 to $6 for each projec-tion, the Veterans Administration could save $750,000 to $900,000 annually by using single-view studies.[151]

On a PA chest, barring scoliosis or other deformities, the medial aspects of both clavicles have a similar relationship to the thoracic spine. Oblique alignment of the x-ray tube or rotation of the patient may cause the distal ends of the clavicle to shift left or right.

The thoracic vertebrae and intervertebral spaces should be faintly visualized through the mediastinum. The scapulae must be rotated forward off of the lateral aspects of the upper lung fields.

TABLE 7-2 The Lateral Chest

Area	Position of Patient/Part	Projection of Central Ray	Demonstrates (View)
Chest (lateral)	Patient erect; left side of chest against film holder (unless right side is area of interest); median plane parallel to film plane; anterior surface of sternum perpendicular to film plane; midaxillary line about 2 in posterior to the midline of the cassette holder; arms above head, grasping elbows	CR directed perpendicular to film plane to enter midline at level of T-4

CR directed perpendicular to film plane to enter at level of T-6/T-7 | Bony thorax; cardiac shadow; lung fields

Heart |
| Chest (esophagus, barium swallow) | Patient in lateral position; anterior surface of sternum perpendicular to film plane; coronal plane of body aligned with midline of table; arms elevated; elbows flexed; forearms beside head | CR directed perpendicular to film plane, to enter coronal plane at level of T-5/T-6 | Opacified esophagus |
| Chest (barium swallow) | See Lateral position | See Lateral projection | Relationship of esophagus to cardiac contours |

In the PA position, the anterior portion of the chest is as close to the detector as possible. A 6 ft FFD is needed to minimize enlargement of the cardiac silhouette caused by the distance of the heart from the image detector. Rotation of the patient influences the appearance of the size and shape of the cardiac silhouette and can cause one lung to appear darker than the other. Patient rotation may also mask a mediastinal shift or a deviation or constriction of an airway, or give the illusion of mediastinal or hilar masses. The cardiac silhouette also changes in size as a result of body position (recumbent, erect, or decubitus), deformities of the thoracic cage, and intrapul-monary or pleural pathology. The Valsalva maneuver and pregnancy also affect the size and shape of the mediastinum.

When imaging the chest of a large patient, it may be difficult to include both costophrenic sulci. There is enough room to center most patients on a 14 in by 17 in cassette, but the dominant hand of the radiographer may tend to push the patient slightly off center, causing unilateral cutoff of one base. A laser positioning device that projects a low level, yet visible, laser beam onto the patient helps precisely to center and align the patient with the image detector. This apparatus is especially useful with dedicated

TABLE 7–3 The Oblique Chest

Area	Position of Patient/Part	Projection of Central Ray	Demonstrates (View)
RAO	PA position; right anterior chest against film holder; body rotated 45 degrees; right arm down, left arm up	CR directed perpendicular to film plane, to enter at level of T-6	Right lung; trachea; bony thorax; heart and aorta anterior to vertebral column
LAO	PA position; left anterior chest against film holder; body rotated 45 degrees; left arm down, right arm up	See RAO projection	Left lung; trachea; bony thorax; heart and aorta anterior to vertebral column
RAO (cardiac series, barium swallow)	See RAO position	See RAO projection	Aortic arch; lungs; mediastinal structures; relationship of esophagus to cardiac contours
LAO (cardiac series, barium swallow)	PA position; left anterior chest against film holder; body rotated 60 degrees; left arm down, right arm up	See RAO projection	See RAO (cardiac series, barium swallow) view
RAO (esophagus, barium swallow)	PA position; right anterior chest against film holder; body rotated 30 to 40 degrees; right arm down, left arm up	See RAO projection	Opacified esophagus
LAO (esophagus, barium swallow)	PA position; left anterior chest against film holder; body rotated 30 to 40 degrees; left arm down, right arm up	See RAO projection	See RAO (esophagus, barium swallow) view

chest film changers restricted to a 14 in by 17 in configuration. See Chapter 2, Fig 2-7.

C A U T I O N : Women with large pendulous breasts, when being positioned for the PA projection, should be asked to lift and separate their breasts laterally, while pressing tightly against the cassette or cassette holder.

The PA chest can also demonstrate anatomy and disease below the diaphragm and herniation of the stomach or bowel into the chest. Gaseous dilatation of the bowel can also be visualized beneath the diaphragm.

Pathological changes in the lower lobes of the lungs are difficult to identify on bedside radiographs since a significant portion of the lower lobes lies behind the diaphragmatic domes. Patients seated in a true upright position for an AP radiograph should be asked to lean forward about 10 degrees for a better visualization of the bases of their lungs.[152]

The lateral erect position images the outline of the heart, aorta, fissures and lobes of the lung, the diaphragm, and pulmonary pathology. The lateral view not only helps visualize vertebral lesions, small areas of pleural effusion, and mediastinal pathology, but sometimes can be used to assess mild cardiomeglia. Overall, the major value of this projection is to confirm or clarify suspicious or abnormal densities seen in the PA view[151] (Fig 7-4).

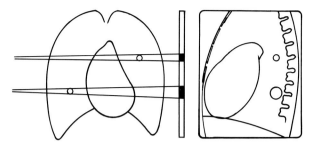

FIGURE 7-4 Lesion in Lateral Chest

Depending on the position of a lesion or foreign body in the thorax, significant enlargement and increased image blur can occur. In the PA sketch, two circles representing the lesions are seen in the right lower and left upper lungs. If the patient were placed in the left lateral position, the lesion imaged in the left lung would be more accurate in size while the lesion imaged in the right lung would be significantly enlarged.

CAUTION: With the arms elevated above the head for the lateral position, the patient may drift forward or backward or rotate when attempting full inhalation. A stabilizing bar suspended above the patient's head helps to avoid positioning and motion difficulties. This is particularly important when using an AEC (Fig 7-5).

DISEASES OR CONDITIONS MERITING SPECIAL CONSIDERATION

Mediastinal Imaging

Demonstration of the bony thorax and associated soft tissue should not compromise the visualization of the lungs or mediastinum. A radiographic technique should be used to balance the abrupt differences between the blackened air-filled lungs, the sometimes chalklike osseous structures, and the mediastinum. Technical adjustments can help demonstrate peripheral vascularity without loss of the mediastinal structures.

With conventional, low to moderate kilovolt/nongrid techniques, demonstration of mediastinal anatomy presents a problem. On nongrid chest radiographs, up to 90% of the photons striking the recording medium behind the mediastinum are non–information-containing photons (scatter). With high kVp/grid radiogra-

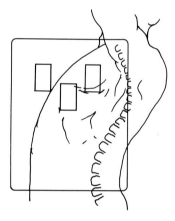

FIGURE 7-5 Use of the AEC for Chest Radiography

The patient must be stabilized for the lateral position to avoid motion when the arms are elevated above the head. If the patient drifts backward when an AEC is being used, a large portion of the imaging frame may be struck by primary radiation, producing significant scatter that may strike the central sensor. The AEC cannot determine whether the radiation striking the sensor is primary or secondary and will terminate the exposure prematurely when the preselected density is reached.

phy of the chest, more information-containing photons help to image the mediastinum.

Wide absorption differences in anatomy or pathology can be overcome by using a scanning equalization device.[153] An advance multiple beam equalization radiography (AMBER) device located in front of the x-ray tube contains a row of 21 beam modulators. Each local slit beam can be changed in height during the scanning procedure. A linear detector array in front of the cassette measures the absorption of the x-ray beam by the patient while raising or lowering the position of the 21 individual beam modulators. A 0.8 second scan time, with a local exposure time of approximately 50 ms, images the mediastinum without overexposing the lungs[154] (Figs 7-6 through 7-8).

Pneumoconiosis

Pneumoconiosis is caused by the inhalation of dust and the tissue reaction to its presence. Inhalation of coal dust can cause pneumoconiosis of coal workers, often called "black lung disease." However, the disease is not limited to coal miners or sandblasters; other potential victims include people who mine stone or ore or work with graphite.

Chest lesions associated with pneumoconiosis can include nodules, cavitations, and/or pleural thickening. Simple pneumoconiosis is asymptomatic and is due to retention of dust in the lungs, with minor fibrosis; it is recognized initially by the appearance of many small nodules, up to 10 mm in diameter. Thickening of the parietal pleura produces plaquelike structures. Calcifications within the pleural thickening often are seen in the later stages of pneumoconiosis.[155,156] The diagnosis is made on the basis of a chest x-ray. Chest radiographs must be of high technical quality since financial compensation to the patient is often determined by the radiographic study.

A special chest-interpretation system devised by the National Institute for Occupational Safety and Health (NIOSH) is used when interpreting these radiographs. For many years, NIOSH has conducted imaging seminars, stress-

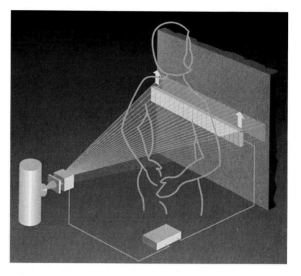

FIGURE 7-6 Scanning Equalization Device

Wide absorption differences in anatomy and pathology are overcome by scanning equalization chest units. The AMBER system contains a row of 21 x-ray beam modulators located in front of the x-ray tube, each able to change the height of the local slit beam during scanning of the chest. A linear detector array in front of the cassette measures variations in the x-ray beam (absorption changes caused by the patient) and adjusts the positions of the individual modulators. Individual strips in the xenon detector measure the x-ray intensity after passing through the patient. (Courtesy Eastman Kodak Company, Rochester, NY.)

ing the value of proper radiographic technique and positioning.

A set of International Labor Office 1980 Standard Reference Radiographs and a copy of guidelines for the classification of pneumoconiosis can be purchased from the regional center of the International Labor Office Publication Center, 49 Sheridan Avenue, Albany, NY 12210.

The resolution characteristics of the newer 300 speed rare earth systems parallel those of the 100 speed calcium tungstate screens originally recommended.

Emphysema

Emphysema is marked by an increase in the size of the air spaces of the terminal bronchioles be-

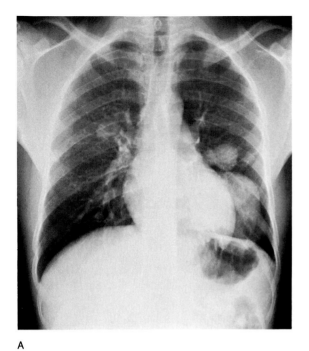

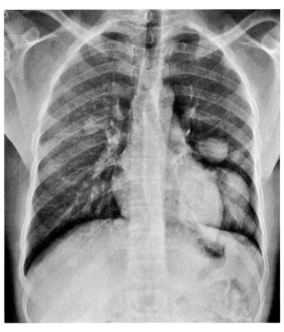

A

B

FIGURE 7–7 Conventional / AMBER Chest Images

(A) A conventional chest radiograph showing multiple lesions within the lungs. (B) A scanning equalization study using an AMBER unit demonstrates the retrodiaphragmatic, retrocardiac, and mediastinal segments of the chest, with an image quality similar to that of the lung fields. The scan requires 0.8 second with a local exposure time of approximately 50 ms. An air–soft-tissue interface, superimposed on the thoracic vertebrae, is well demonstrated through the dense mediastinum. (Courtesy Eastman Kodak Company, Rochester, NY.)

yond their normal capacity. Overinflation of the lung increases the lung volume as the diaphragms move downward. The overexpanded lungs will often flatten the normal curvature of the diaphragm. Because of overinflation, the emphysematous lung is easy to overexpose. The minimum response time limitation of an AEC often results in overexposed radiographs. See Chapter 1.

Compensatory emphysema results when a lobe of a lung is collapsed or has been removed surgically. The remaining lung tissue expands to fill the space.

A localized area of hypertranslucency in the lung indicates that a portion of the lung is overdistended. On occasion, a plug (tumor or foreign body) can cause a partial or complete blockage of the bronchus, thus acting as a valve, allowing air to enter but not to escape the lung ("check valve" disease). Ballooning or overinflation of the lung beyond the blockage may take place. Automatic exposure control devices are designed to produce a preselected density (an overall blackening) of the lung fields and can mask an area of hypertranslucency. After conventional radiographs have been made, an expiration PA image using a manual technique is needed to complete the study. The localized overdistended segment of the lung should be adequately exposed on the conventional expiration study. The remaining lung tissue will not image because of the lack of aeration.

The chest radiograph can be used to determine bronchial obstruction owing to aspirated foreign bodies in young children and infants. Chest radiography can also be used to visualize

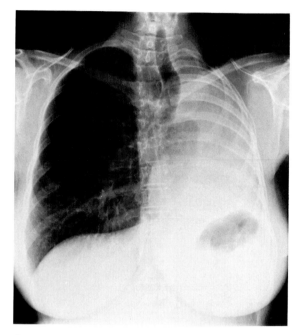

A

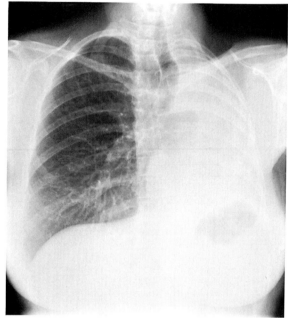

B

FIGURE 7–8   Conventional / AMBER Chest Images

(A) A conventional chest x-ray was made of a patient with significant fluid in the left lung. It is impossible for an AEC to balance the density between the aerated right lung and the opaque, fluid-filled left lung. Imaging is further complicated by the superimposition of the breasts on the costophrenic sulci. (B) A second conventional image was made with a reduction in technical factors to visualize the right lung field better. The result was a lack of information on the fluid-filled left chest, with some loss of detail in the right lung base. (C) A third image was made using the scanning equalization device (AMBER). Note the excellent visualization of details through the thoracic spine, as well as through the fluid-filled lung. The right lung field is adequately exposed, including the right costophrenic sulcus. Pulmonary markings can be seen through the diaphragm in the right lower lung. (Courtesy Eastman Kodak Company, Rochester, NY.)

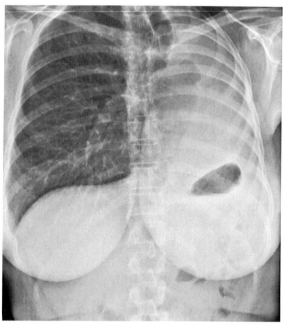

C

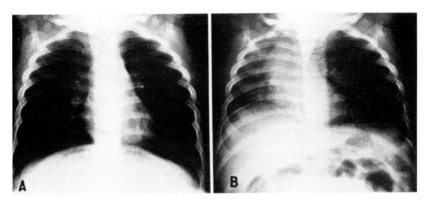

FIGURE 7-9 Assisted Expiratory Chest Radiography

(A) Normal inspiratory radiograph of an 18-month-old boy who had exhibited wheezing and coughing of an abrupt onset several hours earlier. (B) Assisted expiratory radiography demonstrates marked air trapping in the entire left lung. At bronchoscopy, a sunflower seed was removed from the left bronchus. (Courtesy Wessenberg RL, Blumhagen JD: Assisted expiratory chest radiography. *Radiology* 1979; 130: 538-539.)

radiolucent foreign bodies in the cervical airway. While objects such as peanuts, sunflower seeds, nuts, and other food particles are not usually visualized in the chest, they are suspected by indirect signs. Atelectasis or air trapping attributable to partial obstruction can be evaluated by chest radiography.[157]

An expiratory radiograph can be used to demonstrate air trapped in the lung of a child, but is sometimes difficult to accomplish. With the child immobilized, the radiographer can apply gentle pressure to the epigastrium with a lead-lined glove while a second radiographer makes an exposure of the assisted expiratory phase[158] (Fig 7-9).

CAUTION: Patient rotation can mimic the displacement of the mediastinum caused by unilateral overinflation of the lung.

Mediastinal Emphysema. Pneumomediastinum results if there has been a disruption in the esophagus or an air leak from a bronchus with air trapped in the mediastinum. This condition may be spontaneous or may be caused by chest trauma, endoscopy, violent vomiting, or a swallowed foreign body. The air is seen as fine streaks of translucency within the mediastinum, often extending upward into the neck.[89]

CAUTION: Some compensatory filters can produce edge markings resembling a pneumomediastinum or pneumothorax.

Subcutaneous Emphysema. Penetrating trauma to the chest, including surgical procedures, can result in subcutaneous emphysema of the chest wall and neck. It can also occur if a fractured rib punctures a lung. Subcutaneous emphysema can obscure air accumulating in the pleural spaces, masking pneumothoraces on a plain radiograph, especially in supine patients.

Pneumothorax

Air may enter the pleural space from the lungs or through a hole in the chest wall. Pneumothorax occurs when free air is trapped in the pleural space and compresses the lung (Fig 7-10). Common causes of pneumothorax include penetrat-

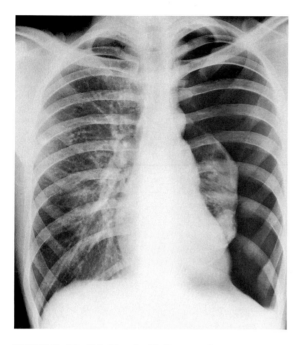

FIGURE 7-10   PA Chest with Pneumothorax

Air in the pleural space has collapsed the left lung.
Note the excellent visualization of bony detail in the
ribs, owing to the lack of pulmonary vasculature.
(Courtesy Eastman Kodak Company, Rochester, NY.)

CAUTION: The use of an AEC is not recommended for the expiration image since the purpose of the control is to produce an image of a specific blackness. The predetermined film-blackening effect of the AEC masks the overaerated segment in the expiration study and can be lost in the overall blackened image. An expiration image made using manual techniques results in visualization of the distended aerated segment since the remainder of the lung fields will be underexposed as a result of the lack of aeration. The pneumothorax is often seen more clearly on the expiratory image because of the increase in the ratio of intrapleural to intrapulmonary gas.[113]

With a patient in the supine position, a pneumothorax commonly is seen in the anteromedial thorax, outlining the right or left heart border. If chest-tube placement is being considered, a decubitus image helps to differentiate an anteromedial pneumothorax from a pneumomediastinum in the pericardiac region.[159]

The following are some of the pitfalls encountered when examining the chest in the recumbent position for a pneumothorax.

• Skin folds may simulate a visceral pleural edge of a lung, resembling a pneumothorax. In the PA projection, the lung markings do not cross the skin fold. A skin fold images as a gradual opacity and a pneumothorax as a fine line[160] (Fig 7-11). A gathering of loose skin against a cassette or table in the AP supine position can give the illusion of a pneumothorax. Some pulmonary vessels often project across a skin fold; an upright or decubitus position can eliminate this gathering of skin. In the lateral projection, skin folds can simulate a lung edge and appear as a broad radiopaque edge rather than as a sharp, thin opaque line. They are difficult to identify since lung markings from the contralateral lung overlap, extending beyond the skin fold.

• Rotation of the chest can cause posterior chest-wall surfaces or the soft tissues of the back to simulate a pneumothorax

• The scapular spine in the lateral view can simulate a lung edge. Pneumothorax is some-

ing chest trauma such as stab and gunshot wounds, fractured ribs, thoracotomy, insertion of a thoracentesis needle or a needle for pleural biopsy, or a spontaneous blowout of a bleb or bulla in the lung.

A tension pneumothorax results when air enters the pleural space and is trapped by a "check valve" mechanism in the fistula.

On the erect PA chest radiograph, when a pneumothorax occurs, pulmonary vessels usually extend to a smooth, thin line representing the visceral pleura bordered by air in the pleural space. A pneumothorax is often seen at the apex of the chest. On occasion, lateral and subpulmonic collections of air can also be visualized. Inspiration and expiration PA chest images are helpful in evaluating this condition.

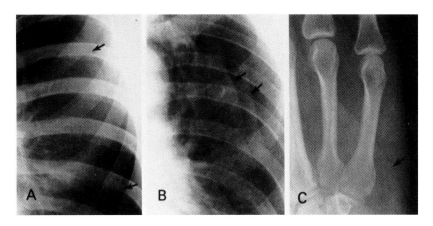

FIGURE 7-11   Skin Fold Versus Pneumothorax

(A) A pneumothorax is represented as a thin, visceral pleural edge (arrows).
(B) Skin folds have a broad opaque edge with an adjacent radiolucent band
and the visceral pleural edge is absent (arrows). (C) Skin-fold effect on
dorsum of hand (arrow). (Courtesy Fisher JK: Skin fold versus pneumothorax.
AJR 1978;130:791-792.)

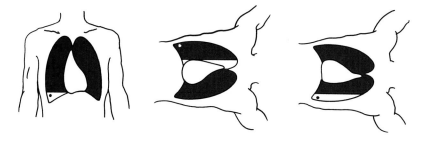

FIGURE 7-12   Effect of Positioning on Chest Imaging

As the position of the patient can affect diagnosis, whenever an unusual
position or tube angle is used, it should be identified with appropriate lead
markers. Left, A patient is shown in the upright position for radiography of the
chest. There is a lesion (black dot) in the right lung obscured by fluid in the
erect position. Center, When the patient is placed in the left lateral decubitus
position, the fluid should gravitate to the medial aspect of the right
hemithorax, clearing the base of the right lung. The lesion is now
demonstrated. Right, If the patient were positioned in the right lateral
decubitus position, the lesion could be obscured as free fluid spills along the
lateral aspect of the chest. (Redrawn from Cullinan JE, Cullinan AM: *Illustrated
Guide to X-Ray Technics.* Philadelphia, JB Lippincott Co, 1980.)

times better demonstrated in the lateral view. In
up to 15% of the patients with a pneumothorax,
a lateral projection can provide additional helpful information.[161]

Hydropneumothorax.   The appearance of air and
blood or some other fluid in the pleural space indicates a hydropneumothorax. On an upright
image, an air–fluid level within the pleural space
generally suggests the presence of blood or another fluid in addition to air. The visualization
of a hydropneumothorax on a supine chest radiograph depends on the amount of air and fluid
present at the time of the exposure. The upright
position or horizontal beam technique is needed
to demonstrate an air–fluid level[162] (Fig 7-12).

Pleural Effusion

Pleural effusion can be caused by inflammation, renal disease, malignancy, surgery, or chest trauma, and it results when excess free or loculated fluid collects in the pleural cavity. A pleural effusion containing blood is called a hemothorax. Free fluid generally gravitates to the most dependent portion of the pleural cavity (Fig 7-12). Pleural effusion, demonstrated by a blunting of the costophrenic angle, is best seen in the erect lateral chest.

It is sometimes impossible to distinguish fluid from thickening on conventional projections, particularly if previous films are not available. The problem can be resolved by utilizing an image made using a horizontal beam. Free fluid within the chest requires that the patient be positioned with the suspected side down to help visualize the fluid and to determine the amount present (Fig 7-12).

On occasion, a fluid-filled lung may be examined in an opposing decubitus position. For example, if free fluid exists in the right lung, the image may be made with the right lung in the superior (nondependent) position. In the decubitus position, with the diseased side up, fluid may shift within the chest, making it easier to visualize pulmonary consolidation, masses, or other abnormalities previously hidden by the fluid (Fig 7-12). Highly viscous free fluid, however, may not move despite repositioning of the patient.[36]

Atelectasis

Atelectasis is a collapsed or airless condition of a lung or a segment of a lung. With atelectasis, there is a loss of volume of some portion of the lung as the result of an obstruction, compression, or contraction attributable to scar tissue.

Aspiration of Fluids

The inhalation of liquids, such as soup, liquid parafin, or vomit, will often produce patchy bronchopneumonia. Irritant gasses such as chlorine can cause bilateral pulmonary edema when inhaled.[157]

Preoperative and Postoperative Chest Imaging

A preoperative chest radiograph may be of value in comparison studies if complications arise after surgery. The decision to perform a preoperative examination is a policy decision and is based on the quality of patient care, cost effectiveness, and a concern for radiation dosage.[163] Baseline radiographs can help in the evaluation and identification of congestive heart failure, pneumonia, and other thoracic abnormalities.

A presurgery workup might include an erect PA and lateral chest as well as a supine AP mobile-technique view of the chest. The supine mobile image can aid in the interpretation of subsequent postoperative studies, which are often performed in the supine position.[164]

Imaging of Cardiopulmonary Devices

Cardiopulmonary devices such as endotracheal tubes, Swan-Ganz catheters, central venous pressure catheters, prosthetic valves, chest tubes, pacemaker wires, and intra-aortic balloon pumps require perfectly positioned radiographs. The precise location of the tip and course of the catheter must be seen.[165]

> C A U T I O N : Although external support devices can mask or mimic disease, these devices should not be removed without the permission of the nursing staff or a physician. If a radiograph is made with a support device in position, that fact should be noted.

Interpretation of a bedside postoperative radiograph, particularly after cardiac surgery, is often complicated by artifacts superimposed on the image. Among devices that may be present are drainage tubes, temporary epicardial wire electrodes, surgical clips, an intra-aortic counterpulsation balloon, atrial pressure monitor catheters, external wires, or a Swan-Ganz catheter.[166]

The superimposition of a large plastic oxygen reservoir rebreathing mask on a postoperative chest radiograph can simulate a pneumothorax. The rounded upper corners of the bag produce a curvilinear white line near the apices

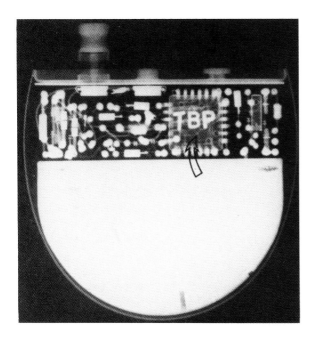

FIGURE 7-13 Pacemaker Visualization

A programmable lithium-powered pacemaker is shown. The radiopaque code TBP (arrow) indicates Teletronic Company (T), model code (B), and programmable (P). The Steiners et al article in *RadioGraphics* listing pacemakers by manufacturer, model number, and code should be consulted for specific information. (Courtesy Steiner RM, Tegtmeyer CJ, Moore D, et al: The radiology of cardiac pacemakers. *RadioGraphics* 1986;6:373-400.)

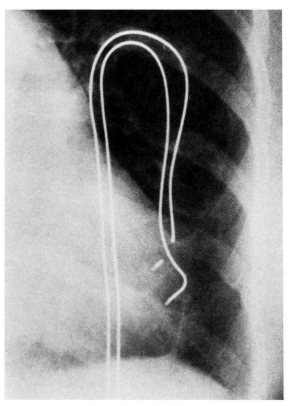

FIGURE 7-14 Pacemaker Lead Fracture

Radiography can be used to demonstrate a lead fracture of a pacemaker. In this illustration, there is a fracture of the epicardial lead. (Courtesy Steiner RM, Tegtmeyer CJ, Moore D, et al: The radiology of cardiac pacemakers. *RadioGraphics* 1986;6:373-400.)

that parallels the apical contour. The seam of the bag is almost indistinguishable from a pneumothorax since there is oxygen within the bag and room air external to it.[167]

Within the past decade, long-lived lithium-powered pacemakers have replaced mercury- and isotope-powered generators. The manufacturer, design, and type of action of a pacemaker can be identified by radiography of the pacemaker generator within a patient. Pacemakers incorporate a radiopaque code that can be seen on properly positioned conventional radiographs (Fig 7-13). Radiography can also demonstrate lead fractures, which occur in approximately 2% to 3% of patients with transvenous pacemakers[168] (Fig 7-14).

SUPPLEMENTARY OR MODIFIED IMAGING OF THE CHEST

Supplementary or modified projections are sometimes needed to demonstrate specific thoracic diseases or conditions. The following describes some variations on routine chest radiographs.

The Supine Position

Pleural effusions are common in critically ill patients. The supine position is often used for bedside chest radiographs since a study in this position is more easily performed than an erect study in this situation. However, the actual size of a pleural effusion is difficult to judge in the supine position.[169]

The Oblique Semisupine Position (Backward Leaning)

An oblique semisupine position with the patient leaning backward helps to collect free pleural fluid in the dorsal costophrenic sinus. The patient sits in a chair with an adjustable back or on a bed. The incline of the dorsal support is 45 to 65 degrees backward from the vertical plane. A 10 cm thick (40 cm by 80 cm) paper pillow is placed behind the patient's back. With the left side nearest to the film, the right side of the patient must be lowered in order to visualize both sides of the thorax simultaneously. The horizontal x-ray beam is centered to image the dorsal half of the thorax (Fig 7-15).

With the patient in the oblique semisupine position, respiration is suspended at full exhalation for the first image; a second image is made at full inhalation. If a pleural shadow shows a change in thickness at exactly the same point in both phases of respiration, or if the thickness of the pleural layer differs from that in the erect lateral view, pleural effusion must be considered.

A small or moderate amount of free fluid will appear to be wedge shaped or to resemble a half crescent as it raises the inferior rim of the lung from the thoracic wall. If the patient suspends respiration at full inhalation, the fluid will appear as a narrow shadow. In general, during the expiration phase, the level of free fluid in the pleural cavity is higher with the patient in the semisupine position than in the lateral decubitus position[170] (Fig 7-16).

Lateral Forward-Leaning Position

On a conventional chest study, it is sometimes difficult to distinguish between free and encapsulated dorsally sited pleural effusions. A lateral view in a forward-leaning sitting position helps to make this distinction. The patient is seated leaning forward with the elbows resting on the knees, positioned so that the dorsal costophrenic sinuses are projected separately.

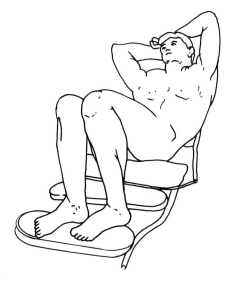

FIGURE 7–15 Oblique Semisupine Position to Demonstrate Pleural Effusion

Patient is seated in the oblique semisupine position, inclined to the right. (Redrawn from Möller A: Pleural effusion: Use of the semi-supine position for radiographic detection. *Radiology* 1984; 150: 245-249.)

With the forward-leaning position, free fluid will shift forward, making it possible to visualize the posterior lung and pleura. This position serves as an alternative for radiographic assessment of lung and pleura obscured by free effusion in conventional images.[171]

Supine Radiography to Demonstrate a Pneumothorax

Critically ill patients in intensive care are difficult to examine. Since many bedside chest radiographs are made in the supine or semirecumbent position, a pneumothorax typically cannot be demonstrated in such areas as those over the lung apices and lateral to the lung. If only supine views are available, the possibility of air in the anteromedial, posteromedial, or subpulmonic pleural spaces must be considered. An early finding helps to avoid progression to a tension pneumothorax.

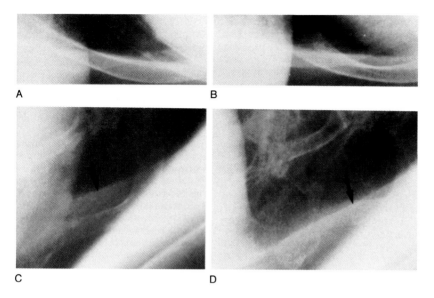

FIGURE 7–16 Pleural Effusion

Radiograph obtained with the patient in the lateral decubitus position and suspending respiration at exhalation (a) shows no pleural effusion. A repeat view, produced with the patient suspending respiration at full exhalation (b), discloses a thin shadow. This repeat image was obtained after radiographs of the patient in the oblique semisupine position and suspending respiration at full exhalation (c) showed a 7 mm thick shadow (arrow). At full inhalation (d), the shadow was extremely thin at exactly the same point (arrow) as in (c), consequently, the shadow represents fluid; pleural thickening is not indicated. (Courtesy Möller A: Pleural effusion: Use of the semi-supine position for radiographic detection. *Radiology* 1984; 150: 245-249.)

Demonstration of the lung bases on bedside radiographs is important, as is the aggressive use of additional radiographic views and CT when feasible.[177]

Air in the anterior medial space of the chest (the least dependent pleural recess) in the supine position could indicate an early subtle radiographic sign of pneumothorax. As the volume of air increases, the pneumothorax extends into the subpulmonic space and then into the apicolateral space.[173]

Early detection of small pleural air collections helps to prevent progression to a tension pneumothorax.[173] Shifting of the midline structures can take place with a tension pneumothorax. Even a slight rotation of the patient can make diagnosis difficult.

Tangential Imaging of the Chest

A 45 degree tangential radiograph of the hemithorax in question can verify the presence of a ventrally located pneumothorax. Extrapulmonary air can be located inside the pleural cavity with this technique[174] (Fig 7-17). A 10 to 25 degree tangential beam radiograph of the chest/abdomen can be used to demonstrate free air in the abdomen[175] (Fig 7-17).

Lordotic Imaging of the Chest

A conventional apical image with shoulders placed against the cassette holder or Bucky positions the ribs horizontally, thus helping to visualize the lungs between the ribs. The clavicles

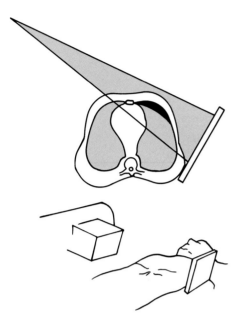

FIGURE 7–17 Tangential Projection to Locate a Pneumothorax

While a supine chest radiograph may be helpful to demonstrate a pneumothorax, the use of a 45 degree tangential radiograph of the hemithorax in question helps to demonstrate extrapulmonary air within the pleural cavity. Top, A 45 degree tube angulation is easy to accomplish with the patient supine. (Redrawn from Galanski M, Hartenauer U, Krumme B: A Roentgendiagnostik des Pneumothorax auf Intensivstationen. *Radiologe* 1981;21:459-462.) Bottom, A 10 to 25 degree tube angle may be used to demonstrate subdiaphragmatic air. (Drawn from Welsh HD, Fleming EG: Radiographic visualization of subdiaphragmatic air. *Med Radiog Photog* 1958;34:78-79.)

project cephalad, avoiding superimposition on the apical area.

While the evaluation of the lung apex benefits from the lordotic position, this position presents an apparent elevation of the diaphragm, poor visualization of the lung bases, a loss of definition of the aortic arch, and apparent widening of the superior mediastinum.[176] A modified AP lordotic view reduces magnification of most of the lung fields. With the upright table tilted

downward approximately 55 to 60 degrees and the footrest in place, the clavicles project away from the apices. The first and second ribs are then parallel with the CR. With the shoulders rolled forward, an exposure is made on deep inspiration.[177] This position can be easily duplicated or modified if additional images are required.

Reverse Lordotic Imaging

A tangential view of the posterior aspect of the diaphragm is suggested to demonstrate the posterior lung bases. The patient must be upright, either sitting or standing, for an AP reverse lordotic view of the chest with caudal angulation (30 degrees) of the beam. A PA view with cephalad beam angulation and with the patient prone can be used, but this increases magnification of the posterior structures of the chest[178] (Fig 7-18).

C A U T I O N : The lateral view of the chest should be evaluated for the position of the diaphragm to determine the exact degree of angulation for each patient.[179]

C A U T I O N : At the bedside, where it is difficult to elevate a patient to the full upright position, 10 to 15 degrees of lordosis can mask or mimic disease in the lower lobe and / or pleural space[179] (Figs 7-19 through 7-21).

The Lateral Chest for Pneumoperitoneum

The demonstration of small amounts of free air beneath the diaphragm depends on proper patient positioning and the imaging sequence.

When the central x-ray beam is parallel to the long axis of the subdiaphragmatic air, the air is easily seen. If the air collects anteriorly, the x-ray beam, now oblique to the air, makes it difficult to demonstrate the free air on a PA radiograph. The lateral projection can be used to show a small curvilinear collection of free intraperito-

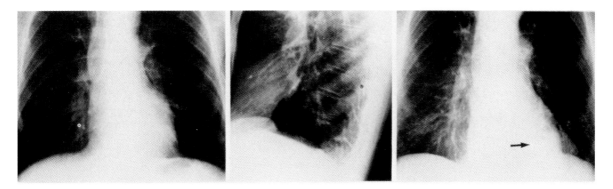

FIGURE 7-18   Reverse Lordotic Position

Three views of the chest are shown. Left, The PA view appears normal. Center, The lateral view demonstrates a vague density in one of the posterior costophrenic angles. Right, The patient was positioned in the 30 degree "reverse lordotic" position to obtain the third view. This image demonstrates a mass (arrow) in the left lung base. A tangential view of the posterior aspect of the diaphragm helps to show the posterior lung bases. The patient can be positioned in the upright position for an AP view of the chest obtained with a caudad tube angle. A PA view can also be obtained with the patient prone, using a cephalad tube angle. (Courtesy Gehl JJ, Johnson LA: Reverse lordotic view for visualization of the lung bases. *AJR* 1987; 148: 651-652.)

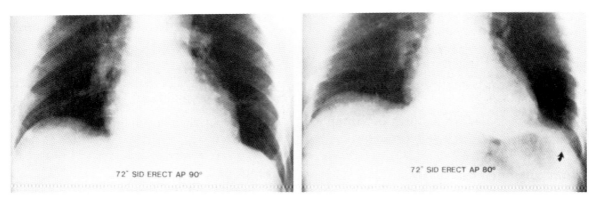

FIGURE 7-19   Left-Lower-Lobe Evaluation at the Bedside

The apex of the left hemidiaphragm is difficult to image owing to cephalad angulation of the CR accompanied by the projection of extrapleural fat on the base of the left lung. A human chest phantom is shown in the erect position. Left, an AP radiograph was obtained with the CR directed perpendicular to the vertical axis of the phantom. This image demonstrates the left lower lobe and pleural space. The diaphragm is sharply depicted. Right, With the phantom in 10 degrees of lordosis, there is a loss of definition of the left hemidiaphragm, simulating a pulmonary consolidation or fluid or both (arrow). (Courtesy Zylak CJ, Littleton JT, Durizch ML: Illusory consolidation of left lower lobe: A pitfall of portable radiography. *Radiology* 1988; 167: 653-655.)

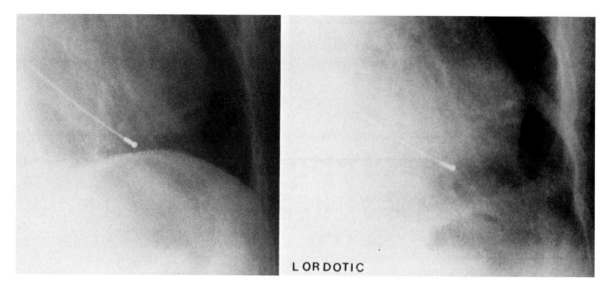

LORDOTIC

FIGURE 7-20   Clinical Image of Left Hemidiaphragm

Left, An AP radiograph of a patient without clinical evidence of chest disease was obtained with the CR perpendicular to the left hemidiaphragm. There is a sharp interface between the left hemidiaphragm and the adjacent lung. Right, Within minutes, a second radiograph was made in the AP position of the same patient, but in 10 to 15 degrees of lordosis. The left hemidiaphragm was obscured, simulating the presence of left-lower-lobe disease. This probably was due to the superimposition of extrapleural fat since the more anterior aspect of the hemidiaphragm is visualized when the patient is imaged in the lordotic position. (Courtesy Zylak CJ, Littleton JT, Durizch ML: Illusory consolidation of left lower lobe: A pitfall of portable radiography. *Radiology* 1988; 167:653-655.)

neal air situated anteriorly beneath a hemidiaphragm[180] (Figs 7-22 through 7-24).

Supine Cross-Table Lateral Chest Radiography for the Detection of Pericardial Effusion

The epicardial fat sign occurs as the result of fluid accumulating between the subepicardial fat and anterior mediastinal fat. Since fatty tissue appears less dense than an effusion on a radiograph, pericardial effusion images as a high density band between two layers of less dense adipose tissue. In the conventional lateral view, large pleural effusions, pulmonary infiltrates, or increased breast tissue makes it difficult to demonstrate the epicardial fat stripe.

Supine cross-table lateral chest radiographs have been shown to have greater sensitivity (51%) for pericardial effusion when compared with conventional lateral chest images with a sensitivity of 31%. With a supine cross-table lateral chest image, the cardiac silhouette tends to move more posteriorly, minimizing structures or shadows that might make detection of the epicardial fat sign difficult.[181]

THE AIRWAY

Because of overlying osseous and soft-tissue structures, it is difficult to demonstrate the larynx, trachea, and bronchi with normal thoracic projections such as the AP, PA, lateral soft-tissue cervical, or overpenetrated upper lateral chest technique.

ANATOMICAL/PATHOLOGICAL OBSERVATIONS

The nasopharynx lies behind the nose above the level of the soft palate. The oropharynx lies between the soft palate and the hyoid bone and the laryngeal pharynx extends with the esophagus

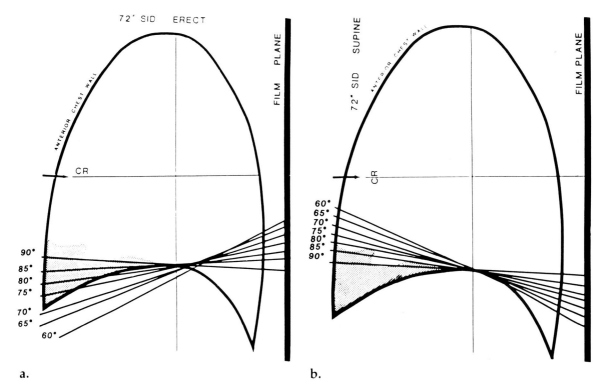

a.   b.

FIGURE 7–21   Schematic of Central-Ray Projection

When the CR is effectively projected 5 to 10 degrees cephalad, the loss of tangential imaging of the apex of the left hemidiaphragm becomes apparent. As angulation is increased, the fat pad projects on to the lower lung, simulating pulmonary consolidation, pleural effusion, or both (a). Conversely, when the CR is effectively directed caudad, it is continually tangential to the curvilinear surface of the diaphragm so that it is always clearly delineated (b). (Courtesy Zylak CJ, Littleton JT, Durizch ML: Illusory consolidation of the left lower lobe: A pitfall of portable radiography. *Radiology* 1988; 167: 653-655.)

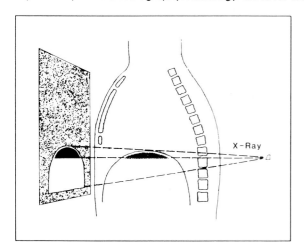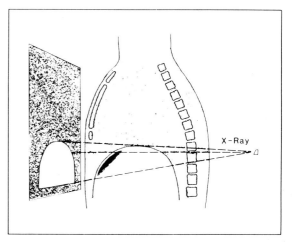

FIGURE 7–22   Schematic Demonstration of Pneumoperitoneum on the Lateral Chest Image

Intraperitoneal free air is usually demonstrated by an erect PA chest radiograph. On occasion, free air can be seen only on the lateral image. Left, With the central x-ray beam parallel to the long axis of the subdiaphragmatic air, it is readily visualized. Right, If the air pockets anteriorly, the same x-ray beam is oblique to the air and a pneumoperitoneum will not be demonstrated on the PA radiograph. (Courtesy of Markowitz SK, Ziter FMH Jr: The lateral chest film and pneumoperitoneum. *Ann Emerg Med* 1986; 15: 425-427.)

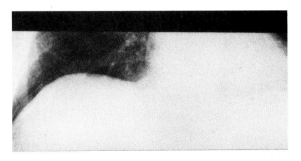 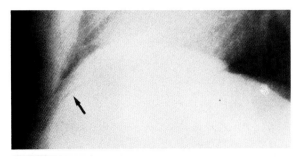

FIGURE 7-23 Free Intraperitoneal Air

Left, A PA chest film in which no free air is demonstrated. Right, A lateral image shows a small curvilinear collection of free interperitoneal air, anterior, beneath the left diaphragm. (Courtesy of Markowitz SK, Ziter FMH Jr: The lateral chest film and pneumoperitoneum. *Ann Emerg Med* 1986;15:425-427.)

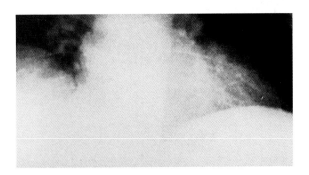 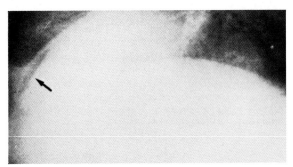

FIGURE 7-24 Postsurgical Collection of Air

Left, A PA radiograph of a postsurgical patient; no free air is seen. Right, In the lateral view, there is a small collection of air beneath the right hemidiaphragm, anteriorly. (Courtesy Markowitz SK, Ziter FMH Jr: The lateral chest film and pneumoperitoneum. *Ann Emerg Med* 1986;15:425-427.)

from the hyoid bone to the lower border of the cricoid cartilage of the larynx.

POSITIONING CONCEPTS

The experienced radiographer must be prepared to step away from the patient if technical duties are superseded by a priority problem such as maintaining an airway.

The nasal and oral pharynges are well visualized in a lateral view of the skull if the exposure is made during the latter phase of inspiration with the patient's mouth closed[182] (Fig 7-25).

Andrus Projection to Demonstrate Trachea and Main-Stem Bronchi

An oblique view of the chest (Andrus method) provides an almost true PA visualization of the trachea and main bronchi and adjacent lymph nodes and retrocardiac regions.[183] The patient and cassette are placed in a 45 degree RAO position with the plane of the cassette against the front of the chest (parallel to the chest) and perpendicular to the median plane of the body (Fig 7-26).

> CAUTION: When this position was first described, grid radiography of the chest was the exception, not the rule. An attempt to produce this image with a grid would require the positioning of the grid lines parallel with the floor, with the CR (top to bottom) centered to the center of the grid to avoid grid cutoff.

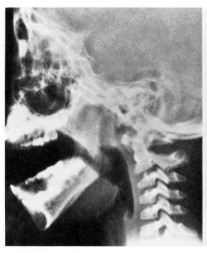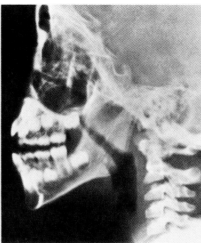

FIGURE 7-25   Nasopharyngeal Visualization

Right, To visualize the nasopharyngeal airway best, the radiograph must be exposed with the mouth of the patient closed, during the later phase of inspiration. Left, On an image obtained with the mouth open, there is a false occlusion of the nasopharyngeal airway. (Courtesy Rivero H, Bender TM, Oh KS: Optimal visualization of the nasopharyngeal airway. *Radiology* 1983;147:877-878.)

Imaging of the Cervicothoracic Inlet

The cervicothoracic inlet can be demonstrated on a supplementary oblique projection with the patient AP and the median plane perpendicular to the cassette. The patient should be rotated 45 to 60 degrees to the left, with the head turned to the true lateral position and the chin slightly elevated. The Valsalva maneuver is required with this exposure to image the larynx, trachea, and bronchi on one radiograph.[184]

A soft-tissue lateral image of the cervical area is used to show foreign bodies in the trachea or esophagus (Fig 7-27).

TECHNICAL CONSIDERATIONS

A "complete" chest radiograph might require more than one exposure or a technical compromise. The dense mediastinum superimposed on the descending aorta, the thoracic vertebrae, the sternum, lung parenchyma, and retrocardiac and subdiaphragmatic structures makes it difficult to select an optimal chest technique. Fluid and radiodense lesions compound this technical

**FIGURE 7-26
Trachea and
Main-Stem Bronchi**

A variation of the oblique position of the chest is required for an almost true PA visualization of the trachea and main-stem bronchi. With the patient positioned in a 45 degree RAO oblique position and the cassette placed against the anterior chest wall, the trachea, main-stem bronchi, adjacent lymph nodes, and retrocardiac area can be demonstrated. The use of a grid for this oblique positioning variation requires that the grid lines be parallel with the floor and that the CR be centered to the center of the grid to avoid grid cutoff.

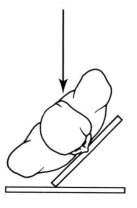

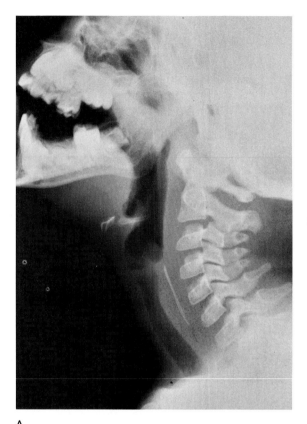 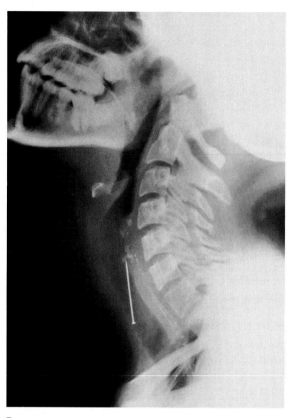

A   B

FIGURE 7–27   Soft-Tissue Lateral Cervical for Foreign Body

(A) Calcific foreign body in the esophagus is identified as a chicken bone. (B) Metallic foreign body (pin) shown in the trachea. (Courtesy Eastman Kodak Company, Rochester, NY.)

problem.[185] On the PA projection of the chest, as much as 40% of the lungs can be projected over the mediastinum and diaphragms. This area is suboptimally imaged (Fig 7-1).

The filling of the lungs with a radiolucent contrast agent (air) is as important as is the use of a radiopaque agent (barium) for a GI study.[185] Full inspiration maximizes imaging of the lung fields. A PA radiograph of the chest made in expiration can cause the heart to appear more transverse in diameter (Fig 7-2). This increases the possibility of artificial findings and may obscure the presence of an underlying disease.

Patients often confuse the holding of their breath with deep inspiration and need instruction on how to take a deep breath.

Kilovoltage Selection

The significant differences in x-ray absorption in the thorax make it difficult to achieve an acceptable density over the entire PA chest radiograph. Mediastinal structures, retrocardiac anatomy, and subdiaphragmatic air are often difficult to evaluate without overexposing the lung fields.

When using a high ratio grid, low kVp and a high contrast film, the mediastinum will image near the sensitometric toe of the film and project as a silhouette, rather than as a detailed segment of anatomy. Use of a high ratio grid, high kVp and a latitude or extended latitude x-ray film improves the imaging of the mediastinum and helps to image linear shadows and mediastinal striping.

A knowledge of mediastinal anatomy is of help to the radiographer in selecting the proper parameters to demonstrate these important diagnostic signs. Thin, linear soft-tissue structures in the lungs are imaged because of the presence of air on each side of the tissue. Stripe effects, the result of an air–soft-tissue interface, represent air-filled lung abutted against a soft-tissue structure.

On occasion, a portion of the stomach can herniate into the thoracic cavity and can be seen on the conventional PA chest view. High kVp, a high ratio grid, and latitude or extended latitude film better visualize the air-filled segment of the stomach superimposed on the mediastinum.

Filtration

Compensatory filters, usually affixed to a thin sheet of plastic and inserted into the external track of a collimator, are designed to help overcome variations in anatomy and to provide a uniform radiographic density. The density-equalizing effect on a chest radiograph exposed with a compensatory filter results because the filter absorbs x-rays over the lung fields.[186] Unfortunately, the use of a filter requires longer exposure times and higher mA or kVp values. This increase in exposure to the mediastinum helps to demonstrate mediastinal and retrocardiac structures that lie out of the toe region of the characteristic curve of the x-ray film.

The choice of the filter used for chest radiography is often a compromise since one size or type of filter cannot fit all sizes and types of patients and cannot overcome variations in pulmonary pathology, heart size, or fluid in the lungs (Fig 7-28). Guilbeau[187] evaluated a shaped filter for use at 140 kVp to detect mediastinal and retrocardiac abnormalities on the PA chest image. He found that there were no significant differences in the analyses of the types or locations of mediastinal lesions when compared with conventional radiographs.

> C A U T I O N : Some compensatory filters can produce edge markings that may resemble pathology, such as a pneumomediastinum or medial pneumothorax.

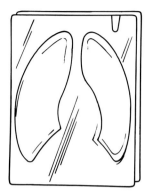

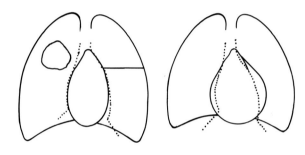

FIGURE 7–28 Compensatory Filtration for Chest Radiography

Top, A compensatory filter for chest radiography permits the penetration of the dense mediastinal area while holding radiation back from the aerated, easy-to-overexpose lungs. Bottom, Illustrations of two atypical chests demonstrate that a single size of opening in a filter is not adequate for all types of body habitus or disease processes. Even if the filter were to match the mediastinal configuration (bottom left), x-radiation would be held back from a lesion in the right upper lung or fluid in the left lung. On the right, the cardiac configuration is larger than the opening in the compensatory filter.

Scoliosis and complex pathological changes or deformities in the thorax make it difficult to evaluate the chest using a compensatory filter. A wedge compensatory filter used for a lateral projection of the chest helps to avoid the imaging differences of the inferoposterior chest (retrocardiac space) as compared with the dense muscular apical area (Figs 7-29 and 7-30).

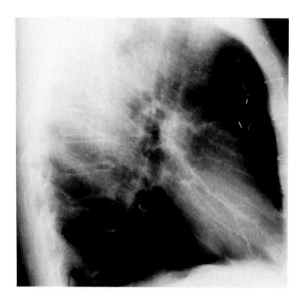

FIGURE 7-29 Lateral Chest Image

Balancing radiographic density in the lateral chest is
not an easy task. An inadequate exposure makes it
difficult to image the apical portion of the chest. The
use of a low to moderate kVp with a high ratio grid
would accentuate this problem since this
combination, when used with normal contrast type
x-ray film, results in an abrupt black and white image.
Note the blackened area in the retrosternal space, as
well as in the retrocardiac space.

Screen-Film Technology

Relatively fast (up to 300 speed) rare earth
screen-film systems have a resolution capability
similar to that of 100 speed calcium tungstate
systems and are recommended for chest
imaging.

The sensitometric limitations of a radiographic film often lead to the use of a filter. A
high contrast radiographic film produces chalklike mediastinal and osseous structures. While of
value in the evaluation of osseous-structure and
contrast medium studies, this type of film is not
optimal for conventional chest radiography. Use
of a high ratio grid with low kilovoltage and a
high contrast film results in extremely short
scale contrast (Fig 7-31).

A high kVp/grid technique using a latitude
film will improve mediastinal imaging. An extended latitude film is designed specifically to
image mediastinal details without compromising the lung fields and without the use of a compensatory filter (Fig 7-32). Kilovoltage must be
matched to the grid ratio.

Nongrid versus Grid Technique

The aerated lungs (spongy, expanded vascular
structures) produce little scatter as compared
with that generated by the spine, descending
aorta, heart, and sternum, which is similar to
that associated with radiography of the
abdomen.

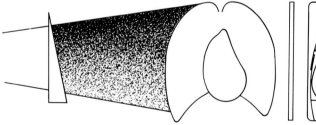
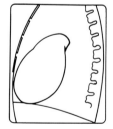

FIGURE 7-30 Use of a Compensatory Filter for Lateral Chest Radiography

A wedge compensatory filter can be used to balance radiographic density in
the lateral chest image. Note that the thinner portion of the wedge (left)
permits a considerable amount of radiation to expose the dense, muscular
apical area of the chest. As the wedge thickens, x-radiation is held back,
helping to avoid overexposure of the lung fields, particularly the retrocardiac
area (right).

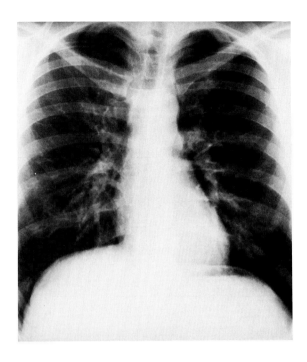

FIGURE 7–31   Low kVp / High Ratio Grid Technique for Chest Radiography

Grid ratio must be matched to the kVp selected for chest radiography. A high ratio grid used with low kilovoltage (particularly with a high contrast film) results in abrupt blacks and whites — chalklike ribs and cardiac silhouette with no mediastinal information available for interpretation. The blackened lung fields may hide small lesions within the lungs.

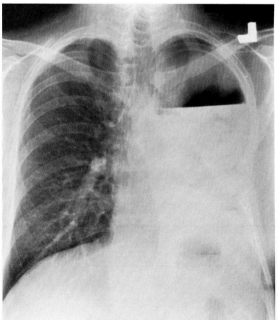

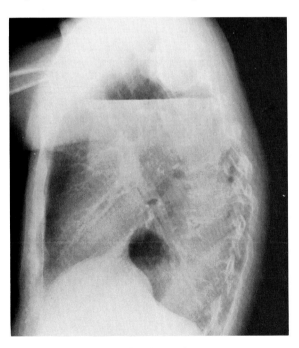

FIGURE 7–32   High kVp / Grid Technique with Extended Latitude Film for Chest Radiography

The use of an extended latitude film results in quality imaging of the lung fields, as well as visualization of the mediastinum or other dense structures. (A) In the PA projection, note the visualization of the right lung as it bows to the left side of the chest. (B) In the lateral projection, the right lung markings can be seen through the fluid-filled left chest. There is a large mass in the posterior apical area. Calcific striations can be seen outlining the mass. This image was made at 140 kVp with a 12 : 1 ratio grid, without a compensatory filter. (Courtesy Eastman Kodak Company, Rochester, NY.)

For many years, the term "Bucky chest" was understood to mean an image obtained with the patient in the supine position and the use of thoracic spine exposure factors to demonstrate mediastinal anatomy, shifting of free fluid, and so on. This was always an additional image made as a follow-up to a PA, nongrid, moderate kVp chest study.

The current literature does not support the use of nongrid/low to moderate kVp techniques for chest radiography that produce short scale contrast images, or abrupt differences in black and white. Today, chest radiographs are usually made in the PA erect position using a Bucky or grid, high kVp values, and an AEC. An increase in kVp (up to 150 kVp) rather than a change in the mAs, produces the latitude effect associated with grid or Bucky chest techniques.

CAUTION: The use of a low ratio grid with high kilovoltage will mask the mediastinum with scatter, giving the illusion of proper exposure (Fig 7-31).

A high ratio grid used with low to moderate kilovoltage (90 kVp or less, particularly with single-phase equipment) produces an abrupt black and white image with chalklike osseous structures, an underexposed mediastinum, and overexposed lungs. The posteroinferior lung segments, poorly imaged through the diaphragm, lack radiographic details (Fig 7-31). Although proper radiographic density, as determined by the AEC, is seen, mediastinal information may be lacking as a result of underpenetration.

High kVp/grid techniques (125 kVp or greater) offer greater exposure latitude—a longer-scale contrast. Specific benefits of high kVp/grid chest radiography include:

1. Decreased bone contrast; suppressed rib details.
2. Better penetration of mediastinal, subdiaphragmatic, and other soft-tissue structures.
3. Decreased radiation to the patient as compared with low kVp/grid techniques.

NOTE: Although more radiation is required to produce a radiograph when using a grid, one should not compare the radiation dosage of a nongrid/moderate kVp study with that of a grid/high kVp study. These studies represent different approaches to imaging. Comparisons made using the same grid at low and high kVp settings (for example, a 12:1 ratio grid using 90 kVp and a 12:1 ratio grid using 130 kVp) are more relevant. Dosage reduction is seen when comparing grid techniques if a higher kVp with a reduced mAs is used for the comparison image.

Most chest grids are positioned for upright radiography, with the grid lines perpendicular to the floor. This means that a shift of the tube to the left or right will result in a unilateral grid cutoff. When a stationary grid is used for a decubitus radiograph of the chest or abdomen, a grid-positioning problem arises. If the grid or grid cassette is positioned in the traditional way (lengthwise), the center of the grid is approximately 7 ins from the tabletop. This implies that every patient being examined is 14 ins wide. One must center to the grid, not to the patient. If the grid is positioned with the grid lines perpendicular to rather than parallel with the floor, then regardless of the size of the patient, one can center to the grid and/or the patient, being careful not to off-center the tube left or right at any height (Fig 7-33).

An artifact-free grid avoids the possibility of masking such pathological conditions as fracture or notching of the ribs, subdiaphramatic air, and subcutaneous emphysema.

The Air-Gap Technique

When an air gap employing an 8, 10, or 12 in OFD is substituted for a high ratio grid, an increased FFD of 8, 10, or 12 ft is required to overcome enlargement of the cardiac silhouette. The air gap, an effective substitute for a grid or Bucky, requires a minimum OFD of 6 in. With an air gap, most of the Compton scatter photons from the patient do not reach the cassette. When examining a large, dense mass, such as an enlarged heart or a chest with a significant amount

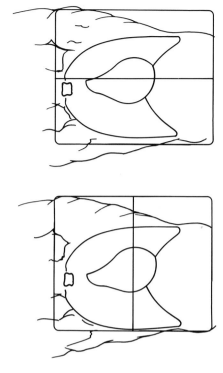

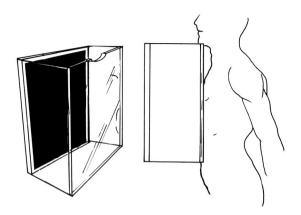

FIGURE 7–34 Positioning Device for Air-Gap Radiography of the Chest

Left, A wall-mounted cassette holder is shown with a sheet of radiolucent plastic mounted either 10 or 12 in from the cassette. Right, The patient is positioned against the low absorption plastic to produce an air gap for high kVp/gridlike chest radiography.

FIGURE 7–33 Use of a Grid for Decubitus Chest Radiography

When a patient is put into the lateral decubitus position for a chest radiograph, a grid cassette is often placed with the grid lines parallel with the x-ray table or floor. Positioning of the grid in this manner assumes that every chest is exactly 14 in wide, with the center of the chest 7 in from the tabletop (top). The grid should be positioned with the lead lines perpendicular to the tabletop (bottom) so that, regardless of the size of the patient, centering to the center of the grid can be achieved.

of fluid, the air gap may not be as effective as a high ratio grid owing to the increase in scatter radiation.

The doubling of the FFD to 12 ft with a 12 in air gap would require an approximate increase of four times the mAs factor. A nongrid technique, however, would permit a reduction in mAs by a factor of four. Theoretically, a 6 ft FFD grid study and a 12 ft FFD nongrid/air-gap study should involve similar technical factors. In prac-tice, however, an air gap usually is not substi-tuted for a grid, but rather for a nongrid tech-nique (Fig 7-34).

AEC for Chest Radiography

Use of an AEC results in a predetermined radio-graphic density when the control is set at its "Normal" position. Each plus or minus setting on the AEC varies exposure times by approxi-mately 25%, thereby increasing or decreasing the preselected density. See Chapter 1, Fig 1-15. If the minus adjustment does not seem to function, especially with small to medium-size patients, the minimum response time of the control must be considered. Let us assume that the normal setting produces a radiograph that is too dark for interpretation. If the exposure time required for the proper density is less than the minimal re-sponse time of the AEC, the minus density ad-justment cannot correct this error because it is not possible for the control to terminate the short exposure since it has reached its minimal response time. As faster screen-film systems be-come more popular, problems of minimum re-sponse times will increase.[7]

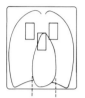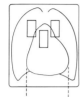

FIGURE 7–35 Automatic Sensor Control Selection for Chest Radiography

Most AECs have three sensing devices for chest radiography, left. The use of one or more of these sensors is determined by departmental preference and/or equipment design. A large heart or consolidated lung positioned over one of the sensors (right) might cause the AEC to lengthen the exposure. The central detector is generally used for lateral chest radiography. For specific information regarding sensor selection, the manufacturer of the unit should be consulted.

CAUTION: With an AEC exposure, adequate film blackening on a chest radiograph can occur even with minimal inspiration. Unfortunately, the elevated diaphragm associated with poor inspiration also widens the heart shadow (Fig 7-2). When a manual timing technique is used, the lack of aeration is apparent on the underexposed image.

The size and shape of the heart, as well as other radiodense pathology, can cause inconsistent operation of an AEC (Fig 7-35). Sensor-selection recommendations for various positions should be provided by the manufacturer of the device.

Mobile Chest Radiography

In some large hospitals, up to 50% of all chest examinations are performed at the bedside using mobile equipment. Technical limitations of such studies include:

1. Poor beam alignment and/or centering.
2. Positioning difficulties, particularly with decubitus or erect positions.
3. Shortened FFD.
4. Grid focus difficulties.
5. Control of scatter.

CAUTION: The shortened FFD and large focal spot often utilized for bedside radiography can cause imaging difficulties, particularly with trauma patients. The demonstration of a wide mediastinum or deviated trachea could indicate a ruptured aorta, but could also be the result of an AP supine radiograph obtained with a shortened FFD or by rotation of the patient.

Images made at the bedside with modern 110 kVp constant potential mobile units and 400 speed, or greater, screen-film systems can be of a technical quality similar to that of conventional images made in the main department.

Modified Dedicated Grid or Bucky Chest Room

A radiographic department that cannot justify the cost of a dedicated chest room or the space required can still produce state-of-the-art chest radiographs. Grid- or Bucky-quality images using high kVp made with an upright chest film holder can duplicate images made on a dedicated chest device.

An automatic cassette loader/unloader and cassettes with dedicated screens make it difficult accidentally to select a film that is not matched to the appropriate speed or emissivity of the intensifying screens.

CHAPTER EIGHT

Mammography

The breasts—accessory organs of the female reproductive system—are studied radiographically by mammography.

There is some patient anxiety even when baseline mammography is performed. Patients fear the results of the test and complain about breast compression and the coldness of the mammographic platform. Patients, however, will allow vigorous compression if its importance is explained prior to the examination. The degree of discomfort associated with compression is thought in part to be related to the use of caffeine. In one study, 60% of the women who were most uncomfortable with the procedure used five or more caffeine-containing products per day.[188]

An ordinary heating pad, at a low setting, placed on the surface of the tray between studies will keep the platform moderately warm.[189]

ANATOMICAL AND PATHOLOGICAL OBSERVATIONS

Breasts (undeveloped in males) develop after puberty in females and usually extend from the second to the sixth ribs and from the lateral border of the sternum to the midaxillary line. The area of the breast known as the axillary tail, or the upper outer portion of the breast, extends upward into the axilla. Axillary and/or internal mammary lymph nodes are often seen on radiographic images.

Composed of fatty, glandular, and fibrous tissue, breasts vary considerably in size, shape, and density among individuals. Age and parity, not necessarily size, influence breast density. Although primarily a female condition, males occasionally develop breast disease and may require mammographic examinations.

Mammographic Screening

The National Council on Radiation Protection and Measurements, at the suggestion of the National Cancer Institute, issued a practical guide for physicians, radiographers, physicists, and engineers titled, *Mammography, A User's Guide* (NCR Report no. 85). Complex dosage information and discussions of the risk/benefit factors in the decision to use mammography and of the practical aspects of the procedure are included in this booklet.[190]

A voluntary accreditation program set up by the American College of Radiology (ACR) should also improve the quality of mammography in the United States. The protocol for accreditation includes quality assurance recommendations for physicists and radiographers. See "Quality Assurance."

POSITIONING CONCEPTS

Optimal imaging of the mammary gland requires special attention to positioning concepts. The breast, thicker at the chest wall than at the nipple area, overlaps the rib cage, making it difficult to image the pyramid-shaped female breast. Images should be made with the patient standing, whenever possible. In the sitting position, the protuberance of the abdomen may make it difficult properly to position the cassette holder close to the chest wall. The erect position minimizes abdominal protuberance, especially in the obese patient.

When using compression, breast thickness should be kept constant over the entire breast. "Whiteout" of the structures near the chest wall results from improper compression.[191] Curved compression paddles may be more comfortable, but they do not compress the breast adequately for screen-film mammography. If breast tissue is pushed above and behind the compression plate, the tissue in the upper, posterior breast will not be seen on the image.[192] The tissue forced backward and upward along the chest wall produces an abrupt difference in breast-tissue thickness at the chest wall, causing a soft-tissue step-wedge effect. Straight-edge compression minimizes the possibility of whiteout[7] (Fig 8-1). To maximize tissue visualization, the radiographer should gently pull the breast forward, lifting the breast tissue onto the support tray.

Multiple projections are necessary to show all portions of the breast. A routine should be established for identifying each view. Generally, ID markers are placed in the upper quadrant with the lateral and lateral oblique positions and in the outer quadrant with the craniocaudal and craniocaudal oblique positions[193,194] (Figs 8-2 through 8-4). A small radiopaque marker should be placed over a palpable lesion to aid in localization at the time of interpretation.[193]

Basic mammographic projections include the following.

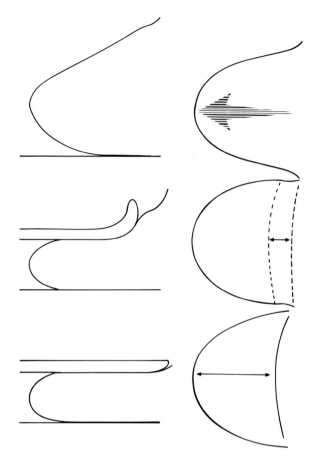

FIGURE 8-1 Mammographic Compression

Because of the thickness of the breast near the chest wall (left top), compression is essential for quality mammography. The arrow represents the difference in radiographic density from the nipple to the chest wall (right top). The darkened portion of the arrow represents the increased radiographic density owing to the thinner segment of the breast. When a curved compression paddle is used to flatten the breast, breast tissue may move backward and upward off the curved surface of the compression paddle (left center). The dotted lines (right center) show an area of "whiteout" at the chest wall, often seen with poor compression. A straight-edge compression paddle will produce an overall even compression from nipple to chest wall (bottom). (Courtesy Cullinan AM: *Producing Quality Radiographs.* Philadelphia, JB Lippincott Co, 1987.)

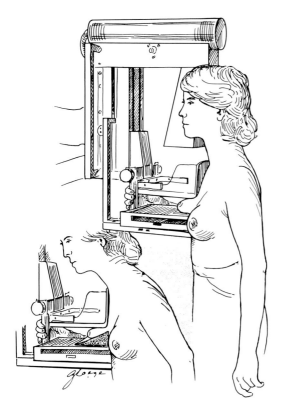

FIGURE 8-2 Craniocaudal Position

This position is obtained by elevating the breast on a support tray, with the medial segment of the breast at the chest wall in close contact with the edge of the film holder. Note the "sponge" craniocaudal position (insert). Lesions deep in the lower hemisphere of the breast may be seen by elevating the rib cage and upper abdomen over the top of the film holder, with the breast lying over the sponge wedge. This helps to visualize the chest wall on the mammographic image. (Courtesy Gormley L, Bassett LW, Gold RH: Positioning in film-screen mammography. *Appl Radiol* 1988 ; 7 : 35-37.)

FIGURE 8-4 Lateromedial Projection

The patient's arm is placed over the cassette holder. The patient is then rotated slightly inward, allowing for ease of positioning and increased visualization of most of the posterior breast tissue. (Courtesy Gormley L, Bassett LW, Gold RH: Positioning in film-screen mammography. *Appl Radiol* 1988 ; 7 : 35-37.)

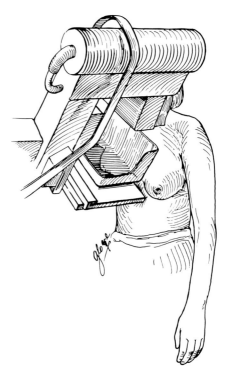

FIGURE 8-3 Mediolateral Oblique

With this projection, the breast is distracted from the pectoralis major muscle and compressed at an angle that runs parallel with muscle fibers of the pectoralis as it enters the axilla. (Courtesy Gormley L, Bassett LW, Gold RH: Positioning in film-screen mammography. *Appl Radiol* 1988 ; 7 : 35-37.)

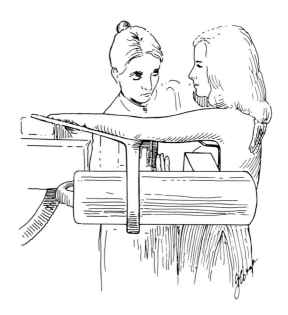

• Craniocaudal. The breast should be lifted onto the support tray so that the medial aspect of the chest wall is in close contact with the edge of the film holder.

CAUTION: In the standard craniocaudal view, the entire lateral aspect of the breast may not be seen (Fig 8-5).

• Mediolateral oblique projection (for visualization of the axillary tail)[195] (Fig 8-3). The lateral juxathoracic portion of the breast, especially the axillary tail of the breast, is best seen in the oblique view, which demonstrates the most breast tissue on a single projection[196] (Fig 8-5). As the breast is pulled away from the pectoralis major muscle, compression should be applied along the plane parallel to the fibers of this muscle as it enters the axilla. The plane of the cassette should be placed along the midaxillary line, with the corner of the cassette in the axilla. If the cassette were positioned along the anterior axillary line, some of the breast tissue might not be visualized. The degree of angulation (of the x-ray tube and/or patient) may vary, depending on patient habitus. A woman with pendulous breasts might require a 40 degree angulation, whereas a tall, thinner woman might require up to 60 degrees of angulation. On average, a 45 degree angulation usually is acceptable.

• Lateral projection. On the lateral and lateral oblique views, the medial and posterior portions of the breast may not be well demonstrated (Fig 8-5). Visualization of the rib cage on the lateral view of the breast does not guarantee that the entire posterior portion of the breast has been imaged. A significant amount of breast tissue adjacent to the chest wall can be missed, depending on the position of the patient[7] (Fig 8-6).

A gentle pull of the breast away from the chest while applying compression helps to image the posterior portion of the breast. The patient's arm should be relaxed, which, in turn, will relax the muscles along the chest wall.

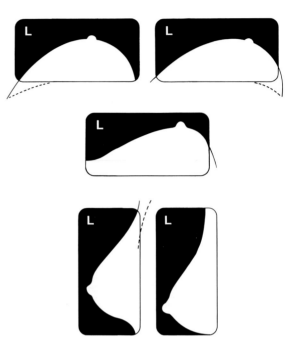

FIGURE 8–5 Need for Additional Positions

Top, Craniocaudal imaging. Because of its configuration, either the medial or lateral aspects of the breast will not be visualized simultaneously in the conventional craniocaudal view. In this illustration of the left breast, when the breast is positioned so that the medial portion is imaged, the outer portion of the breast (axillary tail) is not demonstrated (left). If the patient were rotated to position the axillary tail of the breast on the film, the medial aspect of the breast would be rotated off of the film (right). A modified oblique projection (center) presents even more of the axillary tail. Bottom, In a 90 degree true lateral position (left), the upper portion of the breast is not well seen. If the patient were positioned for a 45 degree lateral oblique projection, the upper breast tissue would be well demonstrated (right). Identification markers are placed adjacent to the outer aspect of the breast in the craniocaudal projections and adjacent to the upper aspect of the breast in the lateral projections.

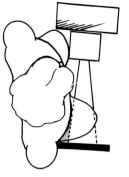

FIGURE 8-6
Visualization of the Chest Wall

The visualization of the chest wall (rib cage) on a radiograph does not always ensure that the posterior portion of the breast has been imaged (shaded area). The mammographer must gently pull the breast forward while it is lifted and placed in contact with the support tray. Vigorous compression should then be applied. If the patient's arm is hyperextended, it is difficult to pull the breast tissue forward. The arm should be relaxed, which, in turn, will relax the muscles along the chest wall. A "whiteout" effect can occur adjacent to the chest wall if proper compression is not used. (Courtesy Cullinan AM: *Producing Quality Radiographs.* Philadelphia, JB Lippincott Co, 1987.)

SUPPLEMENTARY PROJECTIONS

About 15% of asymptomatic patients and about 35% of symptomatic patients require supplementary views on their initial study. On subsequent screening studies, about 1% of asymptomatic patients require supplementary views.[197]

The selective use of a third view should decrease the number of false positives and increase the diagnostic accuracy of the two-view mammographic examination. A symptomatic routine includes:

1. Craniocaudad projection.

NOTE: Sometimes a lesion located far superiorly in the breast will be forced backward, even with straight-edge compression. A modified-compression approach is suggested[192] (Fig 8-7).

2. Mediolateral oblique projection.
3. A 90 degree lateral projection (lateromedial or mediolateral) (Fig 8-8).

When a standard two- or three-view study is inconclusive, the mammographer should be able to decide which additional projections are needed. An additional view may be required to image in full a lesion not seen on the standard projections.[192]

FIGURE 8-7 Breast-Compression Modification

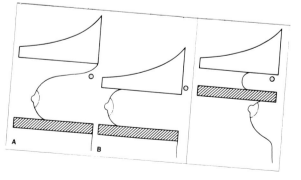

Proper breast compression may prevent the inclusion of a lesion that is high in the chest on the chest wall. (A) Note the lesion located far superiorly in the breast before compression is applied for imaging of the craniocaudal projection. (B) While vigorous compression is being applied, the compression plate has traveled so far down the chest wall that the lesion is not included in the image. The same lesion with imaging of only the uppermost breast tissue ("lumpogram") permits the lesion to be included in the craniocaudal projection while vigorous compression is applied. (Courtesy Sickles EA: Practical solutions to common mammographic problems: Tailoring the examination. *AJR* 1988;151:31-39.)

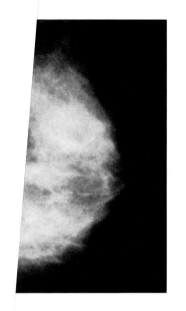

...ferior aspect of the left breast
...ipple of the opposite breast
...A, Destouet JM, Monsees B:
...ram. *Radiology* 1989;170:272.)

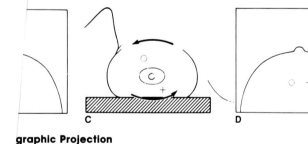

...graphic Projection

...ojection can be achieved by changing the orientation of the ...glandular tissue at the 12 o'clock position (circle) and another at ...rimpose on a standard craniocaudal projection and create a ...he upper part of the breast were "rolled" either medially or laterally ...ger project over each other. A repeat craniocaudal view will show ...esy Sickles EA: Practical solutions to common mammographic ...988;151:31-39.)

...een on two ...additional ...ent projec- ...uity of the ...vith respect ...t image can ...on only one ...overlapping

structures, the projection can be repeated after the breast has been "rolled" slightly in its relationship to the cassette[192] (Fig 8-11).

A tangential oblique projection differs from the standard projection with subsequent rotation of the body in that the breast is compressed in the oblique position. This projection also helps to overcome the summation effect of superimposed focal areas that may be interpreted as a mass[202] (Fig 8-12).

A straight lateral projection may be the most effective way to solve the problem of superimposition of normal breast tissue simulating a mass.[197]

Double-Breast Compression View (Craniocaudal Projection)

A lesion deep in the most medial aspect of the breast close to the sternum may require the double-breast compression craniocaudal view. With the sternum and innermost aspects of both breasts placed against the cassette, presternal tissue between the breasts is pulled forward over the cassette and compression is applied bilaterally. The medial aspects of both breasts are imaged simultaneously.[193]

The Sponge Craniocaudal View

The "sponge craniocaudal" view (Fig 8-2, insert), may help to detect lesions deep in the lower hemisphere of the breast. This noncompressed craniocaudal view is most helpful in detecting deep lesions in the upper hemisphere of the breast, close to the chest wall, that shift posteriorly when compression is used. A triangular sponge placed under the breast elevates the rib cage and upper abdomen over the top of the film holder, helping to demonstrate the chest wall. This technique, however, results in geometric distortion of the breast tissue.[193]

Spot Compression

Increased breast compression helps to spread apart an overlying island of dense breast tissue. Spot compression over an area of interest involves a relatively small part of the breast, separating localized superimposed structures and forcing the segment of the breast in question closer to the detector. As the breast is flattened out over a greater area, the ratio of scatter to primary radiation decreases.

Spot compression helps to (1) better characterize a mass seen on a routine view and (2) distinguish true abnormalities from those caused by superimposition of normal breast tissue.[203]

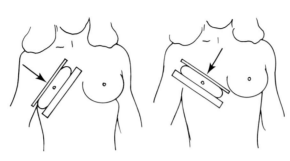

FIGURE 8-12   Tangential Oblique Projections of the Breast

In a tangential oblique projection, the breast is compressed in the oblique position as compared with the standard method, with subsequent rotation of the body. (Redrawn from Hall FM, Berenberg AL: Selective use of the oblique projection in mammography. *AJR* 1978;131:465-468.)

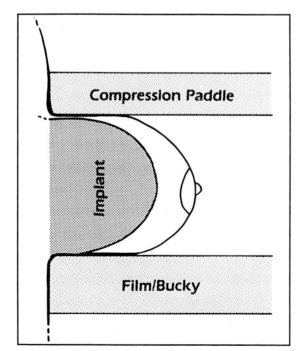

Compression Paddle

Implant

Film/Bucky

FIGURE 8-13   Positioning of the Augmented Breast

Routine positioning technique to include an implant. (Courtesy Brower TD: Positioning techniques for the augmented breast. *Radiol Technol* 1990;61:209-211.)

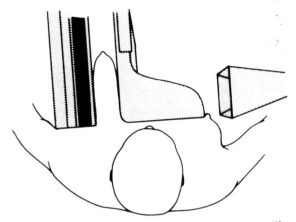

FIGURE 8-9   Technical Difficulty Encountered with the Mediolateral Projection

A diagram of a mammographic unit is shown with the left breast compressed and the nipple of the opposite breast projected into the x-ray field. (Courtesy Gilula LA, Destouet JM, Monsees B: Nipple simulating a breast mass on a mammogram. *Radiology* 1989;170:272.)

view. The entire body must be turned so that additional lateral and/or medial aspects of the breast can be demonstrated on the repeat craniocaudal image.[192]

The craniocaudal oblique position (exaggerated axial view) made with the patient erect and the trunk turned 20 degrees visualizes the extreme lateral breast and the axillary extension not usually seen on a routine craniocaudal view. With the arm raised, the breast becomes a continuation of the pectoral muscle in the caudomedial direction[199] (Fig 8-5). Lundgren[199] described this variation of the craniocaudal oblique position of the outer breast and axillary tail.

Another variation of the craniocaudal oblique position requires that the seated patient lean backward and laterally in a semireclining position, with some lateral rotation of the torso ("Cleopatra" position). The maximum amount of tissue should be spread over the cassette for compression.[200,201]

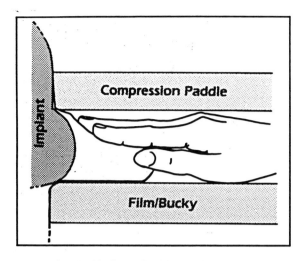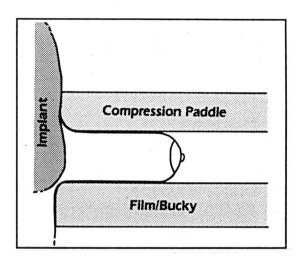

FIGURE 8-14 Modified Positioning Routine of the Augmented Breast

The modified positioning routine pulls the breast tissue forward while pushing the implant backward. (Courtesy Brower TD: Positioning techniques for the augmented breast. *Radiol Technol* 1990;61:209-211.)

Imaging of the Augmented Breast

Implants in the retromammary and subpectoral regions make it difficult to compress the breast tissue. Modified positioning is required to image the augmented breast (Figs 8-13 through 8-15).

Manual shifting of the implant by the radiographer may allow the remainder of the breast to be pulled forward. If the implant is displaced posteriorly against the chest wall and the breast tissue is pulled over and in front of the implant, more tissue can be compressed[204,205] (Figs 8-14 and 8-16).

A routine examination of the augmented breast includes:

1. Standard 45 degree mediolateral oblique projection.
2. Standard craniocaudal projection.
3. Modified compression; mediolateral oblique projection.
4. Modified compression; craniocaudal projection.

Additional views include a 90 degree mediolateral projection, which is recommended for implants that are rigidly encapsulated. With noticeable fibrous encapsulation of the implant (15% to 20% of patients), it is difficult to flatten or displace the implant posteriorly against the

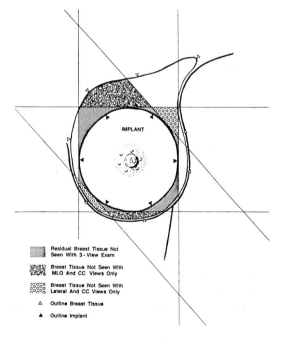

FIGURE 8-15 Limitations of Implant Imaging

The shaded areas on the schematic drawing show the tissue obscured by an implant when standard mediolateral oblique, craniocaudal, and 90 degree lateral compression views are used. (Courtesy Eklund GW, Busby RC, Miller SH, et al: Improved imaging of the augmented breast. *AJR* 1988;15:469-473.)

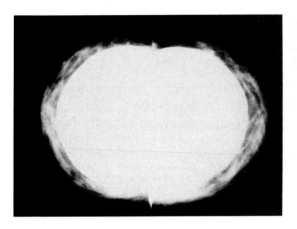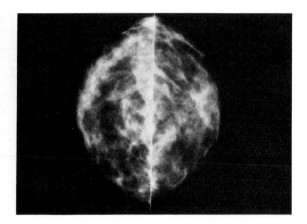

FIGURE 8-16   Routine versus Modified Craniocaudal Views

Craniocaudal views of the augmented breast with routine positioning and compression techniques demonstrate poor visualization of the breast tissue. Left, The implant limits compression. Right, The modified view with the implant excluded demonstrates a marked increase in the degree of compression that can be applied and the amount of breast tissue that can be shown. (Courtesy Brower TD: Positioning techniques for the augmented breast. *Radiol Technol* 1990;61:209-211.)

chest wall. By pulling more breast tissue in front of the implant, a 3 to 5 cm increase in compression is possible if the implant is excluded from compression. A 90 degree lateral view compensates for the lack of imaging of the tissue immediately above and below the implant. Patients with pectoral implants might experience pain upon compression since the pectoral muscle is also compressed.[204]

Eklund[204] states that mammographers should not be reluctant to perform examinations of the augmented breast and should not be concerned about damaging the implant by the modified compression positioning procedure. In response to a report of a collapse of a saline-filled silicone implant following mammography, Eklund concluded that the possibility of damage to an implant by compression exists. However, the implant is usually under less pressure with the modified technique, where it is displaced or flattened against the chest wall, as opposed to direct compression by a compression paddle.

CAUTION: Compression of the augmented breast should be performed with the permission of the radiologist

Another possibility is focal compression or magnified images, if so indicated.

TECHNICAL CONSIDERATIONS

Image Blur

The reduction of image blur in mammography is due partially to improvements in the image chain since improved screen-film technology makes it possible to increase the FFD and to use smaller focal spots and low ratio grids.

In the craniocaudal view, if microcalcifications are present in the superior portion of the breast, these calcifications could be a considerable distance from the detector. The breast tissue and the calcifications, if present, are brought closer to the image detector with compression. The production of scatter is also reduced[7] (Fig 8-17). Localized areas of clinical concern, such as calcifications in patients with implants, are seen better with focal compression, with or without magnification[204] (Fig 8-18).

Vacuum screen-film holders use a single screen and a single emulsion film inserted into a lightproof bag. When the air is evacuated from the bag, which is then sealed by a heat bar, excellent screen-film contact is produced.

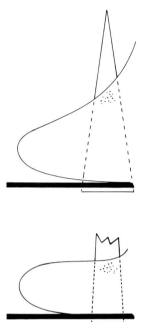

FIGURE 8-17 Effect of Compression on Mammography

Since the female breast is pyramidal in shape, compression is necessary in order to image the breast adequately. Vigorous compression of the breast brings breast tissue closer to the image detector and lessens the production of scatter. Top, The pyramid-shaped breast presents several imaging difficulties. An exposure used to image breast tissue near the chest wall would overexpose the nipple area. Note the presence of the calcifications in the superior portion of the breast and their distance from the detector. This increased OFD would result in significant blur of the calcifications. Bottom, The combination of a small focal spot and vigorous breast compression minimizes image blur as the calcifications are brought closer to the detector. The production of scatter is also reduced. (Courtesy Cullinan AM: *Producing Quality Radiographs.* Philadelphia, JB Lippincott Co, 1987.)

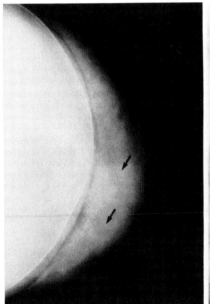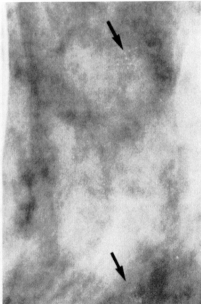

FIGURE 8-18 Benefit of Focal Compression: Magnified Image for Detection of Microcalcifications

Left, Compression of standard craniocaudal view poorly demonstrates subtle calcifications (arrow). Right, A modified-compression magnified image shows two clusters of microcalcifications (arrows). (Courtesy Eklund GW, Busby RC, Miller SH, et al: Improved imaging of the augmented breast. *AJR* 1988;15:469-473.)

Direct Roentgen enlargement is possible with fractional-focal-spot tubes. Minute calcifications or changes in breast stroma are enlarged with this approach.[7] Many modern mammographic units have 1.5× to 2.0× magnification capability.

Benefits of magnification include:

1. Increased resolution.
2. Decreased noise, relative to object size, although the inherent noise of the detecting system does not change.

Disadvantages of magnification are:

1. The possibility of increased image blur.
2. Possible need for focal spots smaller than 0.2 mm.
3. Increased entrance dosage since the breast is closer to the x-ray source.

Kilovoltage Selection

Conventional radiographic equipment is not acceptable for mammographic imaging. A dedicated mammographic unit with a molybdenum target x-ray tube, which at 26 to 30 kVp produces an x-ray spectrum rich in 17.4 and 19.6 keV characteristic x-rays, is recommended for this study. As molybdenum has a K-edge absorption at 20 keV, it strongly absorbs x-rays at and above this energy level.[207] Low-energy x-radiation from an x-ray tube that has a molybdenum anode instead of a tungsten anode improves the contrast between parenchyma, fat, and small calcific densities. Malignant calcifications (numerous, punctate, and closely grouped) are often less than 1.0 mm in size.[196]

Nongrid screen-film images are usually obtained at 25 to 28 kVp with a molybdenum target tube and at 22 to 26 kVp when a tungsten target tube is used. An additional 2 kVp is needed to compensate for the absorption characteristics of a grid.[207]

Filtration

Most dedicated mammographic units with molybdenum targets are equipped with 0.03 mm molybdenum filters. An aluminum filter would cause excessive beam hardening and is not recommended for use with screen-film mammography.[208]

Tungsten target tubes, if used for mammography, should have a beryllium window and minimal aluminum filtration.

> C A U T I O N : The mirror optic system in a conventional collimator has a filtration effect even if all added filtration is removed.

Scatter

With tight beam collimation, scatter radiation is reduced; however, no single mammographic cone can be configured to all breast sizes or shapes. A piece of rubberized lead placed on the mammographic platform and moved forward toward the nipple can reduce scatter and undercutting of the image.[189] Proper collimation will also minimize scatter arising from the chest wall.

Breasts that are difficult to compress or that contain extremely dense glandular tissues benefit from grid techniques (Fig 8-19). Grids used for mammography contain lead strips that are usually separated by carbon-fiber–resin interspacing. These grids have an ultra–high strip density (150 to 200 lines per inch) as compared with conventional Bucky grids (80 or more lines per inch). Stationary grids typically have a 3.5:1 ratio and reciprocating grids have 4:1 to 5:1 ratios.

The use of a reciprocating grid adds a gap of 1 to 2 cm between the lower surface of the breast and the screen-film detector.[208] Irregular grid motion or a problem with the grid drive mechanism can produce artifacts on the image.

The increase in exposure required for grid as compared with nongrid radiography of the breast can be compensated for by higher kilovolt settings and/or a faster recording system.

> C A U T I O N : The grid focal range of stationary grids that fit into standard cassettes must be matched to the FFD of the mammographic unit.

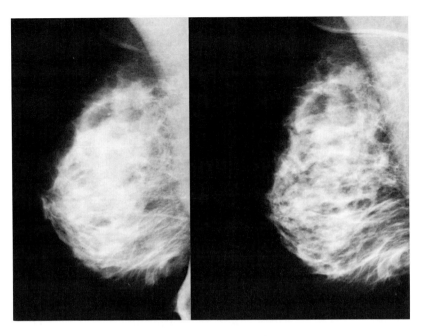

FIGURE 8–19 Grid versus Nongrid Mammography

Visibility of details is improved by grid images of the breast. A nongrid mammogram (left) is compared with a grid image (right). (Courtesy Eastman Kodak Company, Rochester, NY.)

Automatic Exposure Control

Anatomical differences in the breasts can account for inconsistent radiographic density on mammograms. There is considerable variation in fat and glandular and fibrocystic elements among different breasts. The AEC, an option on many units, should be considered essential since this device can overcome differences in density among patients or between the breasts of the same patient. With an AEC, an average of 95% of the exposures are correct, except when the breast is too small to cover the control's sensing area.[209]

> CAUTION: If the breast does not cover the AEC sensor, it may be necessary to use a manual technique.[7]

An AEC can be modified to accommodate screen-film systems of various speeds.[210]

Screen-Film Technology

The small punctate calcifications associated with breast malignancies are difficult to image because of the lack of subject contrast in the breast. Contrast is especially important because of the subtle differences in the densities of the breast, as well as the need to detect microcalcifications and marginal structural characteristics of soft-tissue masses.[208] Early direct-exposure techniques using industrial-type films to improve contrast required 1,800 mAs (300 mA for 6 seconds) at 25 to 35 kVp. Some early investigators used nonscreen (direct-exposure) prepacked films.

Single-screen and single-emulsion films produce higher film contrast and permit an approximately 50 to 100 times reduction in exposure as compared with direct exposure films.[208] Intensifying screens for mammography are made of conventional phosphors (primarily blue-light emitters) or rare earth phosphors (primarily green-light emitters). Blue- or green-sensitive films must be appropriately matched to the screen selected. A special safelight filter (Eastman Kodak GBX) required for green-sensitive films also may be used with most blue-sensitive films.

CAUTION: Intensifying-screen phosphors are often labeled as blue or green emitters, whereas, in actuality, most screens emit blue, green, and ultraviolet light. It is fair to say, however, that a screen is primarily a green or primarily a blue emitter. It is not wise to use a blue-sensitive film with a primarily green-emission screen, and vice versa, since this could reduce the system speed by one half or more.

Dual emulsion, zero crossover films with two screens permit a dosage reduction of approximately 50%, when compared with single-screen, single emulsion film techniques. Flat, tablet-shaped T-grain emulsions, combined with a light absorbing dye on the film base, reduce light crossover to 0%.[211]

If screen-film exposures exceed 1 second in length (depending on the milliampere limitations of the x-ray unit, the screen-film combination, and/or the use of a grid), "reciprocity law failure" must be considered. This falloff in film speed may require an exposure increase of up to 15%.[208] Reciprocity data are available from x-ray film manufacturers.

Although the breast is one of the more radiosensitive organs, the risk of a radiation-induced breast carcinoma is negligible with properly functioning state-of-the-art equipment and modern screen-film techniques.[193]

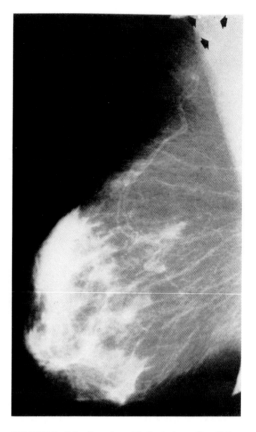

FIGURE 8–20 Foreign Material on the Skin

A mediolateral oblique view of the breast demonstrates several small calcificlike densities in the region of the axilla (arrows). This represents an artifact produced by deodorants, which usually contain a salt of aluminum and may contain talcum powder. Arm motion and moisture in the axilla caused the deodorant to clump into small collections of materials mimicking calcification. (Courtesy Cuomo L: A no sweat artifact. *Radiol Technol* 1988;59:517-518.)

Quality Assurance

The ACR accreditation program, a voluntary program for the evaluation of mammographic screening sites, requires participants to document information regarding the type of x-ray equipment, image receptor, technical factors, and all quality control procedures used. Mammograms and ACR mammographic phantom images must be submitted for evaluation by panels of radiologists and of medical physicists respectively. Radiation dose is also evaluated.[208,212]

The ACR quality assurance procedures to be carried out by physicists include:

1. Entrance exposure and average glandular dose measurements.
2. Testing for kVp accuracy reproducibility.

3. Beam quality (half-value layer) evaluation.
4. Evaluation of system performance of the AEC.
5. Estimation of beam restriction accuracy.
6. Focal spot size measurement (particularly important if image magnification techniques are attempted).
7. Ascertaining of uniformity of image receptor speed.

Quality assurance tests in mammography performed by radiographers include:

1. Processor quality assurance to include replenishment rates, transport time, and archival quality of the images.
2. Screen evaluation for cleanliness and screen-film contact. Dust or dirt on an intensifying screen blocks the light emitted by the screen during an exposure, producing an artifact that may simulate microcalcifications.
3. Exposure of an ACR approved mammographic phantom.
4. Evaluation of darkroom conditions to include cleanliness, lighting, safelighting, and film handling.

With regard to the last quality assurance procedure, cassettes should be cleaned frequently with unsterile gauze and an antistatic cleaner recommended by the manufacturer of the screens. Walls, cabinets, floors, countertops, and the processor also must be cleaned regularly.

A major influence on the quality of mammographic images is the quality of the film processing. Whenever possible, a screen-film mammographic imaging site should have access to a dedicated processor. Time, temperature, and processor maintenance, as recommended by the manufacturer of the screen-film/processor, must be carried out. The chemistry chosen for the processor must be compatible with the film in use.

A major cause of fogged mammograms is the use of the wrong safelight in the darkroom.[212] An Eastman Kodak GBX filter should be substituted for a Wratten series 6B filter for use with orthochromatic films (green-sensitive). The GBX filter can be used with most blue- and green-sensitive radiographic films.

Finally, with regard to patient preparation, patients should be instructed not to use deodorants on the day of the examination.

CAUTION: A talcum powder artifact may be seen on the image if the patient has used a deodorant containing aluminum compounds[213] (Fig 8-20).

Foreign material on the skin, small glass particles in the breast tissue, or adhesive tape used after a thoracotomy can also mimic intramammary microcalcifications.[214] Limiting the use of caffeine prior to the study has been suggested as a way to reduce patient discomfort during compression of the breasts.[188]

References

1. Ballinger PW: *Merrill's Atlas of Radiographic Positions and Radiologic Procedures.* St Louis, CV Mosby Co, 1982.
2. Bontrager KL, Anthony BT: *Textbook of Radiographic Positioning and Related Anatomy.* Denver, Multimedia Publishing Inc, 1982.
3. Eisenberg RL, Dennis CA, May CR: *Radiographic Positioning.* Boston, Little Brown & Co, 1989.
4. McInnes J: *KC Clark's Positioning in Radiography.* Chicago, Year Book Medical Publishers Inc, 1973.
5. Jaffe C: Medical imaging, vision and visual psychophysics. *Med Radiogr Photogr* 1984;60:1-48.
6. Sprawls P: *Physical Principles of Medical Imaging.* Rockville, Md, Aspen Publishers Inc, 1987.
7. Cullinan AM: *Producing Quality Radiographs.* Philadelphia, JB Lippincott Co, 1987.
8. Tuddenham WJ: In defense of opacity, editorial. *RadioGraphcs* 1986;6:171-172.
9. Vezina JA: Compensation filter for shoulder radiography. *Radiology* 1985;155:823.
10. Smith DC, Tidwell J: Adjustable sliding aluminum wedge filter device for angiographic enhancement. *Radiol Technol* 1978;49:459-471.
11. Bushong SC: *Radiologic Sciences for Technologists.* St Louis, CV Mosby Co, 1984.
12. Gratale P, Wright DL, Daughtry L: Using the anode heel effect for extremity radiography. *Radiol Technol* 1990;61:195-198.
13. Sweeney RJ: The use of an inverted Kodak X-Omatic cassette as an improvised grid. *Radiol Technol* 1977;49:257-261.
14. Reynolds J, Skucas J, Gorski J: An evaluation of screen-film speed characteristics. *Radiology* 1976;118:711-713.
15. Logan H, Daly L, Masterson J: A comparison of two different T-grain films in rare-earth screens with a standard film-screen combination for intravenous pyelography and bone examinations. *Br J Radiol* 1989;62:237-240.
16. Hufton AP, Russell JGB: The use of carbon fibre material in tabletops, cassette fronts and grid covers: Magnitude of possible dose reduction. *Br J Radiol* 1986;59:157-163.
17. Murray JP: The chest in critical care. *Radiography* 1978;44:173-178.
18. Straub WF (ed): *Manual of Diagnostic Imaging.* Boston, Little Brown & Co, 1989.
19. Milne ENC: The conventional chest radiograph— does it have a future? *Appl Radiol* March/April 1985, p. 13-14.
20. Kerley P: Anatomical and pathological factors in chest radiography. *X-Ray Technician* 1943;15:89-95.
21. Colson DH: Inventive radiographic positions. *X-Ray Technician* 1942;14:59-62.
22. Daffner RH, Diamond DL: Trauma radiology: An integrated approach. *Appl Radiol* January 1988.
23. O'Rahilly R: Plain words on planes and sections. *Radiol Technol* 1981;52:615-617.
24. American Society of Radiologic Technologists: *Practitioner Educational Package,* contract no. 223-77-6013.
25. Westacott S, Hall JRW: *Key Anatomy for Radiology.* Oxford, Heinemann Professional Publishing, 1988.
26. Sartoris DJ: Musculoskeletal imaging: An evolving subspecialty. *AJR* 1987;148:1186-1187.
27. Keats TE: *Emergency Radiology.* Chicago, Year Book Medical Publishing Co, 1984.
28. Kerr R: Diagnostic imaging of upper extremity trauma. *Radiol Clin North Am* 1989;27:891-908.

29. Yochum TR, Rowe LJ: *Essentials of Skeletal Radiology.* Baltimore, Williams & Wilkins, 1987.

30. Mitchell MJ, Ho C, Resnick D, et al: Diagnostic imaging of lower extremity trauma. *Radiol Clin North Am* 1989;27:909-924.

31. Hendrix RW, Rogers LF: Diagnostic imaging of fracture complications. *Radiol Clin North Am* 1989; 27:1023-1033.

32. Pitt MJ, Speer DP: Radiologic reporting of orthopedic trauma. *Med Radiogr Photogr* 1982;58:14-18.

33. Richardson ML, Kilcoyne RF, Mayo KA, et al: Radiographic evaluation of modern orthopedic fixation devices. *RadioGraphics* 1987;7:685-701.

34. Griswold R: Elbow fat pads: A radiography perspective. *Radiol Technol* 1982;53:303-308.

35. Alexander JE, Holder JC: Fat pad signs in the diagnosis of subtle fractures. *Am Fam Physician* 1988;37:93-102.

36. Jacobs ER (ed): *Medical Imaging, A Concise Textbook.* Tokyo, Igaku-Shoin Medical Publishers Inc, 1987.

37. Gratale P, Burns CB, Murray J: Advantages of a 400 speed image receptor system for cast radiography. *Radiol Technol* 1987;58:401-403.

38. Galasko CSB, Isherwood I (eds): *Imaging Techniques in Orthopaedics.* New York, Springer-Verlag, 1989.

39. de Lacey G, Evans R, Sandin B: Penetrating injuries: How easy is it to see glass (and plastic) on radiographs? *Br J Radiol* 1985;58:27-30.

40. Tandberg D: Glass in the hand and foot. Will an x-ray film show it? *JAMA* 1982;248:1872-1874.

41. Fodor J III, Malot JC: The Min-R system: An alternative to xeroradiography. *Radiol Technol* 1984; 55:41-43.

42. Desautels JEL, Radomsky JW, Erickson LM: Evaluation of mammography unit and rare earth screens for high resolution hand radiography. *J Can Assoc Radiol* 1980;31:185-186.

43. Ngo C, Yaghmai I: The value of immersion hand radiography in soft tissue changes of musculoskeletal disorders. *Skeletal Radiol* 1988;17:259-263.

44. Gratale P, Turner GW, Burns CB: A modified AP projection of the thumb. *Radiol Technol* 1985;56:320-321.

45. Lewis S: New angles on the radiographic examination of the hand — II. *Radiography Today* 1988;54:29.

46. Lewis S: New angles on the radiographic examination of the hand — I. *Radiography Today* 1988;54:44-45.

47. Lewis S: New angles on the radiographic examination of the hand — III. *Radiography Today* 1988;54:47-48.

48. Just SL, Sloth C, Amundsen P-O: Diagnosis of fracture of the carpal scaphoid with 4 oblique projections. *Eur J Radiol* 1989;9:152-154.

49. Lindequist S, Larsen CF: Radiography of the carpal scaphoid: An experimental investigation evaluating the use of oblique projections. *Acta Radiol (Diagn)* 1986;27:97-99.

50. Proubasta I, Lluch A, Celaya F, et al: Angled radiographic view of the wrist for diagnosis of fractures of the carpal scaphoid. *AJR* 1989;153:196.

51. Kindynis P, Resnick D, Kang HS, et al: Demonstration of the scapholunate space with radiography. *Radiology* 1990;175:278-280.

52. Fodor J III, Malott JC, Merhar GL: Carpal tunnel syndrome: The role of radiography. *Radiol Technol* 1987;56:497-501.

53. Balfour GW: Diagnosis of oblique fractures of the distal ulna using an extended pronated view of the wrist. *Orthopedics* 1990;13:247-252.

54. Greenspan A, Norman A: Radial head-capitellum view: An expanded imaging approach to elbow injury. *Radiology* 1987;164:272-274.

55. Cullinan JE: Personal communication.

56. Bangert BA, Pathria MN, Resnick D: Advanced imaging of the shoulder. *Surg Rounds Orthopaed* June 1989, pp 48-57.

57. Clements RW: Adaptation of the technique for radiography of the glenohumeral joint in the lateral position. *Radiol Technol* 1979;51:305-312.

58. Horsfield D: The bicipital groove: A simple technique. *Radiography* 1988;54:109-110.

59. Kilcoyne RF, Reddy PK, Lyons F, et al: Optimal plain film imaging of the shoulder impingement syndrome. *AJR* 1989;153:795-797.

60. Horsfield D, Phillips RR: The zero projection. *Radiography Today* 1990;56:14-16.

61. Sloth C, Just SL: The apical oblique radiograph in examination of acute shoulder trauma. *Eur J Radiol* 1989;9:147-151.

62. Kornguth PJ, Salazar AM: The apical oblique view of the shoulder: Its usefulness in acute trauma. *AJR* 1987;149:113-116.

63. Thomas D, Moody A: The acromioclavicular joint: An alternative view. *Radiography* 1988;54:119-120.

64. Kumar R, Madewell JE, Swischuk LE, et al: The clavicle: Normal and abnormal. *RadioGraphics* 1989; 9:677-706.

65. Funke T: Tangential view of the scapular spine. *Med Radiogr Photogr* 1958;34:41-43.

66. Conklin WA, Atwill JH: Lateral radiography of the scapula with patient supine. *Med Radiogr Photogr* 1959;35:46-47.

67. Brand PW, Coleman WC: A standard for dorsal-plantar and lateral radiographic projections of the feet. *Orthopedics* 1987;10:117-120.

68. Keene JS, Lange RH: Diagnostic dilemmas in foot and ankle injuries. *JAMA* 1986;256:247-251.

69. Cullinan JE, Cullinan AM: *Illustrated Guide to X-Ray Technics.* Philadelphia, JB Lippincott Co, 1980.

70. Mohr R: Oblique view of the lower end of the fibula. Dupont X-Ray News no. 58. *X-Ray Technician* 1962; 34:2.

71. Rijke AM: Acute ankle sprains: What is the role of the radiologist? *Appl Radiol* September 1989, pp 11-16.

72. Funke T: Radiography of the knee joint. *Med Radiogr Photogr* 1960;36:1-67.

73. Singer AM, Naimark A, Felson D, et al: Comparison of overhead and cross-table lateral views for detection of knee-joint effusion. *AJR* 1985;144:973-975.

74. Resnick D, Vint V: The "tunnel" view in assessment of cartilage loss in osteoarthritis of the knee. *Radiology* 1980;137:547-548.

75. Turner GW, Burns CB, Previtte RG Jr: Erect positions for "tunnel" views of the knee. *Radiol Technol* 1983; 55:640-642.

76. Kimberlin GE: Radiological assessment of the patello-femoral articulation and subluxation of the patella. *Radiol Technol* 1973;45:129-137.

77. Daffner RH, Tabas JH: Trauma oblique radiographs of the knee. *J Bone Joint Surg* 1987;69-A:568-572.

78. Bradley WG, Ominsky SH: Mountain view of the patella. *AJR* 1981;136:53-58.

79. Cooperstein LA, in Staub WA (ed): *Manual of Diagnostic Imaging.* Boston, Little Brown & Co, 1989.

80. Eisenberg RL, Hedgcock MW, Akin JR: The 40 degree cephalad view of the hip. *AJR* 1981;136:835-836.

81. Young JWR, Burgess AR, Brumback RJ, et al: Pelvic fractures: Value of plain radiography in early assessment and management. *Radiology* 1986;160:445-451.

82. Martz CD, Taylor CC: The 45-degree angle roentgenographic study of the pelvis in congenital dislocation of the hip. *J Bone Joint Surg* 1954; 36-A:528-532.

83. Farell J: Orthoradiographic measurement of shortening of the lower extremity. *Med Radiogr Photogr* 1953;29:32-38.

84. Horsfield D, Jones SN: Assessment of inequality in length of the lower limb. *Radiography* 1986;52: 223-227.

85. Kumpel K: Bone length radiography. *X-Ray Technician* 1954;25:265-267.

86. McClean PM, Lireka PJ: *Plain Skull Radiography in the Management of Head Trauma: An Overview.* US Dept of Health and Human Services FDA publication 81-8172, Rockville, Md, 1981.

87. Gray AL: Roentgen examinations for head injuries. *AJR* 1988;150:7-10 1988 (reprinted from AJR 1914;1:294-297.

88. Quencer RM: Neuroimaging and head injuries: Where we've been—where we're going. *AJR* 1988;150:13-18.

89. Armstrong P, Wastie ML: *Diagnostic Imaging.* Oxford, Blackwell Scientific Publishers, 1987.

90. de Lacey G, McCabe M, Constant O, et al: Testing a policy for skull radiography (and admission) following mild head injury. *Br J Radiol* 1990;63:14-18.

91. Hough JE: The sphenoid strut parieto-orbital projection. *Radiol Technol* 1968;39:197-209.

92. Leaman AM, Gorman DF, Danher J, et al: Skull x-rays after trauma: Are both laterals necessary? *Arch Emerg Med* 1988;51:18-20.

93. Dixit JK: "No lip" Waters view. *AJR* 1988; 151:839-840.

94. Squire LF, Novelline RA: *Fundamentals of Radiology.* Cambridge, Mass, Harvard University Press, 1979.

95. Dalrymple GV, Slayden JE: *Radiology in Primary Care.* St Louis, CV Mosby Co, 1975.

96. Baker SR: *Diagnostic Challenges in Radiology.* Philadelphia, JB Lippincott Co, 1989.

97. Payne D, Bore R: Skull radiography after recent trauma—a review. *Radiography Today* 1989;55:12-15.

98. Rosenblum J, Yousefzadeh DK, Ramilo JL: Skull radiography in infants: Potential hazards of the use of head clamps. *Radiology* 1986;161:367-368.

99. Heystek HD, Hildreth RC: Radiography of calcified submandibular calculi. An oblique anteroposterior projection. *Med Radiogr Photogr* 1958;34:20-22.

100. Grove AS: New diagnostic techniques for evaluation of orbital trauma. *Trans Am Acad Ophthalmol Otolaryngol* 1977;83:626-640.

101. Brandt C: A shot in the dark: Foreign body localisation. *Radiography* 1987;53:26-27.

102. Lagow ND: Radiography of the skull by tangential projection. *X-Ray Technician* 1953;24:335-336.

103. Kimber PM: Isocentric neuroradiography. *Radiography* 1987;53:201-210.

104. Frank ED, Stears JG, Gray JE, et al: Use of the postero-anterior projection: A method of reducing x-ray exposure to specific radiosensitive organs. *Radiol Technol* 1983;54:343-347.

105. Gehweiler JA Jr, Osborne RL, Becker RF: *The Radiology of Vertebral Trauma.* Philadelphia, WB Saunders, 1980.

106. England AC III, Shippel AH, Ray MJ: A simple view for demonstration of fractures of the anterior arch of C-1. *AJR* 1985;144:763-764.

107. Smith G, Abel M: Visualization of the posterolateral elements of the upper cervical vertebrae in the anteroposterior projection. *Radiology* 1975;115:219-220.

108. Woodford MJ: Radiography of the acute cervical spine. *Radiography* 1987;53:3-8.

109. Tihansky DP, Augustine G: Magnified axial-oblique projection of cervical articular facets. *Radiol Technol* 1987;58:426-430.

110. Vanden Hoek T, Propp D: Cervicothoracic junction injury. *Am J Emerg Med* 1990;8:30-33.

111. Rhea JT, DeLuca SA, Llewellyn HJ, et al: The oblique view: An unnecessary component of the initial adult lumbar spine examination. *Radiology* 1980;134:45-47.

112. Brower AC: Disorders of the sacroiliac joint. *Surg Rounds Orthopaed* 1989;7:47-54.

113. Yankes JR, Solot JA: Radiography in the multiply traumatized patient. *Journal of AOA* 1983;82:331-337.

114. Yelton R: Cervical spine protocol for emergency room use. *Radiol Technol* 1979;50:693-698.

115. Daffner RH: *Imaging of Vertebral Trauma.* Rockville, Md, Aspen Publications Inc, 1988.

116. Holohan F: Simplified positioning of the scoliotic spine. *X-Ray Technician* 1963;34:347-351.

117. Hoffman DA, Lonstein JE, Morin MM, et al: Breast cancer in women with scoliosis exposed to multiple diagnostic x-rays. *J Natl Cancer Inst* 1989;81:1307-1312.

118. Frank ED, Kuntz JI: A simple method of protecting breasts during upright lateral radiography for spine deformities. *Radiol Technol* 1983;55:532-535.

119. Fearon T, Vucich J, Butler P, et al: Scoliosis examinations: Organ dose and image quality with rare earth

screen-film systems. *AJR* 1988;150:359-362.

120. Dillon WP: Myelography: In memoriam. *Perspect Radiol* 1988;1:131-146.

121. Hesselink JR: Spine imaging: History, achievements, remaining frontiers. *AJR* 1988;150:1223-1229.

122. Minken TJ, Ahlgren P: Cross-table cervical myelography: A technique to improve visualization. *AJNR* 1988; 9:874.

123. Pearson GR: Radiographic projection studies. *X-Ray Technician* 1951;23:1-9.

124. Wolfson JJ, Atencio IF: The value of the "silhouetted view." DuPont X-Ray News no. 61. *X-Ray Technician* 1963;34:5.

125. Moore TF: An alternative to the standard radiographic position for the sternum. *Radiol Technol* 1988;60: 133-134.

126. Arnold M, Mills P: The oblique sternum: An alternative projection. *Radiography* 1988;54:159-161.

127. Holly EW: Some radiographic techniques in which movement is utilized. *Radiogr Clin Photogr* 1942;18:78-83.

128. Garber RL, Tossey I: Radiography of the sternum. *Med Radiogr Photogr* 1953;29:93-94.

129. Piper KJ: Reappraisal of the erect abdominal radiograph. *Radiography* 1987;53:19-21.

130. Martinez LO, Freidland JT, Silberman MR: Empty right iliac fossa. *South Med J* 1985;78:958-961.

131. Cullinan JA: Personal communication.

132. Leonard P, Schieb MC: Radiological detectability of surgical swabs and sponges. *Australas Radiol* 1982; 26:97-103.

133. Pinckney LE: *Foreign Bodies in Children.* Eighth Annual San Diego Postgraduate Radiology Course, October 24-28, 1983.

134. Desaga JF: Visualization of the mucosal villi on double-contrast barium studies of the small intestine by using a high molecular fraction of guaran. *Gastrointest Radiol* 1989;14:25-30.

135. Munro TG: Brief communication: A simple model for teaching double-contrast examinations of the gastrointestinal tract. *J Can Assoc Radiol* 1989;40:162-163.

136. Danielson KS, Hunter TB: Barium capsules. *AJR* 1985;144:414.

137. David EFL: Drinking cup for double-contrast esophagography. *Radiology* 1988;168:564-565.

138. Bitterman RA, Paul RI, Poe DS: Foreign bodies: What care is best? *Patient Care* February 15, 1990, pp 109-124.

139. Op den Orth JO: Use of barium in evaluation of disorders of the upper gastrointestinal tract: Current status. *Radiology* 1989;173:601-608.

140. Levin MS, Rubesin SE, Herlinger H, et al: Double-contrast upper gastrointestinal examination: Technique and interpretation. *Radiology* 1988;168: 593-602.

141. De Lange EE, Shaffer HA Jr: Barium suspension formulation for use with the bubbly barium method. *Radiology* 1985;154:825.

142. Maglinte DDT, Lappas JC, Kelvin FM, et al: Small bowel radiography: How, when and why? *Radiology* 1987;16:297-305.

143. *FDA Roundup.* Medical Devices Report, May 18, 1989.

144. Bury RF: *Radiology: A Practical Guide.* Oxford, Oxford University Press, 1988.

145. Ounjian ZJ, Laing FC: Stratification in the gallbladder on intravenous cholangiography. *Radiology* 1976; 121:591-593.

146. Rhinehart DA: *Roentgenographic Technique.* Philadelphia, Lea & Febiger, 1931.

147. Hattery RR, Williamson B Jr, Hartman GW, et al: Intravenous urographic technique. *Radiology* 1988; 167:593-599.

148. Geraghty JA: An approach to the problem of intestinal gas in diagnostic radiology. *Br J Radiol* 1966;39:42-46.

149. Peitzman AB, McGuire SP, Paris PM: Blunt abdominal trauma, in Staub WH (ed): *Manual of Diagnostic Imaging.* Boston, Little Brown & Co, 1989.

150. Riggs W Jr: Errors in radiographic measurements caused by variations in the tabletop/Bucky tray distance. *Radiology* 1977;124:844.

151. Eisenberg RL, Hedgcock MW, Williams EA, et al: Optimum radiographic examination for consideration of compensation awards. *AJR* 1980;136:1065-1069.

152. Peruzzi W, Garner W, Bools J, et al: Portable chest roentgenography and computed tomography in critically ill patients. *Chest* 1988;93:722-726.

153. Wandtke JC, Plewes DB, McFaul JA: Improved pulmonary nodule detection with scanning equalization radiography. *Radiology* 1988;169:23-27.

154. Vlasbloem H, Schultze Kool LJ: AMBER: A scanning multiple-beam equalization system for chest radiography. *Radiology* 1988;169:29-34.

155. Sargent EN (ed): *Technique for Chest Radiography for Pneumoconiosis.* Chicago, American College of Radiology, 1982.

156. Sargent EN, Cullinan JE: Techniques of chest radiology—occupational lung disease. ASRT update. *Radiol Technol* 1986;57:4.

157. Palmer PES, Cockshott WP, Hegedus V, et al: *Manual of Radiographic Interpretation for General Practitioners.* Geneva, World Health Organization, 1985.

158. Wesenberg RL, Blumhagen JD: Assisted expiratory chest radiography. *Radiology* 1979;130:538-539.

159. Mootz AR: Chest radiography in thoracic trauma. *Diagnostic Radiology Update.* University of Texas Southwestern Medical Center, Dallas, October 28-30, 1988.

160. Fisher JK: Skin fold versus pneumothorax. *AJR* 1978;130:791-792.

161. Glazer HS, Anderson DJ, Wilson BS, et al: Pneumothorax: Appearance on lateral chest radiographs. *Radiology* 1989;173:707-711.

162. Chiles C, Ravin CE: Radiographic recognition of pneumothorax in the intensive care unit. *Crit Care Med* 1986;14:677-680.

163. Mendelson D, Khilnani N, Wagner LD, et al: Preoperative chest radiography: Value as a baseline examination for comparison. *Radiology* 1987;165:341-343.

164. Henry DA, Jolles H, Berberich JJ, et al: The post-

cardiac surgery chest radiograph: A clinically integrated approach. *J Thorac Imag* 1989;4:20-41.

165. Thompson MJ, Kubicka RA, Smith C: Evaluation of cardiopulmonary devices on chest radiographs: Digital vs analog radiographs. *AJR* 1989;153:1165-1168.

166. Landy MJ, Mootz AR, Estrera AS: Apparatus seen on chest radiographs after cardiac surgery in adults. *Radiology* 1990;174:477-482.

167. Shapiro MP, Gerzof SG. Oxygen reservoir rebreathing mask simulating pneumothorax. *Radiology* 1987; 164:743-744.

168. Steiner RM, Tegtmeyer CJ, Morse D, et al: The radiology of cardiac pacemakers. *RadioGraphics* 1986;6: 373-400.

169. Ruskin JA, Gurney JW, Thorsen MK, et al: Detection of pleural effusion on supine chest radiographs. *AJR* 1987;148:681-683.

170. Möller A: Pleural effusion: Use of the semi-supine position for radiographic detection. *Radiology* 1984;150:245-249.

171. Möller A: Forward-leaning position for radiographic differentiation between free and encapsulated pleural effusion. *Acta Radiol (Diagn)* 1985;26:519-520.

172. Torcino IM, Miller MH, Fairfax WR: Distribution of pneumothorax in the supine and semirecumbent critically ill adult. *AJR* 1985;144:901-905.

173. Torcino IM: Pneumothorax in the supine patient: Radiographic anatomy. *RadioGraphics* 1985;5:557-586.

174. Galanski M, Hartenauer U, Krumme B: Rontgendiagnostik des Pneumothorax auf Intensivstatiomen. *Radiologe* 1981;21:459-462.

175. Welsh HD, Fleming EG: Radiographic visualization of subdiaphragmatic air: Oblique lateral projection with patient supine. *Med Radiogr Photogr* 1958;34:78-79.

176. Hollman AS, Adams FG: The influence of the lordotic projection on the interpretation of the chest radiograph. *Clin Radiol* 1989;40:360-364.

177. Kinslow WE: A special lordotic position. *X-Ray Technician* 1955;47:108-109.

178. Gehl JJ, Johnson LA: The reverse lordotic view for visualization of the lung bases. *AJR* 1987;148:651-652.

179. Zylak CJ, Littleton JT, Durizch ML: Illusory consolidation of the left lower lobe: A pitfall of portable radiography. *Radiology* 1988;167:653-655.

180. Markowitz SK, Ziter FMH: The lateral chest film and pneumoperitoneum. *Ann Emerg Med* 1986;15: 424-427.

181. Heinsimer JA, Collins GJ, Burkman MH, et al: Supine cross-table lateral chest roentgenogram for the detection of pericardial effusion. *JAMA* 1987;257: 3266-3268.

182. Rivero H, Bender TM, Oh KS: Optimal visualization of the nasopharyngeal airway. *Radiology* 1983; 147:877-878.

183. Felson B: *The Fundamentals of Chest Roentgenology.* Philadelphia, WB Saunders Co, 1960.

184. Wright IP, Fergusson PA: Supplementary projection to demonstrate the thoracic inlet. *Radiography* 1986;52:152-153.

185. Cullinan JE: A "perfect" chest radiograph — or a compromise? *Radiol Technol* 1981;53:121-137.

186. Manninen H, Rytkonen H, Siomakallio S, et al: Evaluation of an anatomical compensation filter for chest radiography. *Br J Radiol* 1986;59:1087-1092.

187. Guilbeau JC, Mazoyer BM, Pruvost P, et al: Chest radiography with a shaped filter at 140 kVp: Its diagnostic accuracy compared with that of standard radiographs. *AJR* 1988;150:1007-1010.

188. Jackson VP, Lex AM, Smith DJ: Patient discomfort during screen-film mammography. *Radiology* 1988; 168:421-423.

189. Schiller I, Knight D, Cromwell E: The practical mammographer. *Appl Radiol* 1988;9:34-36.

190. NCRP Report no. 85, *Mammography — A User's Guide.* National Council on Radiation Protection and Measurements, March 1986.

191. Logan WW, Muntz EP (eds): *Reduced Dose Mammography.* New York, Masson Publishing USA, 1979.

192. Sickles EA: Practical solutions to common mammographic problems: Tailoring the examination. *AJR* 1988;151:31-39.

193. Gormley L, Bassett LW, Gold RH: Positioning in film-screen mammography. *Appl Radiol* 1988;7:35-37.

194. Bassett LW, Gold RH: Breast radiography using the oblique projection. *Radiology* 1983;149:585-587.

195. Vyborny CJ, Schmit RA: Mammography as a radiographic examination: An overview. *RadioGraphics* 1989;9:723-764.

196. Andersson I: Mammography in clinical practice. *Med Radiogr Photogr* 1986;62:1-40.

197. Feig SA: The importance of supplementary mammographic views to diagnostic accuracy. *AJR* 1988; 151:40-41.

198. Gilula LA, Destouet JM, Monsees B: Nipple simulating a breast mass on a mammogram. *Radiology* 1989; 170:272.

199. Lundgren B: The oblique view at mammography. *Br J Radiol* 1977;50:626-628.

200. Goodrich WA Jr: The Cleopatra view in xeromammography: A semi-reclining position for the tail of the breast. *Radiology* 1978;128:811-812.

201. Bassett LW, Axelrod S: A modification of the craniocaudal view in mammography. *Radiology* 1979; 132:222-224.

202. Hall FM, Berenberg AL: Selective use of the oblique projection in mammography. *Am J Roentgenol* 1978; 131:465-468.

203. Berkowitz JE, Gatewood OMB, Gayler BW: Equivocal mammographic findings: Evaluation with spot compression. *Radiology* 1989;171:369-371.

204. Eklund GW, Busby RC, Miller H, et al: Improved imaging of the augmented breast. *AJR* 1988;151:469-473.

205. Brower TD: Positioning technique for the augmented breast. *Radiol Technol* 1990;61:209-211.

206. Hawes DR: Collapse of a breast implant after mammography. *AJR* 1990;154:1345-1346.

207. Feig SA: Mammograph equipment: Principles, features, selection. *Radiol Clin North Am* 1987;

25:897-911.

208. Haus AG, Feig SA, Ehrlich SM, et al: Mammographic screening: Technology, radiation dose and risk, quality control and benefits to society. *Radiology* 1990; 174:628-656.

209. Rose JH Jr, Berdahl CM: An automatic x-ray exposure controller for mammography. *Radiology* 1977; 122: 252-253.

210. Rossi RP, Williams C, Gill D: Modification of an automatic exposure control system for mammography to accommodate multiple-speed screen-film systems. *AJR* 1988;151:685-686.

211. Wojtasek DA, Teixdor HS, Govoni AF, et al: Diagnostic quality of mammograms obtained with a new low-radiation-dose dual-screen and dual-emulsion film combination. *AJR* 1990;154:265-270.

212. Hendrick RE: Standardization of image quality and radiation dose in mammography. *Radiology* 1990; 174:648-656.

213. Cuomo L: Technical query. A no-sweat artifact. *Radiol Technol* 1988;59:517-518.

214. Pamilo M, Soiva M, Suramo I: New artifacts simulating malignant microcalcifications in mammography. *Breast Dis* 1989;1:321-327.

Index

Page numbers followed by *t* indicate tables. Page numbers followed by *f* indicate figures.

ISBN 0-397-51050-0

90000

9 780397 510504